The Physiological Control of Mammalian Vocalization

The Physiological Control of Mammalian Vocalization

Edited by

John D. Newman

National Institutes of Health
Poolesville, Maryland

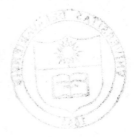

Plenum Press • New York and London

Library of Congress Cataloging in Publication Data

Symposium on the Physiological Control of Mammalian Vocalization (1986: Washington, D.C. and Poolesville, Md.).
    The physiological control of mammalian vocalization / edited by John D. Newman.
        p.   cm.
    "Proceedings of a Symposium on the Physiological Control of Mammalian Vocalization, held November 12–14, 1986, during the Annual Meeting of the Society for Neuroscience, in Washington, D.C. and Poolesville, Maryland"—T.p. verso.
    Includes bibliographical references and index.
    ISBN 0-306-43003-7
    1. Mammals—Vocalization—Regulation—Congresses. I. Newman, John D. II. Society for Neuroscience. III. Society for Neuroscience. Meeting (1986: Washington, D.C. and Poolesville, Md.) IV. Title.
QL765.S96   1986   88-23844
599'.059—dc19   CIP

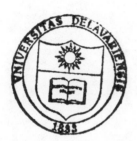

Proceedings of a Symposium on the Physiological Control of
Mammalian Vocalization, held during the Annual Meeting
of the Society for Neuroscience, November 12-14, 1986,
in Washington, D.C., and Poolesville, Maryland

John D. Newman, Ph.D., edited this book as part of his
official duties as a U.S. Government employee.

© 1988 Plenum Press, New York
A Division of Plenum Publishing Corporation
233 Spring Street, New York, N.Y. 10013

This book is dedicated to the
memory of Bryan Robinson and to the memory of Peter Winter.

FOREWORD

To the majority of biologists, the physiological control of mammalian vocalizations is only a small part of the large field of motor physiology. It is indeed a very specialized part, and the number of scientists dealing with it is relatively small. Still, it is an autonomous subject embracing more than the motor control of the body and is, therefore, by far more complex. Anatomically, essential cerebral structures involved in the control of gross and fine movements of the mammalian body seem to participate in the control of the voice as well. The central control system, however, as well as the larynx (the primary effector organ), possess features not found in the remaining motor system. An example is the perfect synergism of the many muscles which control the *m. vocalis*, not to speak of the speed of successions in which this occurs. Furthermore, this muscle, similar to the facial muscles, is segmentally adjustable independently of the joints. The most remarkable feature of the central control area, however, seems to be the effector organ's manifold direct and indirect dependence on the limbic system of the brain. This makes the voice--like no other motor organ (with the partial exception of the facial musculature)--the chief organ for the expression of emotion and the indicator of behavioral states. Except in man, the voice is independent of neocortical control. Animal vocalizations are species-typical and genetically programmed. Ethologically, they belong to the behavioral class of fixed action patterns. Vocalizations are social signals as well, and, thus, communication-directed motor activities. Man, too, has made use of his voice in developing his unique, species-typical form of communication--speech. In the course of ontogeny, the human voice comes under neocortical control, and this makes speech possible. Nevertheless, the human voice is still the most sensitive indicator of behavioral states and serves to express emotions.

Twenty-five years ago, I began my work in this field of research, with the squirrel monkey as test animal. I had been equipped for this type of work--with the exception of sonography, which at that time was still in its early stages--in the laboratory of Paul MacLean. He knew of my ethological interests and had

invited me to spend two years with him at the NIMH as a visiting
scientist. It was in his Section of Limbic Integration and
Behavior that the idea was born of providing psychiatry with a
basic research footing for the study of emotion and communication--
the key issues for psychiatry--by ethological and neurobiological
methods. When establishing the laboratories of primate behavior
at the Max Planck Institute of Psychiatry in Munich, I was lucky.
I met Peter Winter, who at that time was a graduate student of
Johann Schwartzkopff. He investigated medullary acoustic centers
of many bird species, and related them to their species-specific
behavior, such as locating prey in the dark or feeding on seeds.
I convinced him that *Saimiri sciureus* was an ideal test animal for
studying audio-vocal communication, and before long we were in the
midst of our work of classifying the vocal repertoire of the
squirrel monkey and its cerebral representation.

We had come to realize that our search for neuronal mechanisms
would yield results only if based on behavioral analyses. In this
regard, it was most fortunate to have Wolfgang Schleidt nearby.
He was with the Max Planck Institute for Comparative Physiology and,
working in the department of Konrad Lorenz, was concerned with
vocalizations of turkeys. He was kind enough to let us borrow a
sound spectrograph that he had constructed for his own work. This
was in 1962. Around that time, the first sound spectrographs
suitable for bioacoustical research were introduced, and, in
laboratories all over the world, the interest in animal vocaliza-
tions--including primate vocalisations--grew. Within a few years,
the results of laboratory and field studies of various Old World
and New World monkeys were published, different classification
methods developed, and vocalizations investigated in the quest for
natural units of behavior. It soon became clear to us and others
that vocal communication not only influences agonistic and cohesive
intragroup behavior but activities external to the group also, with
alarm calls playing a particularly important role. The function
and meaning of primate signals is a subject which remains to be
settled.

Neurophysiologists studying audio-vocal behavior were also
concerned with the problem of functional units. One typical
question was: "Are there neurons in the auditory cortex specifically reacting to a certain call (e.g., isolation peep, cackle,
etc.)?" It became apparent that the decoding of natural calls is
a highly complex process involving large parts of the cortex and all
of the auditory system. We are still far away from knowing how the
neuronal decoding mechanisms function to enable animals to recognize
a call and "answer" it (e.g., to vocalize in a dialogue). The
understanding of the physiological control of vocalization made
progress with the introduction of new anatomical techniques in the
early seventies. Finally, by means of conventional brain research
methods such as electrical brain stimulation and brain lesioning,
together with the new neuronal staining techniques, it became

possible to give a more or less rough description of the brain
circuitry involved in audio-vocal behavior. However, the key
questions regarding the physiological control of audio-vocal
behavior remain to be answered. What about the neuronal mechanism
of analyzers and sensory trigger systems controlling vocal signals,
or the central pattern generators organizing call-specific motor
programs? What about the system that selects the appropriate call
from the animal's repertoire or regulates motivated behavior
according to the internal state and acquired information? Unsolved
in particular is the sensorimotor coordination problem, i.e., the
search for specific feedback and feedforward mechanisms, an issue
of utmost importance for research on audio-vocal behavior. The
specific circuitry and function of such reafferent or corollary
discharge mechanisms is not yet known, and may be different at
the various operating levels of the nervous system. Today, the
question is not whether such cybernetic mechanisms do, in fact,
exist, but rather precisely in what structures are they embedded
and how they work at different levels within a hierarchically
organized system of vocal communication. These physiological
control mechanisms most certainly serve as prerequisites for the
evolution of human speech.

                              Detlev Ploog

                              Max Planck Institute for Psychiatry
                              Munich, Germany

PREFACE

   This book is based on a two-part symposium held in November,
1986 at the Society for Neuroscience Annual Meeting in Washington,
DC and at the NIH Animal Center in Poolesville, MD. The idea for
the symposium and this volume arose with the realization that a
growing body of new information on the evolution and physiological
control mechanisms underlying expression of mammalian vocalizations
had not been summarized either in print or in a public forum.
Discussions with several prospective participants met with enthusi-
astic agreement, and plans for the symposium were set in motion.
A number of invited participants agreed to include new data from
their work not previously published in detail. Three of the contributors (Bryan, Gooler, and Kehoe) based their chapters on
doctoral dissertation research, thereby providing early perspectives
on new research directions. Several contributors unable to attend
the symposium nevertheless graciously agreed to prepare chapters
for the book.

   Inclusion of this symposium in the Society for Neuroscience
program was noteworthy, in that this annual meeting returned to the
venue of the inaugural meeting of the Society. The Poolesville
part of the symposium was the first such gathering of invited
scientists at the new NIMH/NICHD research facility, and provided
the opportunity to test the logistics of shuttling a group of
symposium participants from their hotels in Washington and Bethesda
to the Animal Center, some 30 miles into the countryside. The
Editor is grateful to the National Institute of Child Health and
Human Development for supporting the Poolesville meeting. Local
assistance was ably provided by Donna Adderly, NICHD Administrative
Officer, and by Kitty Compton, Judy Newman, and Sharon Rozek.

                                        John D. Newman
                                        Poolesville, Maryland
                                        May, 1988

CONTENTS

INTRODUCTION AND BRAINSTEM MECHANISMS

FOREBRAIN MECHANISMS

INVESTIGATING THE PHYSIOLOGICAL CONTROL OF MAMMALIAN VOCALIZATIONS

John D. Newman

Laboratory of Comparative Ethology
National Institute of Child Health and Human Development
NIH, Bethesda, Maryland

INTRODUCTION

Studies of the physiological factors regulating the occurrence and physical characteristics of mammalian vocalizations have a long history. The end organ of phonation in mammals, the larynx, has been the object of many anatomical and physiological investigations. Major emphasis has been given to the comparative anatomy of the larynx and accessory organs, and to the role of particular laryngeal intrinsic muscles and their associated cartilages and nerve branches in regulating the quality of emitted sounds. Historically, studies of brain physiology and neuroanatomical substrates related to vocal behavior have reflected the traditional view that vocalizations are a behavioral measure of emotional expression. This is evident in the early reference to "pain cries" and "distress vocalizations" produced by electrical stimulation of the brain in conscious animals. More recently, the contributions made by zoologists and others familiar with the communicative behavior of social mammals have documented a rich array of vocal signals used in an equally rich variety of social contexts. With this new information has come a growing appreciation for the value of studying the neural representation and physiological control mechanisms of specific vocalizations in specific mammalian species.

THE ISOLATION CALL

One category of vocalization that has received particular attention is the isolation call. Also referred to as 'separation calls' and 'lost calls,' isolation calls have attracted the attention of behavioral neurobiologists for several reasons. First, they are given by the infants of all mammals when separated from their littermates or parents. This fact permits comparisons of controlling mechanisms between species, with the assurance that the same functional category of behavior is being measured in each case. Second, isolation calls are readily produced in a laboratory setting, simply by removing the infant from its home environment and placing it by itself in an observation enclosure. The robustness of this behavior also extends to the

1

adults of some mammals, who similarly emit isolation calls when visually and acoustically separated from familiar conspecifics. Although not yet fully exploited, another attribute of isolation calls described for some mammals, their simple and stereotyped acoustic structure, makes them an excellent neurobehavioral probe. This attribute permits more ready comparison of the morphology of this behavior under different experimental protocols, and enables identification of experimental manipulations that cause the behavior to take a form that falls outside of the normal range of variability. This fact is of value, for example, in interpreting the effects of experimental brain damage or a novel drug on this category of vocal behavior.

Isolation calls generally are grouped together in the acoustic sub-category of "tonal" or "voiced" vocalizations, possessing the acoustic property of continuous tonal pitch over the main course of the call, with little obscuring broad band energy or abrupt frequency changes. The acoustic details that distinguish isolation calls from other tonal calls in a given species' vocal repertoire have been worked out for only a few species. In some primates, tonal calls are given not only by separated individuals but also when the same individuals are in contact with social companions. These vocalizations, then, are part of a larger category of 'contact calls,' and in at least 3 primate species, measureable differences in structural details have been shown to correlate with the contextual details of the social contact, including circumstances where social contact is interrupted (Green, 1975; Lillehei and Snowdon, 1978; Boinski and Newman, 1988). Thus, not only must a vocalizer recognize when it is separated from familiar conspecifics, but more subtle details of social contact must be correctly interpreted in order for the appropriate variant of the 'contact call' category to be emitted. In addition, there is evidence in macaques that the pitch and duration of tonal 'coo' calls can be modified under experimenter control by differentially rewarding the vocalizer (Larson et al., 1973). These facts suggest a significant level of conscious control over the functional category of vocalizations to which the isolation call belongs, at least in some nonhuman primates.

NEURAL SUBSTRATES

It has been known for more than 3 decades that certain brain structures now grouped within the limbic system have an important relationship to vocal expression in mammals. Evidence for this relationship has come both from electrical stimulation of circumscribed brain areas through indwelling electrodes and from experiments in which all or parts of these same brain areas are experimentally destroyed. Less clear has been the relationship between specific brain structures and specific vocalizations. However, in a pioneering brain stimulation study in unanesthetized rhesus macaques, Bryan Robinson (1967; cf. Fig. 1) provided the first clue as to the location of the neural substrate underlying the production of isolation calls. Robinson reported that a "soft, high-pitched descending call similar to the separation call" (1967:349) was evoked by stimulation of sites in the anterior cingulate gyrus or its immediate vicinity. The anterior cingulate sites from which vocalization could be elicited were "centered on the frontal extension of the anterior cingulate gyrus and its subadjacent white matter and extend posteriorly into that part of the anterior cingulate gyrus overlying the genu

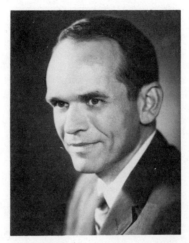

Figure 1. Bryan W. Robinson (1929-1979).

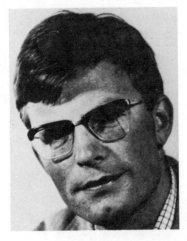

Figure 2. Peter Winter (1935-1972).

of the corpus callosum and into the subcallosal region" (1967:348). Since a sound spectrographic analysis of the calls studied by Robinson was not performed, it is not possible to compare the evoked vocalizations with naturally elicited calls, and thereby confirm the structural properties of the evoked calls. However, Peter Winter (Fig. 2) and his co-workers at the Max Planck Institute for Psychiatry in Munich, Germany, have provided this level of information for the squirrel monkey. Jürgens and Ploog (1970) determined that electrical stimulation of the ventral part of the cingulate gyrus produced a structural class of calls which included the species-typical isolation call. By reference to an earlier descriptive analysis of the vocal repertoire in captive squirrel monkeys (Winter et al., 1966), it was possible to demonstrate that electrical stimulation of the forebrain elicited sounds identical to naturally produced sounds (Jürgens et al., 1967). Of particular interest in the present context is the fact that 'peep' calls associated with the species-typical genital display were elicited along with genital erection from electrode sites in the septum. Peep calls given in the context of display and excitement, while differing in quantifiable details, are structurally similar to 'isolation peeps' (Newman, 1985a; Boinski and Newman, 1988).

As a general principle, the physiological mechanisms controlling the expression of a particular class of vocalizations have evolved under selection pressures that promote the efficient exchange of information between vocalizer and potential listeners. In the case of isolation calls, the listeners of importance to the vocalizer are the caregiving parent (if the vocalizer is an infant), other familiar conspecifics, and potential predators. Isolation calls have evolved to provide adequate cues to permit a parent or social companion to determine the general location of the vocalizer, without providing more precise localization cues (such as acoustic transients) that would make the vocalizer particular vulnerable to a predator (cf. Newman, 1985b). On the other hand, alarm calls directed by a social group toward a slow-moving, terrestrial predator possess acoustic properties that promote localization of the vocalizer, an adaptation that permits recruitment and coordination of group 'mobbing' behavior toward a potential predator (cf. Vencl, 1977; Klump and Shalter, 1984). Given the different selection pressures on isolation and alarm calls shaping the acoustic properties of the signal and the differentiation of the behavioral contexts in which these 2 classes of vocalization are produced, it would not be surprising if different neural mechanisms mediated their production. Evidence in support of this comes both from brain stimulation studies (cf. Jürgens and Ploog, 1970; Jürgens, 1982) and from behavioral pharmacology studies (cf. Newman, in press).

CONCLUSIONS

As the study of the physiological control of mammalian vocalizations has reached a certain level of maturity, it seems timely to consider the future of this subdiscipline and its probable role in the larger discipline of behavioral neuroscience. Whatever name one wishes to assign to it (e.g., "comparative neurolinguistics," Newman, 1988), investigations of the neural mechanisms underlying the perception of auditory communication signals is likely to continue to serve as an important driving force for considerations of the probable evolutionary history of human speech mechanisms from earlier antecedents.   Earlier, I have referred to the need for models of human brain mechanisms underlying language functions that take into consideration a general primate neurobehavioral plan out of which the cerebral control of human language has evolved (Newman, 1983).   This evolutionary perspective may appropriately be extended to all extant mammals, due to the growing evidence for shared neuroanatomical substrates and related neurochemical mechanisms that mediate vocal production in a wide range of species.

REFERENCES

Boinski, S., and Newman, J.D., 1988, Preliminary observations on squirrel monkey (Saimiri oerstedi) vocalizations in Costa Rica. Amer. J. Primatology, 14:329.

Green, S., 1975, Variation of vocal pattern with social situation in the Japanese monkey (Macaca fuscata), in: "Primate Behavior," volume 4, L.A. Rosenblum, ed., Academic Press, New York.

Jürgens, U., 1982, Amygdalar vocalization pathways in the squirrel monkey. Brain Research, 241:189.

Jürgens, U., and Ploog, D., 1970, Cerebral representation of vocalization in the squirrel monkey. Exp. Brain Res., 10:532.

Jürgens, U., Maurus, M., Ploog, D., and Winter, P., 1967, Vocalization in the squirrel monkey (Saimiri sciureus) elicited by brain stimulation. Exp. Brain Res., 4:114.

Klump, G.M., and Shalter, M.D., 1984, Acoustic behaviour of birds and mammals in the predator context. Z. Tierpsychol., 66:189.

Larson, C.R., Sutton, D., Taylor, E.M., and Lindeman, R., 1973, Sound spectral properties of conditioned vocalizations in monkeys. Phonetica, 27:100.

Lillehei, R.A., and Snowdon, C.T., 1978, Individual and situational differences in the vocalizations of young stumptail macaques (Macaca arctoides). Behaviour, 65:270.

Newman, J.D., 1983, On models, mechanisms, and the evolution of human language. The Behavioral and Brain Sciences, 6:217.

Newman, J.D., 1985a, Squirrel monkey communication, in: "Handbook of Squirrel Monkey Research," L.A. Rosenblum and C.L. Coe, eds., Plenum, New York.

Newman, J.D., 1985b, The infant cry of primates: an evolutionary perspective, in: "Infant Crying: Theoretical and Research Perspectives," B.M. Lester and C.F.Z. Boukydis, eds., Plenum, New York.

Newman, J.D., 1988, Primate hearing mechanisms, in: "Comparative Primate Biology, vol 4 (Neurosciences)," H.D. Steklis and J. Erwin, eds., Alan J. Liss, New York.

Newman, J.D., in press, Ethopharmacology of vocal behavior in primates, in: "Primate Vocal Communication," D. Todt, P. Goedeking and D. Symmes, eds., Springer, Berlin.

Robinson, B.W., 1967, Vocalization evoked from forebrain in Macaca mulatta. Physiology and Behavior, 2:345.

Vencl, F., 1977, A case of convergence in vocal signals between marmosets and birds. Amer. Naturalist, 111:777.

Winter, P., Ploog, D., and Latta, J., 1966, Vocal repertoire of the squirrel monkey (Saimiri sciureus), its analysis and significance. Exp. Brain Res., 1:359.

ON THE MOTOR COORDINATION OF MONKEY CALLS

Uwe Jürgens and Detlev Ploog

Max Planck Institute of Psychiatry
Munich, FRG

INTRODUCTION

Vocalization is a complex motor pattern made up of essentially three components, namely, vocal fold adduction, respiratory
activity (usually of the expiratory type) and movements of supralaryngeal structures, such as the lower jaw, lips, tongue and soft
palate. According to this composite character, the motoneurons involved in vocalization are widely dispersed. The motoneurons responsible for vocal fold adduction lie in the nucl. ambiguus, a long,
slender cell column in the ventrolateral medulla oblongata. The
motoneurons responsible for the expiratory component lie in the
thoracic and upper lumbar ventral horn of the spinal cord. The motoneurons involved in supralaryngeal movements are found in the lateral pons (trigeminal motor nucleus), ventrolateral and dorsomedial
medulla (facial and hypoglossal nucleus, respectively). From this,
the question arises of how these widely scattered motoneuron pools
are coordinated in their activity to finally accomplish a full-
blown species-specific vocalization.

ANATOMICAL STUDIES

As a first step to approach this problem, we have tried to
find out from which brain areas the phonatory motoneuron pools
receive their input. We were especially interested in the question
of whether there is an area which is connected with all phonatory
motoneuron pools conjointly. Theoretically, such an area would be
in an ideal position to coordinate the activity of the different
phonatory muscles and, thus, act as a phonatory motor center. In

a recent study in the squirrel monkey (Thoms and Jürgens, 1987),
we therefore injected horseradish peroxidase (HRP) in one animal
into the nucl. ambiguus, that is, the site of the laryngeal motoneurons.   In another animal, the trigeminal motor nucleus innervating the jaw muscles was injected.   A third animal received HRP
into the facial nucleus which controls lip movements; and a fourth
animal was injected into the hypoglossal nucleus which is responsible for tongue movements (Fig. 1).   As HRP is known to be taken
up by axon terminals and being transported retrogradely back to
their perikarya, it allows to trace the afferent input of the
injected nuclei.

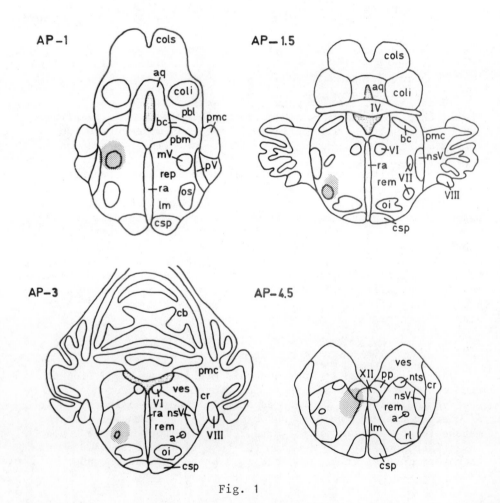

Fig. 1

When we compared the areas containing retrogradely labeled cells in the four animals, we found that there were indeed some areas common to all four animals. These areas are shown by stippling on the right side of the brain diagrams in Figs. 2 and 3.

In order to be sure that these areas do project in fact to all phonatory cranial motor nuclei and are not due to spread of the HRP injection into structures surrounding them, we made control injections with radioactive leucine into the retrogradely labeled areas. As leucine, in contrast to HRP, is exclusively transported anterogradely and is only taken up by nerve cell bodies but not axons, it allows to trace the efferent projections of an injection site.

Fig. 1.   Stippling indicates HRP injection sites in four squirrel monkeys. Abbreviations: a - nucl. ambiguus; an - nucl. anterior thalami; anl - ansa lenticularis; aq - periaqueductal gray; bc - brachium conjunctivum; ca - nucl. caudatus; cb - cerebellum; cc - corpus callosum; cen - nucl. centralis superior Bechterew; cent - centrum medianum; ci - capsula interna; cin - cingulum; cn - nucl. cuneatus; coli, cols - colliculus inferior, superior; cr - corpus restiforme; csp - tractus corticospinalis; dbc - decussation of brachium conjunctivum; dv - dorsal motor nucleus of vagus; f - fornix; gl, gm - lateral, medial geniculate body; gp - globus pallidus; gpm - periventricular gray; h - field H (Forel); ha - habenula; hi - tractus habenulo-interpeduncularis; hip - hippocampus; hl - lateral hypothalamic area; hv - ventromedial hypothalamic nucleus; in - nucl. interpeduncularis; lm - lemniscus medialis; m - mammillary body; md - nucl. medialis dorsalis thalami; mt - tractus mammillothalamicus; mV - trigeminal motor nucleus; nsV - spinal trigeminal nucleus; nts - nucl. tractus solitarii; oi, os - oliva inferior, superior; p - pedunculus cerebri; pbl, pbm - nucl. parabrachialis lateralis, medialis; pmc - brachium pontis; po - pontine gray; pp - nucl. praepositus; pu - pulvinar; put - putamen; pV - principal sensory trigeminal nucleus; ra - raphe; re, rem, rep - midbrain, medullary, pontine reticular formation; rtp - nucl. reticularis tegmenti pontis; rub - nucl. ruber; sm - stria medullaris; sn - substantia nigra; st - stria terminalis; su - subthalamus; va - nucl. ventralis anterior thalami; ves - vestibular complex; vl, vpl, vpm - nucl. ventralis lateralis, ventralis posterolateralis, ventralis posteromedialis; zi - zona incerta; II - tractus opticus; III - nucl. and nervus oculomotorius; IV - nucl. and nervus trochlearis; VI - nucl. abducens; VII - nucl. and nervus facialis; VIII - nucl. cochlearis; XII - nucl. hypoglossus.

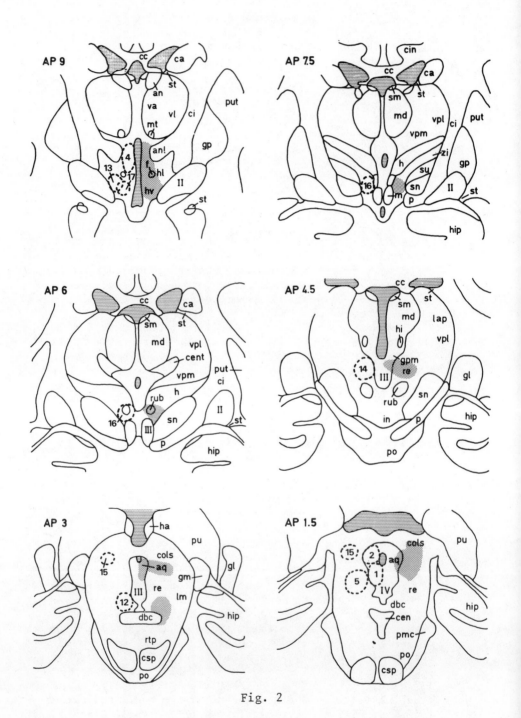

Fig. 2

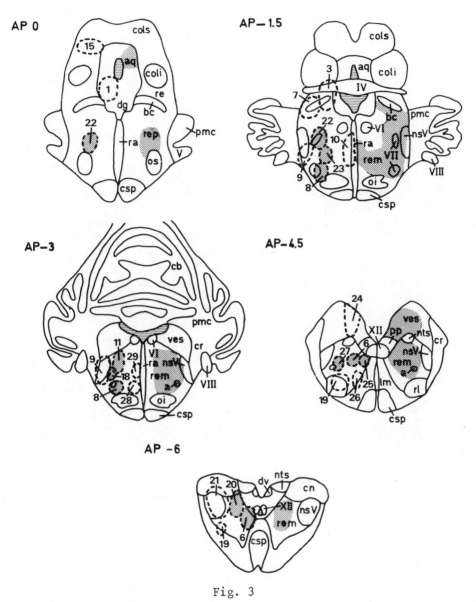

Fig. 3

Figs. 2 and 3.   Stippling on the right side of the brain diagrams
                 indicates areas retrogradely labeled after HRP in-
                 jections into the nucl. ambiguus, trigeminal motor,
                 facial and hypoglossal nucleus. Dashed outlines
                 on the left side indicate ³H-leucine injection
                 sites; those projecting to all four phonatory
                 cranial motor nuclei are filled with stippling.
                 Numbers refer to animals. Abbrev. see Fig. 1.

The control injections revealed that a number of the retrogradely
labeled areas do not project to all four phonatory nuclei, but to
only two or three of them. These injections are indicated on the
left side of the brain diagrams of Figs. 2 and 3 by dashed outlines.
This finding did not come completely unexpected as the nucl. ambiguus and hypoglossal nucleus are so small in diameter that it is
virtually impossible to restrict an HRP injection to these nuclei
without invading the surrounding reticular formation.

Some leucine injections, however, did yield projections to all
four phonatory cranial motor nuclei. These injections are shown
in Fig. 3 by dashed outlines filled with stippling. The most
rostral positive injection site lies in the lateral reticular formation of the caudal pons, near the anterodorsal edge of the superior
olive. From here, effective injection sites can be followed continuously through the reticular formation of the lower brain stem
down to its caudal end. As there are several studies (Feldman et
al., 1985; Holstege and Kuypers, 1982; Jones and Yang, 1985; Miller
et al., 1985) indicating that part of the medullary and caudal
pontine reticular formation also projects into the ventral horn of
the thoracic and upper lumbar spinal cord (harboring the expiratory
motoneurons), we may conclude that this structure probably is
directly connected with all essential motoneuron pools involved in
phonation and thus seems to be in a suitable position to coordinate
the different components underlying vocalization.

LESION STUDIES

Coordinated activity of motoneurons in the nucl. ambiguus,
facial nucleus, hypoglossal nucleus, trigeminal motor nucleus and
anterior horn does not only take place during vocalization but
also in a number of other motor patterns, such as coughing, swallowing, vomiting, panting, etc. In order to find out whether the
reticular formation of the lower brain stem projecting to these
motoneurons is indeed involved in phonatory functions, we have made
a lesioning study in which the effects of stereotactically placed
coagulations in different regions of the squirrel monkey's brain
stem were tested on vocalization (Kirzinger and Jürgens, 1985).
Fig. 4 gives a summary of the results of this study.

In this figure, hatching from the upper right to the lower left
corner indicates brain areas the bilateral destruction of which
has no effect on the acoustic structure of the squirrel monkey's
calls. Hatching from the upper left to the lower right corner,
in contrast, indicates lesions causing a deterioration of the
calls. A comparison with Fig. 3 reveals that all brain areas
connected with the four phonatory motor nuclei conjointly show
phonatory deficits when damaged. The deficits in most cases consisted of a reduction in fundamental frequency, together with an
increase of non-harmonic, that is noise-like, energy in the power
spectrum.

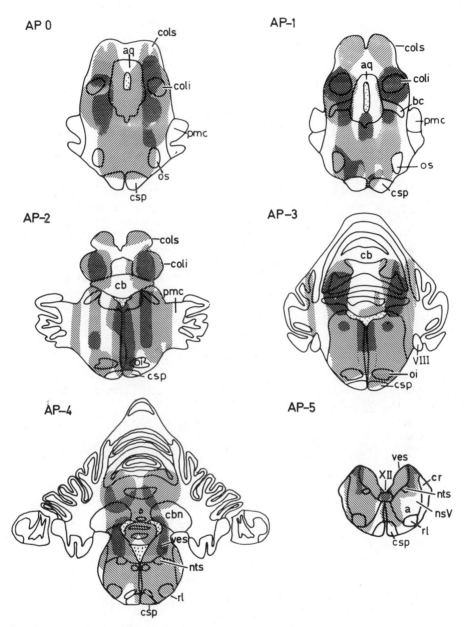

Fig. 4.   Hatching from the upper right to the lower left corner
          indicates brain areas the bilateral destruction of which
          has no effect on the squirrel monkey's calls. Hatching
          from the upper left to the lower right corner demarcates
          lesions which cause a deterioration of the calls. The
          hatched areas are the result of a superposition of the
          lesions made in altogether 44 animals. Abbreviations
          see Fig. 1. (From Kirzinger and Jürgens, 1985)

STIMULATION STUDIES

Electrical Brain Stimulation

Another observation which suggests that parts of the medullary and posterolateral pontine reticular formation are involved in phonatory motor coordination comes from electrical
brain stimulation studies. It is known since quite a long time
that a number of brain structures yield vocalization when electrically stimulated (for reviews see Jürgens, 1979, and Ploog, 1981).
Among those are the posterolateral pontine and medullary reticular
formation. What distinguishes the latter two from the rest of
vocalization-eliciting areas, however, is that the acoustic structure of the elicited calls is clearly abnormal. An example is
given in Fig. 5. In this case, the call was obtained by stimulating the dorsolateral medullary reticular formation just
beneath the solitary tract nucleus. The stimulation frequency
used was 33 pulses per sec. It can be seen from the sonagram
that the elicited vocalization bears a frequency and amplitude
modulation of 33 Hz. A call of this type is never uttered spontaneously by the squirrel monkey and also cannot be obtained from
vocalization-eliciting areas in the forebrain and midbrain. The
call thus clearly bears an artificial character, showing a stimu-
lation-controlled acoustic structure. This suggests that in such
areas the stimulation interferes directly with phonatory motor-
coordinating mechanisms.

Chemical brain stimulation

In order to clarify whether the artificial character of the
calls is due to activation of interneurons or fibers-en-passage,
such as axons of laryngeal motoneurons coursing through the
reticular formation on their way from the nucl. ambiguus to the
vagal rootlets, we have used chemical brain stimulation with
glutamate (Jürgens and Richter, 1986). Glutamate is a putative
neurotransmitter which is known to activate not only gluta-
matergic neurons but also neurons working with other transmitters
(Fonnum, 1984; Watkins, 1981). In fact, current knowledge suggests that glutamate has an excitatory effect on all types of
neurons. This excitatory effect is limited, however, to those
regions of the neurons containing synapses, that is, it neither
activates axons nor nerve cell bodies free of synapses, such as
dorsal root ganglion cells (Fries and Zieglgänsberger, 1974).
Glutamate thus allows to distinguish those electrical stimulation sites from which vocalization can be obtained by activation of synaptic relays from those producing vocalization by
activating fibers-en-passage.

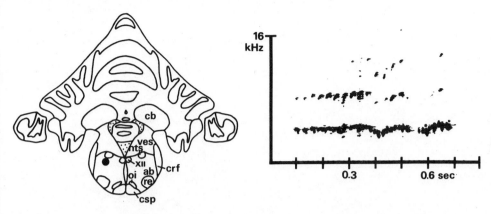

Fig. 5.   Cross-section through the lower brain stem of the
          squirrel monkey indicating a site (black circle) which
          yields abnormal calls when electrically stimulated.
          The type of call obtained is shown in the sonagram on
          the right. Abbreviations: ab - nucl. ambiguus; cb -
          cerebellum; crf - corpus restiforme; csp - tractus
          corticospinalis; nts - nucl. solitarius; oi - oliva
          inferior; re - nucl. reticularis lateralis; ves -
          vestibular complex; XII - nucl. hypoglossus (from
          Jürgens and Pratt, 1979).

       In our study (Jürgens and Richter, 1986), we injected gluta-
mate into a number of brain sites yielding normal and abnormal
vocalization when electrically stimulated and compared the effects
of chemical and electrical stimulation. All circles in the brain
diagrams of Fig. 6 represent sites the electrical stimulation of
which yielded vocalization. The white circles represent sites the
glutamate stimulation of which did not produce vocalization. The
black circles indicate sites the glutamate stimulation of which
produced normal species-specific calls. The asterisk-marked
circles represent sites which yielded abnormal calls with both
glutamate and electrical stimulation. It can be seen from Fig. 6
that only a part of the sites producing vocalization with electrical stimulation also produce vocalization when glutamate-
injected. This was to be expected from the fact that electrical
stimulation activates bypassing fibers as well as synaptic relay
areas, while glutamate activates only the latter. Fig. 6, furthermore, shows that there are several sites in the reticular formation
of the lateral pons and medulla which yield abnormal calls with
glutamate. Such calls, of course, do not show the rhythmic
frequency modulation typical for the electrically elicited calls
from the same site - as glutamate acts continuously, not rhythmically, on the substrate. The acoustic structure of the elicited
calls, nevertheless, is clearly abnormal and never occurs in
spontaneous utterances (Fig. 7).

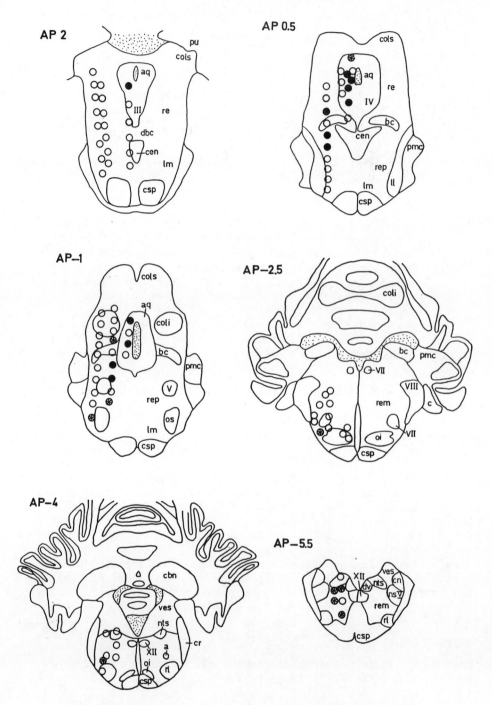

Fig. 6. For explanation see text. Abbrev. see Fig. 1

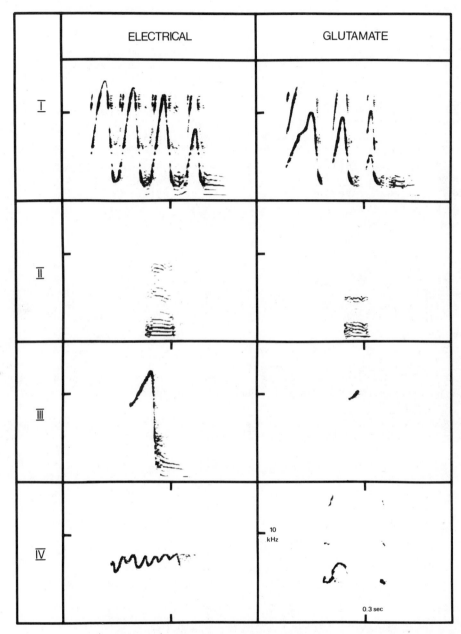

Fig. 7.   Sonagrams of electrically and glutamate-induced vocalizations from four different sites. I to III: normal
species-specific calls elicited from forebrain and midbrain. IV: abnormal calls obtained from the lateral
pontine reticular formation (from Jürgens and Richter,
1986).

CONCLUSIONS

   As glutamate-induced abnormal vocalizations can be obtained
from regions often far away from the phonatory motor nuclei, it
must be assumed that production of these calls is due to activation of a higher level than that of the "final common pathway".
On the other hand, the artificial character of the calls suggests
that the stimulation, in these cases, impinges on the phonatory
motor-coordinating mechanisms and not on motivation-controlling
areas triggering vocalization indirectly - as it seems to be the
case in the forebrain and most parts of the midbrain from which
normal species-specific calls can be obtained. We suggest,
therefore, that the lateral pontine and medullary reticular formation contain interneurons playing an essential role in the
motor coordination of vocalization.

REFERENCES

Feldman, J. L., Loewy, A. D., and Speck, D. F., 1985, Projections
      from the ventral respiratory group to phrenic and intercostal
      motoneurons in cat: an autoradiographic study, J. Neurosci.,
      5:1993.
Fonnum, F., 1984, Glutamate: a neurotransmitter in mammalian
      brain, J. Neurochem., 42:1.
Fries, W., and Zieglgänsberger, W., 1974, A method to discriminate
      axonal from cell-body activity and to analyse "silent calls",
      Exp. Brain Res., 21:441.
Holstege, G., and Kuypers, H. G. J. M., 1982, The anatomy of brain
      stem pathways to the spinal cord in cat. A labeled amino
      acid tracing study, in: "Progress in Brain Research", Vol.
      57, H. G. J. M. Kuypers and G. F. Martin, eds., Elsevier,
      Amsterdam.
Jones, B. E., and Yang, T.-Z., 1985, The efferent projections from
      the reticular formation and the locus coeruleus studied by
      anterograde and retrograde axonal transport in the rat,
      J. Comp. Neurol., 242:56.
Jürgens, U., 1979, Neural control of vocalization in nonhuman
      primates, in: "Neurobiology of Social Communication in
      Primates: An Evolutionary Perspective", H. D. Steklis and
      M. J. Raleigh, eds., Academic Press, New York.
Jürgens, U., and Pratt, R., 1979, Role of the periaqueductal grey
      in vocal expression of emotion, Brain Res., 167:367.
Jürgens, U., and Richter, K., 1986, Glutamate-induced vocalization
      in the squirrel monkey, Brain Res., 373:349.
Kirzinger, A., and Jürgens, U., 1985, The effects of brain stem
      lesions on vocalization in the squirrel monkey, Brain Res.,
      358:150.

Miller, A. D., Ezure, U., and Suzuki, J., 1985, Control of abdominal muscles by brain stem respiratory neurons in the cat, J. Neurophysiol., 54:155.

Ploog, D., 1981, Neurobiology of primate audio-vocal behavior, Brain Res. Rev., 3:35.

Thoms, G., and Jürgens, U., 1987, Common input of the cranial motor nuclei involved in phonation in squirrel monkey, Exp. Neurol., 95, in press.

Watkins, J. C., 1981, Pharmacology of excitatory amino acid transmitters, in: "Amino Acid Transmitters. Advances in Biochemical Psychopharmacology", Vol. 29, F. V. DeFeudis and P. Mandel, eds., Raven Press, New York.

FUNCTIONAL NEURAL PATHWAYS FOR VOCALIZATION IN THE DOMESTIC CAT

Nihal C. de Lanerolle and Frederick F. Lang

Section of Neurosurgery
Yale University School of Medicine
New Haven, Connecticut

INTRODUCTION

The domestic cat has been a companion of man for a very long time. However, until very recently, little was known about the structure, function and natural history of the vocalizations of the domestic cat. This is particularly surprising as animal vocalizations in general have been the subject of intensive research by ethologists, and very significant advances have been made with respect to the neural mechanisms of avian vocalization (Konishi, 1985; Andrew, 1974).

A study of the ethology and neural control of vocalization in a mammalian species such as the domestic cat, apart from being of much interest in itself, can provide valuable information for at least two other areas of study. Firstly, it could help understand the etiology of speech and voice disorders manifested in a range of neurological disorders such as Tourette syndrome, Parkinson disease, spasmodic dysphonia, essential voice tremor and several other disorders (Aaronson et al., 1968; Harcherik et al., 1984; Van Woert et al., 1976; Hartman, 1984). Secondly, since in the cat and other species of animals vocalizations are an expression of emotional state (Andrew, 1974; Jurgens, 1979), a study of the neural control of vocalizations could provide a better appreciation of the nature and underlying mechanisms of emotional states. In this chapter we will review what is known to date about the neural mechanisms underlying the causation of vocalization in the cat.

DESCRIPTION OF DOMESTIC CAT VOCALIZATIONS.

The earliest comprehensive report of domestic cat vocalizations was by Moelk (1944), an amature naturalist, who described in detail and classified cat vocalizations using phonetic notations. Since then 3 studies have described cat vocalizations on the basis of sound spectrograms -- Hartel (1975), Brown et al. (1978) and McKinley

(1982). The most comprehensive of these studies is that by McKinley. On the basis of several techniques of cluster analysis applied to a variety of characteristics of the sound spectrograms of cat calls, she recognized 23 different types of calls. These 23 types can be divided into 2 major groups: (1) Pure calls -- purr, murmur, growl, squeak, shriek, hiss, spit, mew, moan, (2) Complex calls -- meow, growl-moan, murmur-moan, murmur-mew, murmur-squeak, squeak-murmur-mew. The pure calls are essentially homogeneous vocalizations with no major changes in frequency range, harmonic structure or pulse modulation characteristics over their duration. The complex type calls are seen as composed of 2 or more pure subunits linked together (McKinley, 1982). However, such a classification may be splitting cat calls into an unnecessarily large number of groups, because hierarchical cluster analysis applied to an extensive series of calls from one cat revealed that the complex type calls do not emerge as separate clusters. In most cases they cluster into groups with one of their subunits. A complex call may thus be assigned to the group with its predominant component. The analytical data presented in this paper (McKinley, 1982) suggest that, in particular, the meow need not be separated from a mew. Both calls have a harmonic structure. Further, the meows do not fall into a separate group, but rather some cluster with short mews and the others resemble long mews in duration, dominant frequency and noise proportion. Our own analysis of vocalizations with a harmonic structure, evoked by electrical brain stimulation, support a division of these calls into 2 groups based on duration (de Lanerolle, in press).

In the identification of vocalizations, non-vocal features associated with the sound may also have to be taken into consideration. Leyhausen (1979) has demonstrated that the position of the ears, size of the face, piloerection etc. may modulate the meaning of the vocal signal. Hunsperger and Bucher (1967) in a study of brain stimulation evoked calls with a harmonic structure (referred to as mews by them) recognized 3 types of mews -- uneasy mews, protest mews and plaintive mews. During uneasy mewing the cat was described as having its jaws half opened, the corners of the mouth not fully retracted, the upper lips slightly pursed and pupils moderately dilated. In protest mewing the chin was pushed forward, the jaws were almost fully opened drawing the ears downward and sideways and the corners of the mouth were retracted. In plaintive mewing, the chin was pushed forward, the jaws were almost fully opened, the corners of the mouth are barely retracted, and the upper lip remained pursed. Since no sonograms are presented, it is not possible to determine if these mews are spectrographically different. However, from our observations it seems that the uneasy mew may be a short duration mew. At the present time it seems practical to refer to all calls with a harmonic structure by one name, either mews or meows. This is further warranted as these two terms are used interchangably in the older literature. The term meow will be adopted in this paper. Subtypes of meows such as short and long meows may be recognized until future work justifies the recognition of further subtypes.

The function of vocalizations in the behavior of the domestic cat has received even less attention. Two papers by Moelk published 35 years apart (1944, 1979) provide the most comprehensive description of the contexts in which domestic cats emit vocalizations. Leyhausen (1979), in the course of wide ranging studies of a variety of Felid species, has also made careful observations on the use of calls by domestic cats. Experimental analyses testing the validity of the observations made by these authors are still extremely few. Some tentative generalizations could be drawn from the above observational studies and other anectodal accounts of cat behavior. Growls, hisses, spits and shrieks occur in situations of defensive threat and attack such as tom cat duals; when a cat encounters a strange cat or other strange animal (including humans); and in establishing territorial rights and rank. Shrieks may also be used by the female during courtship behavior, and by cats subject to intense pain. The murmer and purr like calls are used in friendly approach and contact, and during mother-kitten relations. The meow type call is the most common of a cat's vocalizations and is given in a wide range of situations. An appreciation of the types of cat vocalizations and their meaning and function is necessary to properly investigate the neural mechanisms underlying cat vocalizations.

NEURAL MECHANISMS OF CAT VOCALIZATIONS

Historical background

Despite the rather slow progress in ethological studies of cat vocal behavior, greater progress has been made concerning the neural substrate underlying vocalization. Much of this information has been generated in the course of studies whose primary objectives were other than the study of vocalization. Information about the causation of vocalization obtained through this early work has provided the foundation of our current work, and will therefore be reviewed briefly here.

(i) Decerebration studies: In very early studies Woodworth and Sherrington (1903) found that in cats in whom the cerebral hemispheres and thalamus were removed, vocalizations angry in tone and sometimes plaintive could be evoked by stimulation of the sciatic, brachial and splanchnic nerves. These vocalizations were associated with other pseudoaffective responses. The vocalizations were blocked by various spinal transections which blocked ascending inputs to the brain. It is not clear whether the hypothalamus was intact in these preparations. In an extensive series of short-lived chronic decerebrate preparations, Bazett and Penfield (1922) observed vocalization in only 10 out of 124 animals. Most of the vocalizations observed were not repeatable except purring. Purring occurred in 4/10 animals. Purring was generally, though not always, associated with feeding, and sometimes given spontaneously or on handling, and mostly evident in young animals or females. The brain transections were through the upper or lower midbrain. In one animal (No.19), the plane of transection was through the anterior half of the superior colliculi dorsally to 2mm in front of the pons ventrally. In this animal, in addition to purrs two loud meow-like angry calls were elicited on handling. Growling occurred in 3 male cats with transections between the superior and inferior colliculi dorsally to a couple of millimeters in front of the pons ventrally. One of the cats also gave a few meows. The problems involved in keeping these animals alive made it difficult for the authors to explore fully the behavioral capacities of these animals. Keller (1932) too has demonstrated that typical rage responses including growling and hissing can be obtained by nociceptive stimuli and sometimes handling of animals with low midbrain transections which left the spinal cord, medulla, pons and small caudolateral portions of the midbrain intact.

The best study of chronic decerebrates is that by Bard and Macht (1958). These animals survived the longest. The decerebration was accomplished by first ablating all brain structures rostral, lateral and dorsal to the olfactory tubercles and the ventral diencephalon, and then removing a 3 to 5mm wedge of tissue at one of 3 brainstem levels. In pontile or bulbospinal cats the wedge of tissue removed consisted of the most caudal segment of the hypothalamus, the rostral third of the tectum, the entire mesencephalic tegmentum and the rostral fourth of the pons. The interpeduncular and red nuclei were completely removed. The application of strong nociceptive stimuli elicited a growl-like vocalization, but no hissing, along with other non-vocal responses. In response to the blast of a whistle, these cats never vocalized, though they seemed to perceive the sound. In low mesencephalic cats, the plane of transection passed dorsally through the rostral portion of the superior colliculi to the level of the exit of the third cranial nerves ventrally. Much of the interpeduncular nucleus was spared, but only the caudalmost part of the substantia nigra remained, while the red nucleus was completely removed. Such animals responded to painful tactile stimuli by hissing, growling and tail lashing, whereas very strong nociceptive stimuli evoked a loud shrill cry like the pain call. In response to an auditory stimulus such as a high pitched whistle, the immediate response was to right itself and meow. This was followed a few seconds later by plaintive meowing. In high mesencephalic preparations the transection was through the rostral portion of the midbrain running through the rostral part of the superior colliculus down to a position behind the mammillary bodies. The response to nociceptive and auditory stimuli was as in low mesencephalic cats. However, as these animals recovered from surgery, their response to nociceptive stimuli increased to include hissing as well as loud growling.

Certain inferences about the neural control of vocalization can be drawn from these decerebration studies. (i) The elicitability of calls in pontile or bulbospinal preparations suggests that the motoneuron groups essential for the coordination of vocalization lie below the level of the midbrain, probably in the pons/medulla region (Bard and Macht, 1958; Keller, 1932). (ii) Pontile preparations produced only growls (Bard and Macht, 1958) whereas low and high mesencephalic preparations were able to emit a wider range of calls -- growls, hisses, meows, purrs (Bard and Macht, 1958; Bazett and Penfield, 1922; Keller, 1932; Bignall and Schramm, 1974). This suggests that midbrain mechanisms are necessary for the patterning of a wider variety of calls. In the hypothalamic preparation the types of calls produced were similar to those in the mesencephalic preparation but they were better integrated into normal call associated behavior patterns of the cat such as escape and defensive threat (Keller, 1932). (iii) The calls produced from these brainstem preparations are more reflex-like in occuring separated from well coordinated behavioral responses. In pontile or bulbopontine preparations only tactile and nociceptive stimuli appear capable of evoking a vocal response, whereas in midbrain preparations other stimulus modalities such as auditory (Bard and Macht, 1958) and those resulting from feeding (Bazett and Penfield, 1922) can elicit a vocal response. Thus midbrain regions seem necessary for completion of the circuits linking these latter stimulus modalities and motor coordinating centers for vocalization.

Does the neocortex play any role in vocalization? Bard and Mountcastle (1948) observed that in cats with only neocortical ablations and the rhinencephalon intact, strong nociceptive stimuli evoked vocalizations -- plaintive meows, screams and sometimes growling and hissing. If in addition to the neocortex the hippocampus, entorhinal cortex and amygdala were removed, the animals growled, spit and bit more readily. This observation suggests an inhibitory role for these latter forebrain areas in the causation of vocalization.

(ii) Selective lesion studies: Localized experimental brain lesions in the cat either make them mute or appear to facilitate vocalization. The muting lesions appear to involve the periaqueductal gray matter (PAG) and perhaps adjacent tegmental areas. Bailey and Davis (1942) reported that with small lesions of the PAG, the cats on awaking from anesthesia became "very wild. They stare vacantly into space with pupils widely dilated, and spit, snarl, mew and strike as though seeing imaginary menaces"; but paid no attention to actual objects in their environment. However, with larger lesions, the animals are said to "lie inert, silent and flaccid as a wet rag." Kelly, Beaton and Magoun (1946) also reported that large midbrain lesions destroying much of the PAG and adjacent tegmentum beneath the superior colliculus produced muting or a marked reduction of vocalization. Their animals did not exhibit the postoperative akinesia observed by Bailey and Davis (1942). Lesions confined to the very rostral part of the PAG, pretectum and adjacent tegmentum; those destroying the hypothalamus at the level of the mammillary bodies; bilateral destruction of thalamic regions where somatosensory fibers are thought to end; and bilateral tectal lesions or transection of the brainstem at the midbrain-diencephalic junction did not make cats mute or abolish pain induced vocalization (Kelly et al., 1946). Kelly et al. concluded that the alteration in facio-vocal behavior by their muting lesions is not due to the interruption of pathways in the region, but is due to the destruction of structures intrinsic to the region.

In another series of lesioned cats, Skultety (1958) observed that mutism was produced in the animals with extensive destruction of the PAG. Lesions limited to the anterior two thirds or posterior third of the PAG did not mute. He therefore concludes that "... mutism is dependent upon the quantity of the periaqueductal gray matter destroyed rather than any particular portion." This conclusion may find support in the earlier lesion studies mentioned above. However, it differs from the conclusions reached in Adametz and O'Leary (1959). These workers found that it is not necessary for the entire PAG to be destroyed for mutism to result. They even reported that unilateral or otherwise incomplete lesions produce mutism. It is not possible on the basis of available information to reconcile this difference from previous studies.

Based upon the observation that midbrain muting lesions did not eliminate all components of the affective response -- the cats still bit, struggled, struck, attempted to escape, and piloerected in response to nociceptive or frightening stimuli -- Kelley et al. (1946) suggested that "the midbrain facio-vocal mechanism is not concerned with integrating the sequence of activities in the component bulbar nuclei innervating cranial and respiratory musculature during vocalization --which probably is managed by interneurons at the bulbar level -- but rather is concerned with precipitating their integrated performance at times when it forms an appropriate part of the behavior of the animal as a whole."

Lesions of the lateral portion of the upper midbrain, which included the medial, lateral, spinal and trigeminal lemnisci, produced a syndrome in which one of the characteristics was a lack of affect; where the cats were mute, lacked facial expression and showed minimal autonomic responses. Along with the lack of affect was also a marked sensory deficit characterized by sensory inattention and poor localization of sensory stimuli (Sprague et al., 1961). Sprague and co-workers suggest that the facio-vocal deficits in these animals may be due mainly to deprivation of afferent sensory input to subcortical structures such as the PAG.

Lesions of parts of the thalamus and amygdaloid complex appear to facilitate vocalization. Lesions of the mediodorsal thalamic nucleus increased the cat's reactivity to non-noxious tactile stimuli, to the degree that even gently removing animals from their cages, cleaning or feeding them resulted in immediate yowling and struggling which continued until they were released. After a while the mere opening of the cage doors or removing and replacing feed bowls resulted in withdrawal of the animal to the rear of the cage, displaying a defense reaction with hissing and low growling interrupted periodically by explosive spitting. Even light pinching of the tail evoked growling and aggressive responses (Schreiner et al., 1953). On the other hand, anterior thalamic nuclear lesions (with some encroachment upon adjacent structures) reduced the reactivity of cats to noxious stimuli, and made them docile. They solicited petting and responded to it by purring loudly and with friendly head-rubbing movements.Only very rough handling made these cats spit and growl; such responses ended as soon as the stimulus was terminated (Schreiner et al., 1953). Lesions of the above two parts of the thalamus thus seem to facilitate different types of vocalizations.

The pyriform lobes containing the amygdaloid complex was removed by Schreiner and Kling (1953). Four to 14 months post-operatively the animals were overly alert and exhibited extreme interest in the activity going on around them. From the second post-operative week they exhibited excessive vocalization, which in many instances had characteristics strikingly similar to those given by cats during the mating season. During these periods of vocalization, the cats directed their attention and activities towards movements in the room, and vocalizations became most intense when an uncaged animal and its handler were in view (Schreiner and Kling, 1953). On placing a female in view of the operated male cats, the males came to the front of their cages, directed their attention to the uncaged animal and vocalized while engaging in treading movements. Females, and males to a lesser extent, engaged in rolling on their sides or backs, squirming and playfully pawing their feeding bowls and other objects, and accompanied such activity with meows. Lesioning of the hypothalamus 4 months after amygdaloid damage, abolished the previously produced increase in vocalization and motor activity in response to visual stimuli. A general feature of all the above mentioned call facilitating lesions is that along with the facilitation of calls there is also an increased responsivity and attention to sensory stimuli.

(iii) Electrical brain stimulation studies: Hess (1928) first described the evocation of vocalizations (hisses) by electrical stimulation of "deep parts of the diencephalon" in an awake unrestrained cat. The hisses were accompanied by other affective responses. Since then there have been several reports of brain stimulation evoked vocalizations. These are summarized in Table I.

A review of these studies reveals several features about the neural control of vocalization in the cat. An important point to recognize from these studies is that while vocalizations are reported to be evoked from various brain areas such as the PAG, hypothalamus etc., the entire nucleus or area did not yield vocalizations; only

Table 1. Call Sites Identified by Electrical Stimulation

Vocalization	Anatomical Locus	Authors
Hiss	PAG and adjacent ventrolateral tegmentum; Hypothalamus (subfornical part of MFB; anterior commissures to ventromedial part from level of supraoptic hypothalamic nucleus; nu. supraopticus diffusus; nu. perifornicalis; nu. dorsomedialis); Amygdala; Olfactory tubercle; Lower rostral hippocampus; Tract and bed nucleus of stria terminalis.	de Molina & Hunsperger (1956); Magoun et al. (1937); Masserman (1941-1942); MacLean & Delgado (1953); Nakao et al. (1968); Ranson & Magoun (1933).
Growl	PAG (medial part); *Lateral tegmentum (near Reils band); Tegmentum (at level of superior colliculus); Reticular formation throughout lower brainstem; Hypothalamus (dorsomedial; ventromedial supraoptic nuclei); Amygdala; Olfactory tubercle; Lower rostral hippocampus; Tract and bed nucleus of stria terminalis.	de Molina & Hunsperger (1959, 1962); Hunsperger (1956); *Kanai & Wang (1962); MacLean & Delgado (1953); Nakao et al. (1968).
Piercing Cry (Loud scream, Wail, Screech)	PAG (*ventral part near level of nu. III; central & lateral part); Ventrolateral tegmentum adjacent to PAG; Reticular formation at level of inferior colliculus; Hypothalamus (dorsomedial, ventromedial & supraoptic nuclei); Wall of infundibulum from anterior region of wall of 3rd ventricle.	*Hunsperger (1956);Kanai & Wang (1962); Karplus & Kreidl (1909); Magoun et al. (1937); Nakao et al. (1968); Spiegel et al. (1954).
Purr	Septum (1 site); Infundibular region (3/400 sites); Anterior lateral portion of hypothalamus (1 site).	Gibbs & Gibbs (1936);Magoun et al. (1937); Meyer & Hess (1957).
Meow	PAG (ventral part);*Tegmentum adjacent to PAG at superior colliculus; Reticular formation adjacent to ventral PAG; *Sites around the medial lemnicus in pons and medulla; Hypothalamus near amygdala; Septum and precommissural fornix; Thalamus near and along stria medullaris.	Hess et al. (1945-6); *Hunsperger (1956, 1963, 1967); *Kanai & Wang (1962); Magnus & Lammers (1956); Nakao et al. (1968).

*Denotes sites from which only vocalizations were elicted. MFB=Medial forebrain bundle.

certain sites within these areas yielded vocalizations when stimulated. Thus, in considering the neural pathways associated with call sites, it is insufficient to assume that they are the same as the connections of the entire nucleus in which the call site resides. The neural pathways associated with call sites may be more specific and need to be traced relative to a functional call site. Further, past studies reveal that there are certain brain areas where electrical stimulation evokes only vocalizations, whereas at other sites vocalizations are associated with other overt behavior and autonomic responses.

Sites from which only vocalizations were obtained have been localized in the ventral part of the PAG near the level of the oculomotor nuclei (piercing cry -- Hunsperger, 1956); in the lateral tegmentum near Reils band (growl -- Hunsperger, 1956); in the tegmentum adjacent to the PAG at the level of the superior colliculus and sites around the medial lemniscus in the pons and medulla (soft mewing cry -- Kanai and Wang, 1962); lateral preoptic and anterior hypothalamic area (mews -- Hunsperger and Bucher, 1967). Stimulation at all other sites evoked in addition to vocalization other behavioral responses as well, most often those associated with the defensive threat display (Leyhausen,1979).

Kanai and Wang (1962) have shown that unilateral lesions placed at call sites near the medial lemniscus in the medulla block the evocation of calls from rostral ipsilateral pontine call sites. However, stimulation of contralateral call sites evoked vocalizations. When corresponding areas were destroyed on the contralateral side too, no vocalizations were obtained. The authors suggest that this pathway for vocalization may be distinct from those mediating the defensive threat response.

Some of the areas from which growling and hissing were obtained associated with other defensive threat responses also seem to form a system. This system includes the growl/hiss sites in the amygdala, stria terminalis, hypothalamus and PAG (de Molina and Hunsperger, 1962). These authors showed that unilateral coagulation of the call sites in the stria terminalis, hypothalamus or PAG abolished amygdala stimulation evoked calls. These sites form a hierarchical system such that coagulation at any particular level abolished calls evoked from more rostral sites but not the caudal ones on the same side. Contralateral lesions abolished calls evoked only from the contralateral sites. The interrelationships and points of interaction between the call only and call plus defensive threat system are as yet poorly defined. The PAG may be an area of importance in this regard.

Brain stimulation studies, like the lesion studies, identify the PAG as an important locus for vocalization. In a study that systematically explored the entire PAG, Nakao and co-workers (1968) found that vocalization sites were located in the caudal two thirds of the PAG, but mainly in the central third. Most of the major calls (meows, growls, hisses and screeches) could be evoked from these areas. Some sites in the PAG seem exclusively concerned with vocalization, yielding only a vocal response on stimulation (Hunsperger, 1956).

A final feature worthy of note in these stimulation studies is the observation that brain stimulation evoked vocalizations are commonly associated with various attentive responses. De Molina and Hunsperger (1959) described a state of focussed attention accompanying growling. Upon stimulation the cat turned its head towards the experimenter, its eyelids opened wide and pupils dilated, fixed its eyes on the experimenter and then began to growl. The growling got stronger and stronger as the stimulation continued. On the other hand, stimulation at a meow site resulted in a state of scanning attention accompanying meows -- the cats pupils were dilated and it showed continuous "movements of inspection" as it looked attentively at its surroundings, then began and continued to mew (Hunsperger, 1963).

(iv) Neurochemical studies: There are no studies as yet that have attempted to analyze directly the neurochemical basis of vocalization in the cat. However, studies of the effects of various drugs on cat behavior provide the basis for some inferences. Injection of d-amphetamine (a drug which causes the release and prevents the reuptake of dopamine) made cats hiss, meow and spit without interrupting the head movements they showed (Jones et al., 1977; Randrup and Munkvard, 1967). Cats

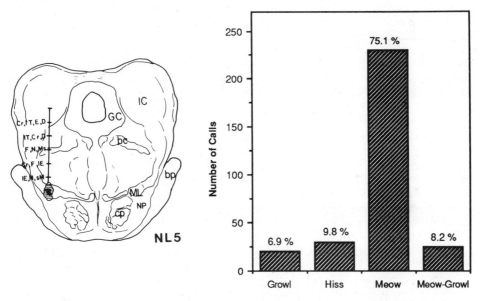

Fig. 1.   Left: An outline drawing of a cat brain section through the midbrain/pons junction to show the location of the ventrolateral pontine call site (hatched with dark center) in one cat of a series studied. This is the typical location of this site. The behavior evoked at points along the trajectory to the call site are given by the following abbreviations: Cr=crouch; D= pupils dilated; E=escape; F= ears flattened; IE=ipsilateral eye shut; IT=ipsilateral turning; Ms= moves in semicrouch; N=pupils narrowed; sM=soft meow. Abbreviations for brain structures: bc= brachium conjunctivum; bp= brachium pontis; CA= anterior commissure; CH= optic chiasm; cp= cerebral peduncle; GC= periaqueductal gray; GP= globus pallidus; IC= inferior colliculus; ML= medial lemniscus; NC= caudate nucleus; NP= basal pontine nucleus. Right: A histogram showing the total number of different call types evoked from the ventrolateral pontine call site in a group of 10 cats. The frequency of each call type expressed as a percentage of the total number of calls recorded is given on the top of each column.

injected bulbocapnine (a dopamine receptor blocker) were reported to vocalize readily and loudly in response to any slight movements in their visual field or any other disturbances (Ernst, 1969). The involvement of dopaminergic systems in vocalization can be inferred from such studies. Acetylcholine may also play a part in the causation of vocalization. The application of carbachol to the preoptic region of the cat evoked a vocal response -- strong growling with some hissing (Brudzynski, 1981a; 1981b). The vocalizations produced were accompanied by eye movements, attentive head movements and arousal. The vocal response alone has been shown to result from the activation of muscarinic cholinergic receptors in the hypothalamus (Gralewicz, 1983).

Current studies

The review of past work points to several important areas in which information is lacking. Most of the experimental studies have not provided a complete and accurate description of vocalizations using objective methods such as sound spectrography. This makes it difficult to evaluate the various call sites as to their role in vocalization. Further, the course of the neuroanatomical pathways linking up the various call sites and through which vocalizations are produced have not been described. Finally while many of the early studies suggest a close relationship between vocalizations and attentional mechanisms and emotions, the neural substrate through which this occurs remains poorly defined. The studies undertaken in our laboratory are aimed at providing information in these three areas.

(i) Vocalizations evoked by brain stimulation: Since the studies of Kanai and Wang (1962) had reported that sites around the medial lemniscus were rather specific for vocalization, we examined these sites in order to describe more fully the vocalizations evoked from them (de Lanerolle, in press). The call sites we examined were located in the ventrolateral pons, in the region of the medial lemniscus at the transition of the tegmentum and pes pontis (Fig. 1). Vocalization was the principal behavior elicited by electrical stimulation at these sites. Spectrographic and quantitative analysis of the evoked vocalizations revealed 4 types of calls -- growls, hisses meows, and meow-growls (Fig. 2). The growl was a rather long call (modal duration 2.8 sec) of low frequency. Its fundamental frequency component was the strongest and below 1KHz and the highest frequency never exceeded 2KHz. The hiss was characterized by a relatively uniform distribution of sound frequencies up to 8KHz. The sound began and ended sharply and had a modal duration of 0.8 sec. The meow was a call that had many frequency bands of sound over a frequency range of 0.6 to 8 KHz. Frequency bands represent a fundamental and its harmonics. The mean fundamental frequency of meows was 0.8 KHz and the median number of harmonics per call was 3. The meow-growl was a single call composed of a meow and growl component. It was a long call with a modal duration of 3.2 sec. The duration of 70% of all meows were less than the modal duration for growls, and 75% of them had durations less than the modal duration for meow-growls. The meows were the calls that showed the greatest variation in form (Fig. 3). They can be divided into 2 groups, short and long meows, on the basis of their duration. They were also the type of call most likely to be associated with another call type to form complex calls (McKinley, 1982) such as meow-growls (de Lanerolle, in press). Seventy five percent of all calls elicited by electrical stimulation of the ventrolateral pontine call site were meows, and the remaining 25% comprised the other call types in about equal proportions (Fig. 1).

The various vocalizations were accompanied by facial activity. The mouth showed the greatest changes in shape for the meow. The mouth was held open during meowing; the degree of opening being related to the intensity of the sound. The three types of meow described by Hunsperger and Bucher (1967) -- uneasy, plaintive and protest meows -- were elicited from the ventrolateral pontine call site by varying the intensity of stimulation. When the cat growled, the mouth was almost closed, and when it hissed the mouth was held wide open and the lips were drawn back so that the canines were visible. During the hiss the eyes were almost closed appearing as narrow slits. Most of the cats remained lying on their bellies with limbs held close to the body as they vocalized during electrical stimulation. Their general posture resembled that of a normal undisturbed cat. Electrical stimulation at this site did not induce the cat to attack a rat or feed on cat chow when either stimulus was presented. These data, in contrast to those of Kanai and Wang (1962), suggest that a wider range of vocalization trypes can be evoked from a site similar to that of their study.

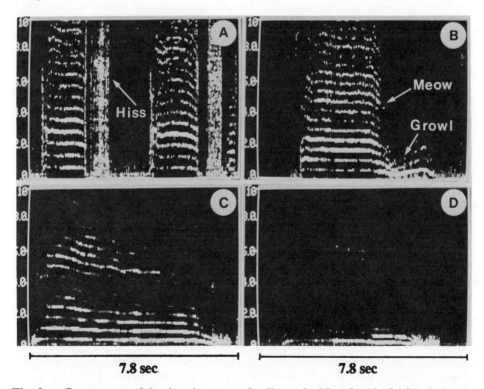

Fig. 2.   Sonograms of the 4 main types of calls evoked by electrical stimulation at the ventrolateral pontine call site. (A) Meow and hiss calls. In this case the hiss immediately followed the meow. However, they are also produced independently. (B) Meow-growl call. (C) A meow of long duration. (D) Growl.

In preliminary studies we have also localized call sites in the PAG and preoptic area. In both of these areas we have found call sites from which calls were elicited without any obvious components of defensive threat behavior. In the preoptic area meow and hiss-growl sites were located, while in the PAG also meow, growl and hiss sites were localized. It therefore seems that growl and hiss sites are not invariably associated with defensive threat responses. Further, stimulation at preoptic and PAG meow sites showed that before the cat began to vocalize it moved its head to look at some part of its visual field and then showed attentive head movements while it vocalized. Growl and hiss site stimulation was associated with focussed attention on the experimenter or if the experimenter could not be seen the cat focussed on a point in front of it. Thus our observations too, like those in earlier studies, support a relationship between vocalization and attentional processes, that is, somewhat different attentional states being associated with different call types. This interaction is being further analysed.

(ii) Tract tracing studies: In order to study the neural pathways associated with the ventrolateral pontine call site, we placed small electrolytic lesions at the call site so as to abolish stimulation-evoked vocalization at 3 times threshold, and traced the resulting axonal degeneration with a silver staining method (de Lanerolle, in press). The degeneration resulting from lesioning these call sites could be traced caudally through the trapezoid area into the magnocellular tegmental field, ipsilateral facial nucleus and to an area which corresponded to the retrofacial nucleus. Degenerating fibers and terminal-like processes were found in all parts of the ipsilateral facial nucleus -- mediodorsal, intermediate, lateral and ventromedial areas, and on the contralateral side in the medio-dorsal facial nucleus. Ascending degenerating fibers passed close to the medioventral edge of the medial geniculate nucleus and into the thalamus; numerous degenerating fibers and terminals were observed in the ipsilateral ventroposterolateral nucleus (VPL) and the zona incerta. An ascending pathway was also traced to the ipsilateral inferior colliculus. The ventrolateral pontine call site thus seems to be connected with brain regions capable of at least some control over all major mechanisms (orofacial, laryngeal and respiratory) necessary for sound production. The facial nucleus innervates the buccinator and buccolabial muscles (Courville, 1966); the retrofacial region innervates the laryngeal muscles (cricothyroid and posterior cricoarytenoid; Gacek, 1975). The retrofacial nucleus also projects to the nucleus ambiguus which in turn innervates laryngeal muscles (Bystrzycka, 1980). The magnocellular tegmental field is also the area in which respiratory centers have been reported (Haber et al.,1957; Nagi and Wang, 1957). The facial nucleus can also control expiratory movements (Pitts et al.,1939).

In order to study the pathways afferent to the ventrolateral pontine call site, the enzyme horseradish peroxidase (HRP) was injected at the call site identified by electrical stimulation, and the retrograde distribution of HRP was examined (de Lanerolle and Lang, in preparation). This study showed that the PAG region of the midbrain had the largest number of labelled neurons (Fig. 4). The neurons were located in those areas of the PAG where Nakao et al. (1968) localized call sites by electrical stimulation. The location of labeled neurons in the PAG suggests that the PAG is likely to be the primary location of neurons projecting to the call coordinating centers in the medulla via the pontine call site. The association of the PAG with

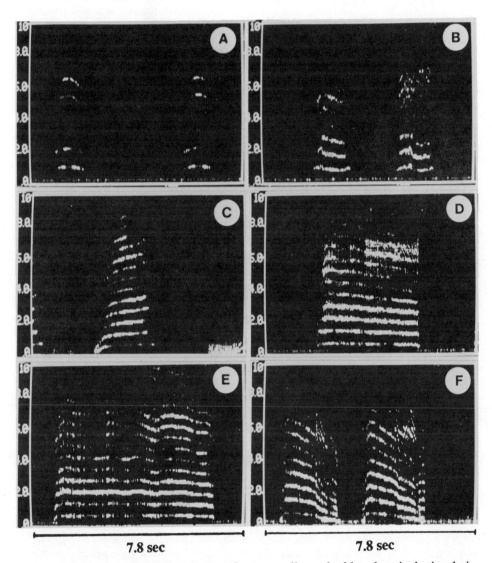

7.8 sec   7.8 sec

Fig. 3.   Sonograms of various types of meow calls evoked by electrical stimulation
at the ventrolateral pontine call site. (A) Short meows which are also soft. (B) Short
meows. (C) Short meows showing a greater number of bands of sound frequency
(harmonics). (D) Long meow. (E) Long meow of longer duration than (D).
(F) Long meows showing a rapid drop in frequency at the end of the   call. This type
of call is also given as a pain response.

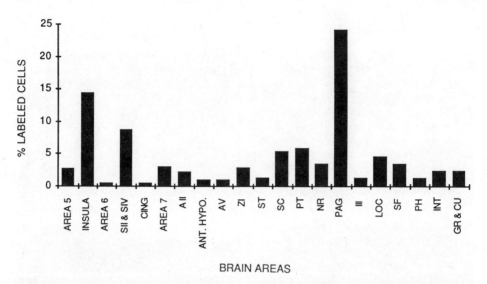

Fig. 4.   Histogram showing the percentage of cells in various brain regions that were retrogradely labeled following an injection of horseradish peroxidase at the ventrolateral pontine call site in a cat. Note that the largest proportion of cells are in the periaqueductal gray area (PAG).

vocalizations through this study adds to the weight of the evidence derived from early studies (reviewed above) implicating the PAG in an important way in vocalization. Retrogradely labeled neurons were also found in several other areas of the brain, notably cortical areas such as the insula, somatosensory areas SII and SIV, area 7, and in other brainstem areas especially the deep layers of the superior colliculus and a pretectal area immediately rostral.

       (iii) Glucose metabolism mapping studies: Conventional tract tracing methods are limited to tracing neural pathways from the site of stimulation to one synapse away. A proper appreciation of the causation of vocalization requires a precise knowledge of all neuroanatomical areas concerned with vocalization, that is, sensory pathways through which relevant stimuli could activate vocalization, motivational/emotional systems involved with the behavior as well as the pathways for motor coordination. The 2-deoxyglucose (2DG) method (Sokoloff, 1978) can in theory provide much of this information because it can detect changes in metabolic activity which occur simultaneously at many levels of the brain, and thus detect areas polysynaptically connected with a stimulated call site. Consequently, we carried out studies in which the 2DG method was combined with electrical brain stimulation of vocalization sites in the cat. To date, the most extensive 2DG studies have been carried out at call sites located in the PAG, with preliminary investigations of ventrolateral pontine (VLP) and preoptic (PO) call sites.

       In the PAG studies, awake unanesthetized cats stimulated with bipolar electrodes at 1 1/2 times threshold or greater were found to give the most reproducible results. Analysis of the resulting autoradiograms involved quantitative methods using two different currently accepted transformations, namely, the relative optical density

(ROD) and the grey white ratio (GWR) value (Eilbert, 1986). Since electrical stimulation was unilateral, metabolic activity on the stimulated side was compared with that on the contralateral side of each animal. In addition, separate control animals were subjected to the same conditions as the experimental animals, including surgical procedures, localization of a call site, and handling conditions. These controls, however, were stimulated at subthreshold currents (1/3 times threshold) and did not vocalize during the 2DG experiment. Changes in 2DG metabolic activity which occurred in all experimental animals on the stimulated side compared to the non-stimulated side were considered most accurate. Findings that were evident only when compared to external controls were considered accurate if they occurred bilaterally in all animals when compared to controls. In all cases both ROD and GWR values had to show the same change for a brain region to be considered altered.

Using these strict standards, several brain areas were found to be important for PAG stimulation evoked vocalization in the domestic cat. Increased activity was observed around the electrode tip as well as within a larger area of the PAG beyond the electrode tip when comparing the stimulated side in vocalizing animals to both the non-stimulated side of the same animal and the stimulated side of the controls (Fig. 5A and 5B). In addition, increased activity was noted in the lateral and ventrolateral tegmentum (Fig. 5A and 5B). This area of tegmental activity extended caudally to an area just beyond the inferior colliculus and in front of the superior olive. Moreover, the superior colliculus showed an altered pattern of activity in the deep layers. More caudal brainstem areas showed bilaterally reduced activity, including the facial nucleus, the vestibular/cochlear nucleus, and the superior olive.

Areas rostral to the PAG also showed altered 2DG activity. In particular, the caudate nucleus had decreased activity bilaterally. The visual cortex (area 17) showed increased bilateral activity which was very strong when compared to controls (Fig. 5E and 5F). Finally, a very well demarcated band on the superior bank of the superior sulcus was evident bilaterally in all experimental animals, but was absent in controls (Fig. 5C and 5D). This band extended from the level of the posterior aspect of the head of the caudate to just behind the anterior aspect of the thalamus. The areas in which this band was located corresponds to cortical area 7 (Reinoso-Suarez, 1984).

From these studies several pieces of information can be gleaned about both rostral and caudal brain areas involved in vocalization. Firstly, a descending pathway from the PAG into the ventrolateral tegmentum might be an important pathway for vocalization in the cat. This pathway as defined by 2DG methods corresponds to the midbrain/pontine regions that produced vocalization by electrical brain stimulation (Kanai and Wang, 1962; Jurgens and Ploog, 1970), and correlates with the extent of lesions needed to produce muting in the cat (Skultety, 1958). The pathway ends in a region near the VLP call site defined above. Secondly, several areas active during vocalization are also involved in processing visual information.

Concluding comments

Some generalizations can be made from what is known at the present time about the neural pathways for vocalization in the cat. The functional and anatomical data we have would suggest that there may be a common route or pathway in the

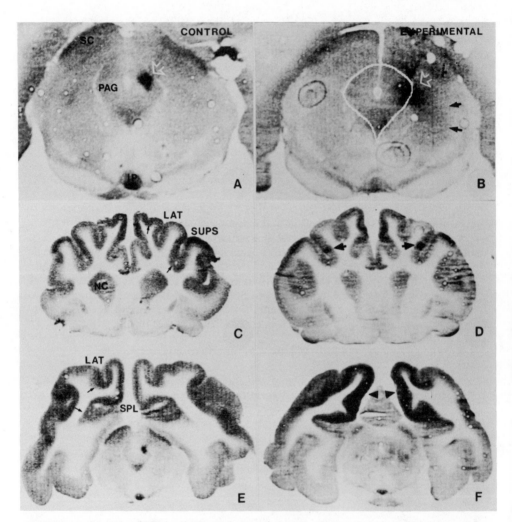

Fig. 5.   (A), (C), (E). 2-deoxyglucose autoradiograms from a cat stimulated at a
periaqueductal gray (PAG) call site at subthreshold current intensity so as not to
evoke vocalizations -- Control. (B), (D), (F). Autoradiograms from a cat stimulated
vocalizations -- Experimental. Comparison of (A) and (B), sections at the stimulation
site (open arrow) shows a greater region of metabolic activity in (B) which extends
into the lateral and ventrolateral tegmentum (arrows pointing to the region.) At a
more rostral region in the same cats in sections (C) and (D) a distinct band of
metabolic activity can be seen in cortical area 7 (middle suprasylvian gyrus) in the
experimental animal (arrows in D). The cross-sectional extent of area 7 at this level is
between the two small arrows in (C). (E) and (F) are sections through area 17
(primary visual cortex) the extent of which is between the small arrows in (E). Note
were given 200 uCi/kg of 14C-2-deoxyglucose intraperitoneally and stimulated for 45
min. with trains of pulses, 60 pps square waves of 1 ms duration. Abbreviations:
SC= superior colliculus; PAG= periaqueductal gray; IP= interpeduncular nucleus;
NC= caudate nucleus; LAT= lateral sulcus; SUPS= suprasylvian sulcus.

caudal brainstem for the motor coordination required to produce a majority of
vocalization types in the cat. This pathway passes through the call sites in the
ventrolateral pons, for stimulation here evokes most of the calls, and lesions here
(Kanai and Wang, 1962) abolish calls evoked from more rostral call sites. HRP
studies suggest that the PAG may be an important source of afferents to this pathway.
Additional evidence for a close PAG/VLP link is that the same range of calls are
produced by stimulation of both these areas. The brainstem system may be the
primary coordinating system for call evocation because early decerebration studies
suggest that calls can be evoked from it even when isolated from more rostral brain
regions. However, when separated from the diencephalon and forebrain areas, only
a very limited number of stimulus types can evoke vocalization from this system, in
particular noxious tactile stimuli. Brain areas rostral to the brainstem vocal pathways
may be necessary for the mediation of vocalizations in response to a wider range of
stimuli. This is supported by the lack of vocal expression in response to visual
stimuli and other non-tactile stimuli in decerebrates, and muting resulting from lesions
of the lateral portion of the upper midbrain which interrupts several ascending
sensory pathways (Sprague et al., 1961). How these sensory systems interact with
the brainstem call coordinating mechanism needs further elucidation. However, it
seems likely that many of these systems may interact eventually at the PAG, for PAG
lesions result not only in muting but also in profound sensory neglect.

Another theme that emerges from the studies reviewed above is the association
of attentional processes with vocalization, most strikingly processes of visual
attention. The neural mechanisms subserving this interaction also need further study.
However, retrograde tract tracing studies and 2DG studies point to certain areas as
likely participants in these processes. HRP studies reveal many labeled neurons in
the deep tectal layers and pretectal areas. 2DG studies have shown increased
metabolic activity in the caudate, superior colliculus, visual cortex (area 17),
association cortex area 7 and possibly prefrontal cortex (in VLP cats). Physiological
studies have shown that many of these areas, identified as related to vocalization, not
only process visual information but also play an important role in the generation of
ocular, head and orienting movements of the types that are a part of the attentional
behavior associated with vocalization. In the cat area 7 has been shown to be
associated in the integration of many different types of sensory inputs (Cavada and
Reinoso-Suarez, 1985). In particular, this area has been shown to receive its vast
majority of afferent fibers from the visual cortex (Cavada and Reinoso-Suarez,
1985). Further, its main efferent projections are to the cortex of the frontal eye fields
(Cavada and Reinoso-Suarez, 1985). Consideration of these connections has led to
the hypothesis that area 7 plays a significant role in the organization of ocular
movements in response to visual cues. More specifically, this cortical region may
integrate visual sensory information, in relation to other sensory information, and via
the frontal eye field cortex (in prefrontal cortex) direct the eyes to focus on the most
behaviorally significant visual stimulus. This hypothesis gains support when
considering that area 7 in the cat is similar to the posterior parietal lobe regions in the
monkey which have been shown in electrophysiological studies to contain neurons
whose electrical activity increases when the monkey detects, looks at, and reaches
toward a motivationally relevant object. In the monkey, this posterior parietal region
also connects with the frontal eye fields as well as the superior colliculus and caudate
nucleus. It has been postulated that a circuit involving these nuclei would be ideal for
carrying out the complex process of focussing and reacting to pertinent visual stimuli,

i.e. attention mechanisms (Mesulam, 1983). To reiterate, nearly all of the areas involved in these attentional mechanisms were implicated in vocalization of the cat through the 2DG studies, and taken in conjunction with the behavioral observations of attentional behavior such as scanning and focussed attention during various vocalizations, reinforces the close relationship between vocalization and attentional processes.

Even the ventrolateral pontine area from which vocalizations can be evoked may have visually responsive cells related to head, eye and body movements (Mower et al., 1979). Such studies thus suggest that an examination of the physiology of some of these areas in relation to vocalization may provide new insights on the relationship of attentional processes to vocalization; a relationship that is of importance even in human speech and language. The study of the neurobiology of vocalization in the cat through the application of modern research methods in neuroscience, holds the promise of new and exciting discoveries in the future.

ACKNOWLEDGEMENTS

This paper is dedicated to the late Professor John P. Flynn for the encouragement and support given to N de L to pursue research on cats, and to Professor Richard J. Andrew who introduced him, as a graduate student, to the study of the neural basis of vocalization in animals. The work was supported by NIH grant NS19919.

REFERENCES

Aaronson, A. E., Brown, J. R., Litin, E. M., and Pearson, J. S., 1968, Spastic dysphonia II. Comparison with essential voice tremor and psychogenic dysphonias, J. Speech Hearing Dis., 33: 219.
Adametz, J., and O'Leary, J. L., 1959, Experimental mutism resulting from periaqueductal lesions in cats, Neurology., 9: 626.
Andrew, R. J., 1975, Midbrain mechanisms of calling and their relation to emotional states, in:"Neural and Endocrine Aspects of Behaviour," P. Wright., P. G. Caryl., and D. M. Vowles, eds., Elsevier Scientific Publishing Company, Amsterdam.
Bailey, P., and Davis, E. W., 1942, Effects of lesions of the periaqueductal gray matter in the cat, Proc. Soc. Exp. Biol. Med., 51: 305.
Bard, P., and Macht, M. B., 1958, The behavior of chronically decerebrate cats, in: "Neurological Basis of Behavior," Ciba Symposium, Little Brown, London.
Bard, P., and Mountcastle, V. B., 1948, Some forebrain mechanisms involved in expression of rage with special reference to suppression of angry behavior, Res. Publ. Ass. ner. ment. Dis., 27: 362.
Bazett, H. C., and Penfield, W. G., 1922, A study of the Sherrington decerebrate animal in the chronic as well as the acute condition, Brain, 45: 185.
Bignall, K. E., and Schramm, L., 1974, Behavior of chronically decerebrated kittens, Exptl. Neurol., 42: 519.
Brown, K. A., Buchwald, J. S., Johnson, J. R., and Mikolich, D. J., 1978, Vocalization in the cat and kitten, Dev. Psychobiol., 11: 559.
Brudzynski, S. M., 1981a, Carbachol induced agonistic behavior in cats: Aggressive or defense behavior, Acta. Neurobiol. Exp., 41: 15.
Brudzynski, S. M., 1981b, Growling component of vocalization as a quantitative

index of carbachol-induced emotional defensive response in cats, Acta Neurobiol. Exp., 41: 33.

Bystryzycka, E. K., 1980, Afferent projections to the dorsal and ventral respiratory nuclei in the medulla oblongata of the cat studied by the horseradish peroxidase technique, Brain Res., 185: 59.

Cavada, C., and Reinoso-Suarez, F., 1985, Topographical organization of the cortical afferent connections of the prefrontal cortex in the cat, J. Comp. Neurol., 242: 293.

Courville, J., 1966, The nucleus of the facial nerve: the relation between cellular groups and peripheral branches of the nerve, Brain Res., 1: 338.

de Lanerolle, N. C., In press, A pontine call site in the domestic cat: Behavior and neural pathways, Neuroscience.

de Molina, A. F., and Hunsperger, R. W., 1959, Central representation of affective reactions in the forebrain and brain stem: electrical stimulation of amygdala, stria terminalis and adjacent structures, J. Physiol., 145: 251.

de Molina, A. F. and Hunsperger, R. W., 1962, Organization of the subcortical system governing defense and flight reactions in the cat, J. Physiol., 160: 200.

Ernst, A. M., 1969, The role of biogenic amines in the extrapyramidal system, Acta Physiol. Pharmac. Neurol., 15: 141.

Gacek, K. E., 1975, Localization of laryngeal motoneurons in the kitten, Laryngoscope, 85; 1841.

Gibbs, E. L., and Gibbs, F. A., 1936, A purring center in the cat brain, J. Comp. Neurol.,64: 209.

Gralewicz, S., 1983, Relationship between some behavioral and electroencephalographic changes induced by intrahypothalamic injections of carbachol in the cat, Acta. Neurobiol. Exp. 43: 311.

Haber, E., Kohn, K. W., Nagy, S. H., Holaday, D. A., and Wang, S. C., 1957, Localization of spontaneous respiratory neuronal activities in the medulla oblongata of the cat: A new location of the respiratory center, Am. J. Physiol., 190: 350.

Harcherik, D. F., Leckman, J. F., Detlor, J., and Cohen, D. J., 1984, A new instrument for clinical studies of Tourette's Syndrome, J. Am. Acad. Child Psychiat., 23: 153.

Hartel, R., 1975, Zur struktur und funktion akustischer signale in pflegesystem der Hauskatze (Felis catus L.), Biol. Zentralbl., 94: 187.

Hartman, D. E., 1984, Neurogenic dysphonia, Ann. Otol. Rhinol. Laryngol., 93: 57.

Hess, W. R., 1928, Stammganglien-Reizversuche. (Verh. Dtsch. physiol. Ges., Sept., 1927), Ber. ges. Physiol., 42: 554.

Hess, W. R., Brugger, M., and Bucher, V., 1945-46, Zur physiologie von hypothalamus, area praeoptica und septum, sowie augrenzender Balken- und stirnhirnbereiche, Mschr. Psychiat. Neurol., 3:17.

Hunsperger, R. W., 1956, Affekreactionen auf elektrische reizung im hirnstamm der katze, Helv. Physiol. Acta, 14: 70.

Hunsperger, R. W., 1963, Comportements affectifs provoques par la stimulation electrique du tronc cerebral et du cerveau anterieur, J. Physiol. (Paris), 55: 45.

Hunsperger, R. W., and Bucher, V., 1967, Affective behavior produced by electrical stimulation in the forebrain and brainstem of the cat, Progress in Brain Res., 27: 103.

Jones, B. E., Harper, S. T., and Halaris, A. E., 1977, Effects of locus coeruleus lesions upon cerebral monoamine content, sleep-wakefulness states and the response to amphetamine in the cat, Brain Res., 124: 473.

Jürgens, U., 1979, Vocalization as an emotional indicator, Behaviour, 69: 88.

Kanai, T., and Wang, S. C., 1962, Localization of central vocalization mechanisms in the brainstem of the cat, Exptl. Neurol., 6: 426.

Karplus, J. P. and Kreidl, A., 1909, Gehirn und sympathicus. I: Zwischenhirnbasis und halssympathicus, Pflug. Arch., 129: 138.

Keller, A. D., 1932, Autonomic discharges elicited by physiological stimuli in midbrain preparations, Amer. J. Physiol, 100: 576.

Kelley, A. H., Beaton, L. E., and Magoun, H. W., 1946, A midbrain mechanism for facio-vocal activity, J. Neurophys., 9: 181.

Konishi, M., 1985, Birdsong: From behavior to neuron, Ann. Rev. Neurosci., 8: 125.

Leyhausen, P., 1979, "Cat Behavior," Garland STPM Press, New York.

MacLean, P. D., and Delgado, J. M. R., 1953, Electrical and chemical stimulation of fronto-temporal portions of limbic system in the waking animal, Electroenceph. clin. Neurophysiol., 5: 91.

Magnus, O., and Lammers, H. J., 1956, The amygdaloid nuclear complex. Part I: Electrical stimulation of the amygdala and the periamygdaloid cortex in the waking cat, Fol. Psychiat. Neurol. Neurochir. Neerl., 55: 555.

Magoun, H. W., Atlas. D., Engersoll, E. H., and Ranson, S. W., 1937, Associated facial, vocal and respiratory component of emotional expression: An experimental study, J. Neurol. Psychopath., 17: 241.

Masserman, J. H., 1941-42, The hypothalamus in psychiatry, Amer. J. Psychiat., 98: 633.

McKinley, P. E., 1982, Cluster analysis of the domestic cat's vocal repertoire, Unpublished Ph.D. thesis, University of Maryland.

Mesulam, M. M., 1983, The functional anatomy and hemispheric specialization for directed attention, TINS, September, 384.

Meyer, A. E., and Hess, W. R., 1957, Diencephal ausgelostes sexualverhalten und schmeicheln bei der Katze, Helv. Physiol. Acta., 15: 401.

Moelk, M., 1944, Vocalizing in the housecat: A phonetic and functional study, Amer. J. Psychol., 57: 184.

Moelk, M., 1979, The dvelopment of friendly approach behavior in the cat: A study of kitten-mother relations and the cognitive development of the kitten from birth to eight weeks, Advances in the Study of Behavior, 10: 163.

Mower, G., Gibson, A., and Glickstein, M., 1979, Tectopontine pathway in the cat: Laminar distribution of cells of origin and visual properties of target cells in dorsolateral pontine nucleus. J. Neurophysiol., 42: 1.

Nagai, S. H., and Wang, S. C., 1957, Organization of central respiratory mechanism in thebrainstem of the cat: Localization by stimulation and destruction. Am. J. Physiol., 190:343.

Nakao, H., Yoshida, M.m and Sasaki, T., 1968, Midbrain central gray and switch-off behavior in cats, Jap. Journal Physiol., 18: 462.

Pitts, R. F., Magoun, H. W., and Ranson, S. W., 1939, Localization of the medullary respiratory centers in the cat, Am. J. Physiol., 126: 673.

Randrup, A., and Munkvad, I., 1967, Stereotyped activities produced by amphetamine in several animal species and man, Psychopharmacologia, 11: 300.

Ranson, S. W., and Magoun, H. W., 1933, Respiratory and pupillary reactions induced by stimulation of the hypothalamus, Arch. Neurol. Psychiat. Chicago, 29: 1179.

Schreiner, L., and Kling, A., 1953, Behavioral changes following rhinencephalic injury in cat, J. Neurophysiol., 16: 643.

Schreiner, L., Rioch, D. McK., Pechtel, C. and Masserman, J. H., 1953, Behavioral changes following thalamic injury in cat, J. Neurophysiol. 16: 234.

Skultety, F. M., 1958, The behavioral effects of destructive lesions of the periaqueductal gray matter in adult cats, J. Comp. Neurol., 110: 337.

Sokoloff, L., 1978, Mapping cerebral functional activity with radioactive deoxyglucose, TINS, September, 75.

Speigel, E. A., Kletzkin, M., and Szekely, E. G., 1954, Pain reactions upon stimulation of the tectum mesencephali, J. Neuropath. exp. Neurol., 13: 212.

Sprague, J. M., Chambers, W. W., and Stellar, E., 1961, Attentive, affective and adaptive behavior in the cat, Science, 133: 165.

Van Woert, M. H., Jutkowita, R., Rosenbaum, D., and Bowers, M. B., 1976, Gilles de la Tourette's Syndrome: Biochemical approaches, in " Basal Ganglia," M. D. Yahr, ed., Raven Press, New York.

Wilson, J. S., and Goldberg, S. J., 1980, Inputs of the pulvinar and lateral posterior nucleus into the abducens nucleus of the cat, Exp. Neurol., 68: 72.

Woodworth, R., and Sherrington, C., 1904, A pseudoaffective reflex and its spinal path, J. Physiol., 31: 234.

STUDIES ON THE RELATION OF THE MIDBRAIN PERIAQUEDUCTAL GRAY, THE

LARYNX AND VOCALIZATION IN AWAKE MONKEYS

Charles R. Larson, John D. Ortega, Elizabeth
A. DeRosier

Departments of Communication Sciences and Disorders
and Neurobiology and Physiology
Northwestern University
Evanston, IL 60201

INTRODUCTION

Mammalian vocalization is a complex behavior involving
muscles of the respiratory and laryngeal systems and usually
muscles of the pharynx, tongue, palate, jaw and lips. Moreover,
it is not uncommon to observe animals moving their ears or
altering their stance when vocalizing. Thus, vocalization may
involve the coordination of a large number of muscle systems of
the body. In this context, vocalization should be considered a
part of a larger behavioral repertoire that is often seen as a
response to an external motivating stimulus, e.g., aggression, or
an internal drive state, e.g., sexual arousal. However,
vocalization can occur without the involvement of many of the
other muscular systems. In fact, the only essential muscular
processes necessary for vocalization, or sound production are
respiratory and laryngeal. Respiratory muscles contract to assist
passive recoil forces in the generation of subglottal pressure,
and laryngeal adductors and tensors contract to place the vocal
folds in the appropriate biomechanical state for responding to
exhaled air and thus producing periodic bursts of air above the
glottis. When such bursts occur with sufficient intensity and
periodicity, a tonal quality is perceived, which we term
vocalization.

The interest in mammalian vocalization has grown
considerably in recent years due in part to interests in animal
communication systems and human speech production. Through the
study of mammalian vocalization, or the structures involved in
producing it (Davis & Nail, 1984; Yoshida et al., 1985; Ueda et

43

al., 1971; Sapir et al., 1981), we have learned a great deal about physiological mechanisms of vocalization. Until recently, there has been a comparative lack of research on the neural mechanisms of vocalization, despite previous studies on the peripheral mechanisms of vocalization.

The majority of the research on neural mechanisms of vocalization has been conducted on anesthetized animals, largely due to the difficulty of studying central neural mechanisms in awake animals. By inserting electrodes or cannula into different areas of the brain and either passing electrical currents or chemicals, it has been determined that certain areas elicit vocalization when stimulated. Magoun et al., (1937) reported that electrical stimulation of the midbrain periaqueductal gray (PAG) of anesthetized monkeys, cats and decerebrate cats produced vocalizations that sounded similar to those naturally produced. Subsequently, other investigators have reported similar findings in a wide variety of animals (Kennedy, 1975; Robinson, 1967; Suga et al., 1973: Jürgens & Ploog, 1970). It has also been determined that lesions involving the PAG render an animal mute (Adametz & O'Leary, 1959).

More recently, studies on the relation of other neural areas to vocalization have also been done. Jürgens & Ploog and their colleagues have carried out a number of studies on squirrel monkeys in which they have shown that the entire vocal repertoire of these animals may be artificially reproduced by electrical stimulation of various limbic system structures. Moreover, not all limbic structures yield the same call when stimulated (Jürgens & Ploog, 1971; Ploog, 1981; Ploog, 1986; Robinson, 1967). Lesions of the anterior cingulate gyrus leads to a reduction in the frequency of emission of some types of calls (Sutton et al., 1974; Kirzinger & Jürgens, 1982). These observations have led to the speculation that electrical stimulation of limbic system structures induces a rather specific motivational change in the animal, and a particular type of call is emitted as a response to that motivational change. When the limbic system is altered through experimental lesions, the call repertoire of the animal changes. The most caudal region of the brain in which stimulation elicits natural sounding vocalizations is the PAG. Since anatomical studies have shown that the above limbic system structures project to the PAG (Jürgens & Pratt 1979a and b; Jürgens, 1982), it has been suggested that the PAG serves as the descending output of the limbic system.

Neuroanatomical tracing studies have shown fibers descending from the PAG along the lateral tegmentum through the pons and into the medulla. Many of these fibers terminate within the reticular formation, but some project directly to the nucleus

tractus solitarius and nucleus ambiguus. The latter is the site
of laryngeal motoneurons and respiratory related neurons (RRNs).
The RRNs show phasic activity with respiration (Cohen, 1981;
Kalia, 1981) and project to cervical and thoracic areas of the
spinal cord where they influence respiratory motoneurons.
Afferent sensory fibers from the larynx and pharynx terminate in
the nucleus tractus solitarius, which projects to the PAG and
nucleus ambiguus (Yoshida et al.1985). Thus, the PAG is
anatomically related to other neural elements important in
controlling vocalization.

The PAG surrounds the 4th ventricle and extends from the
hypothalamus rostrally to the pons caudally. It consists of small
cells with soma diameters ranging from 8 to 35 μm and dendrites
extending for several hundred μm in several directions. PAG cell
types have been described as multipolar, stellate, pyramidal,
bipolar and fusiform (Mantyh, 1982; Beitz & Shepard, 1985). Most
axons within the PAG are non-myelinated or only thinly myelinated
(Beitz, 1985), and maximum conduction velocities of action
potentials within the PAG are about 2.7 m/s (Sandner et al.,
1986). Many axons also branch off to provide collaterals to
nearby cells (Tredici et al., 1983; Gioia et al., 1985), and it is
through these collaterals that PAG cells may excite or inhibit one
another (Sandner et al., 1986). In this context, it has been
suggested that the axon collaterals may provide interconnections
between PAG cells allowing them to function as groups (Gioia et
al., 1985). Notwithstanding that PAG cells may function as
groups, evidence for discrete nuclei within the PAG does not
exist. However, there are regional differences in the sizes and
shapes of PAG cells (Beitz & Shepard, 1985; Gioia et al., 1984;
Mantyh, 1982; Gioia et al., 1985), which may underlie
physiological differences in cell activity.

Despite the extensive anatomical studies of the PAG and its
connections with other areas of the brain, comparatively few
studies have been done on its physiology. For this reason, we
began a series of studies a few years ago designed to improve our
understanding of these mechanisms. We chose to study the PAG since
it seems to serve an important role in the neural control of
vocalization. In our studies, we have analyzed the activity of PAG
neurons during vocalization in awake monkeys (Larson & Kistler,
1984, 1985, 1986). More recently we have begun a series of studies
utilizing microstimulation techniques in order to refine our
understanding of PAG function. The present chapter will review
our earlier findings and present some of our more recent
observations. These data when combined with observations made by
others lead us to suggest that the PAG may not only link higher
and lower areas of the brain, but also may be involved in
coordination of muscular activity during vocalization.

METHODS

The methodology has been described elsewhere. In brief, nine
monkeys, five male macaca nemestrina, one male macaca
fascicularis, and three female macaca fascicularis, have been used
thus far. Each animal was trained to enter a primate restraining
chair and sit quietly. Six of the monkeys used for unit recording
were also trained to vocalize to obtain a fruit juice reward.

Following a training period, which in some cases lasted 6
months, surgeries were performed on the animals to implant chronic
electromyogram (EMG) electrodes in several laryngeal muscles (and
respiratory muscles in one animal), fuse the cervical vertebrae
with the skull and implant a recording chamber and stabilization
lugs on the skull. All surgeries were done under general
anesthesia using aseptic techniques, and two weeks were allowed
for recovery between the surgeries.

For the recording studies, a tungsten microelectrode
insulated with epoxylite, except for the tip, was hydraulically
advanced into the PAG while the monkey vocalized. Each isolated
cell was noted for its relationship to vocalization, and those
that changed their firing rate before or during vocalization were
recorded on magnetic tape along with the voice and EMG signals. In
some cases, after recording from a cell, the electrode was
connected to an electronic stimulator (Grass S-88) through
constant-current isolation units, and microstimulation was
performed. Rectified EMGs were averaged following 20 trains of
pulses (0.1 ms biphasic square wave, 200 pps, train duration 20
ms, at 20, 40 and 60 μA)

For the stimulation studies, the same type of electrode was
advanced into the PAG. On the initial days, the electrode was
connected to an amplifier and unit activity of the superior
colliculus, mesencephalic nucleus of the trigeminal nerve and PAG
were used to identify the location of the PAG. On subsequent days,
the recording step was eliminated, and the electrode was lowered
to a predetermined depth. At this depth, 20 trains of pulses (0.1
ms biphasic square wave, 200 pps, train duration 20 ms, 150 μA)
were passed between the microelectrode and an indifferent
electrode over the dura. A synch pulse from the stimulator
triggered an averaging computer which sampled rectified EMGs for
50 ms prior to the pulse and 100 ms following. Activity from the
20 trains of stimuli was averaged. If changes in the EMGs were
noted, the current was dropped to 80, 60, 40 and 20 μA and
stimulation done at each current level. The electrode was then
advanced 500 μm, and the procedures replicated. Using an X-Y
micrometer stage on the recording chamber, the electrode was moved
horizontally on successive days by 0.5 or 1 mm steps. The chamber
diameter was 9 mm, which allowed us to investigate a 9 mm rostral-

caudal and lateral segment of the PAG. At the conclusion of the
experiments, the animals were anesthetized with Nembutal, an
electrode was lowered to previous stimulation and recording sites
and a lesion was made by passing cathodal current of 20μA for 30
sec. The electrode was then withdrawn, the animal was perfused
through the left ventricle with normal saline followed by 10%
formalin, the brain removed, and the muscles dissected to locate
the EMG electrodes. Histological processing of the brain was done
to locate the marking lesions.

The single unit data were analyzed in several ways. Spike-
triggered averaging of laryngeal EMGs was done with about one half
of the cells (Fetz & Cheney, 1980). Firing rate patterns of cells
were determined by making raster displays of unit activity along
with ensemble averages of rectified voice, EMGs and unit firing
frequency for several vocalizations. Unit, EMG and vocal activity
was digitized onto magnetic tape, and measurements of these
parameters were made on a trial-by-trial (vocalization-by-
vocalization) basis for several vocalizations. From the
measurements of activity related to a single cell, Pearson product
moment correlations were performed between measures, the data were
plotted in scatter plots and lines of linear regression were
fitted to the data by a computer algorithm. This analysis
technique will be referred to as "parametric correlations".

RESULTS

From the six animals used for recording, activity from 250
units was recorded and found to be temporally related to
vocalization. Many other units were observed that were not
temporally related to vocalization. Almost all units, whether or
not they were related to vocalization, showed irregular, slow
(e.g., less than 50 s/s) spontaneous firing rates. Many units
increased their firing rates after vocalization and could possibly
be involved in gustation. One area of the PAG was located in which
the cells gave bursts of activity related to eyeblink. Some cells
responded to auditory stimulation. Many additional units were
sporadically active but could not be related to any specific
behavior on the part of the monkeys. Thus, based on firing rate
patterns, it appears the PAG is composed of cells with a multitude
of functional relationships.

With respect to vocalization, 66% of the 250 cells were
either silent or fired sporadically in the absence of vocalization
and then increased their rate of discharge before or during
vocalization, 31% decreased their rate before vocalization, and
3% exhibited increases and then decreases in firing rate. Although
it was not uncommon to observe cells completely silent in the
absence of vocalization, most cells displayed intermittent

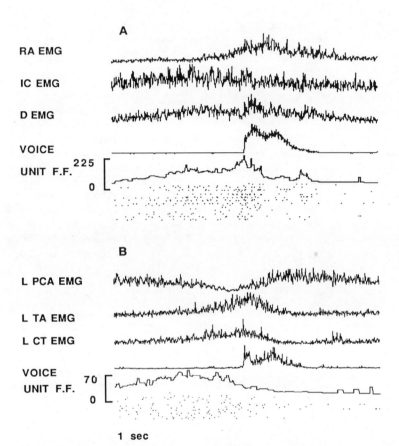

Fig. 1. A. Ensemble averages of rectified activity from rectus
        abdominus (RA), intercostal (IC), and diaphragm (D) muscles,
        voice, and averaged instantaneous unit firing frequency for
        20 vocalizations. B. Similar data for another cell along
        with left posterior cricoarytenoid (L PCA), left
        thyroarytenoid (L TA) and left cricothyroid (L CT)
        muscles. The line up point for averaging is at the beginning
        of the vocalization. Time scale is 1 sec for the entire
        display.

activity and then consistently increased or decreased their rate
before vocalization.

Figure 1 A and B illustrate ensemble averages of rectified
EMG and voice traces, unit firing frequency and dot-raster
displays of units that are typical of many of the units that we
recorded. Figure 1A represents a unit that increased its rate
before vocalization and then decreased its rate just after onset
of vocalization. In this example, the temporal pattern of
discharge frequency resembles the temporal change in diaphragm (D)
EMG. Most of the units that increased their rates before
vocalization displayed a temporal pattern like that in Fig. 1 A.
Although one might suggest, based on the temporal pattern of unit
activity, that the unit was correlated with diaphragm muscle, note
in (B), from a different monkey, that the thyroarytenoid (TA) and
cricothyroid (CT) muscles display a very similar temporal pattern
to that of the diaphragm. It was not always possible to record
from the same muscles in each monkey, however, by comparing muscle
activity patterns from different monkeys, we are certain that the
muscles behave similarily in different animals. One may suppose,
then, that the CT and TA muscles from the monkey whose data are
depicted in (A) would behave like those in (B). Therefore, the
temporal pattern of unit activity in Figure 1A is similar to the
diaphragm, cricothryoid and thyroarytenoid muscles. It also is
likely that other muscles may demonstrate a similar temporal
pattern.

The unit illustrated in Figure 1B increased its firing rate
at about the time that the TA and CT began increasing their
activity. Then the unit decreased its activity at the same time
that the posterior cricoarytenoid (PCA) muscle decreased its
activity. In this case, the temporal changes in unit firing
frequency resemble changes in two different types of muscles.
Although it is possible that single PAG units influence the
activity of more than one muscle, it is hazardous to make
statements as to unit function based on such data. Because of
these similarities, it becomes difficult to use temporal activity
patterns as a basis for determining the function of a particular
cell.

An important feature of PAG cell activity is that changes in
firing rate generally occurred before vocalization and the
beginning of EMG changes accompanying vocalization. The time
between onset of firing rate change and onset of vocalization was
measured from records such as those in Figure 1 for 149 cells and
are plotted as a histogram in Figure 2. It is clear that the vast
majority of cells exhibit rate changes before onset of
vocalization or the beginning of EMG changes (indicated by arrow).
These findings suggest that most PAG cells were not responding to
sensory stimuli associated with vocalization.

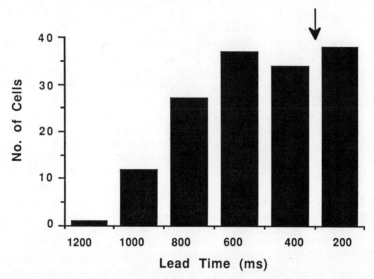

Fig. 2. Histogram illustrating time between onset of unit activity
and vocalization (Lead Time) for 149 cells. Arrow indicates
approximate onset of EMG before vocalization.

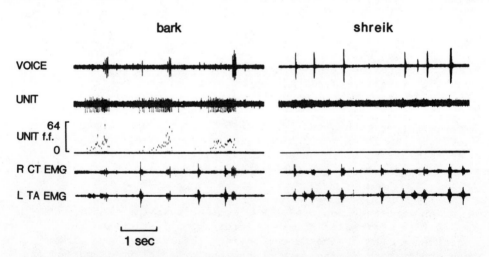

Fig. 3. Single event traces for a unit that was active for "bark"
vocalizations but not for "shreik" vocalizations. Trace
identifications: Voice, Unit potentials, Unit firing
frequency, right cricothyroid (R CT) and left thyroarytenoid
(L TA) muscles. This figure was reproduced with permission
from Experimental Brain Research, 1986, vol. 63, page 601.

Although the monkeys normally emitted a single type of vocalization, such as a bark or a coo, one could elicit shrieks by displaying a frightening object to them (capture gloves used to catch loose monkeys). In so doing, we noticed that a few cells, such as that in Figure 3 would discharge for one of the vocalization types but not for another. Not shown in Figure 3 is the fact that with the shriek vocalizations, the monkeys also displayed other signs of fear such as retraction of the angle of the mouth.

Because of the problems mentioned above in determining unit function from ensemble averages, parametric correlation analyses were performed on 146 of the 250 cells. Parametric correlations were not done on those cells for which only a few vocalizations were recorded or on those cells that exhibited only slight changes in firing rate with vocalization. From the 146 cells, 91 had correlation coefficients (r) significant at the .02 level of confidence. Some cells were correlated with a measure of vocalization (duration, maximal loudness, or fundamental frequency), some with a measure of muscle activity (duration of activity, mean EMG level, or the EMG integrated over the duration of its enhanced activity), and some with both vocalization and EMG. Figure 4 A & B shows scatterplots depicting the relationship between unit activity and measures of vocalization, while C & D are scatterplots depicting the relationship between unit activity and EMGs. In most cases, the lines of linear regression had positive slopes indicating the tendency for units to increase their activity as the output parameter increased in magnitude. In fewer cases, e.g., Figure 4 C, lines of regression had negative slopes indicating the opposite relationship between cell and output parameter.

Both the temporal and parametric correlation analyses imply that some PAG cells are involved in vocalization. Other forms of analysis were used to more firmly establish the function of these cells. One technique that has been used with success in other motor systems is spike-triggered averaging (Fetz & Cheney, 1980). This technique was attempted with 82 cells in the present investigation, and Figure 5 illustrates an example of one of the better results. In this case, an increase in EMG of the L TA muscle may be seen following the discharge of the cell. There are not similar changes in the other muscles. We did not observe EMG changes following most of the units studied. Despite the fact that the change in the L TA muscle of this figure is clear, it is probably the best example we have obtained and is not as clear a response as may be seen using the same technique for motor cortex cells. One reason why spike-triggered averaging was not more effective is that PAG cells typically fire at a relatively low rate, and it is therefore not usually possible to average the EMG 5,000 or 10,000 times, as has been done for motor cortex cells (Fetz & Cheney, 1980). Also, it may be that the PAG cells affect

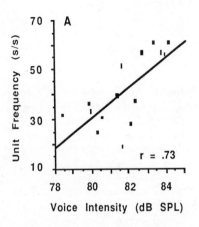
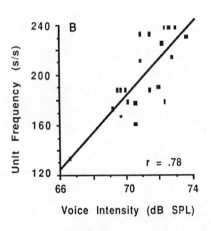

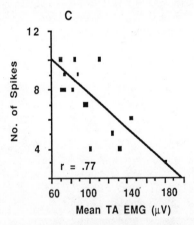
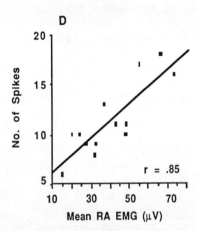

Fig. 4. Scatterplots between measures of unit activity, measures
of vocalization (A & B), mean thyroarytenoid (TA) and rectus
abdominus (RA) EMGs (C & D). The lines of linear regression
and correlation coefficients (r) were determined by a
computer program.

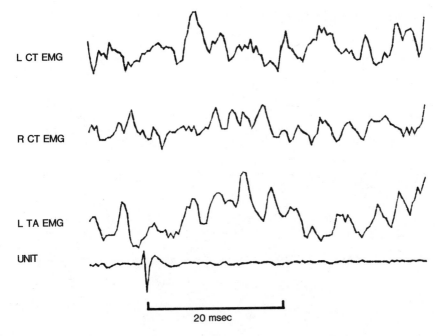

Fig. 5. Results from spike-triggered averaging. A computer was
triggered from a unit potential (bottome trace) and
rectified cricothryoid (CT) and thyroarytenoid (TA) EMGs
were averaged.

laryngeal motoneurons through one or more interneurons. In that
case, the temporal jitter associated with multiple synapses would
reduce the time synchrony necessary to show clear effects from
spike-triggered averaging.

Another technique that was used to help define the function
of PAG cells was microstimulation. After recording the activity
of a cell, the electrode was used for microstimulation by
connecting it to a stimulator and passing 20 ms trains of
electrical pulses. Figure 6 illustrates two examples from the 34
successful attempts in which microstimulation resulted in a change
in laryngeal or respiratory muscle activity. In this and other
examples of microstimulation, the timing of the 20 ms stimulus
trains is indicated by the time bar at the bottom. In each case,
20 trains of stimuli were delivered and the rectified EMGs
averaged. Figure 6A illustrates an instance in which
microstimulation elicited an increase in diaphragm muscle EMG,
with a possible excitation in the intercostal muscle as well. This
observation was made after recording from a cell that increased
its activity before vocalization. Figure 6B illustrates an

increase in cricothyroid EMG following microstimulation, also from
a cell that increased its activity before vocalization. These
examples illustrate our most frequent observations, that
microstimulation adjacent to a cell that was temporally related to
vocalization generally caused excitation of one or two muscles.

   From the histological examination of the brains of the
monkeys following their sacrifice, it was clear that most cells
related to vocalization were located in the dorsolateral PAG.
Figure 7 illustrates coronal sections from the brains of two
animals and shows the locations of marking lesions made in the
areas from which vocalization-related cells were located. Note in
monkey M1 that vocalization-related cells were located in the
dorsolateral and ventrolateral PAG. In the other monkeys, cells
related to vocalization were only located in the dorsolateral
region. A few cells related to vocalization were found in
isolation in other parts of the PAG. We examined all cells to see
if their discharge properties bore some relationship to their

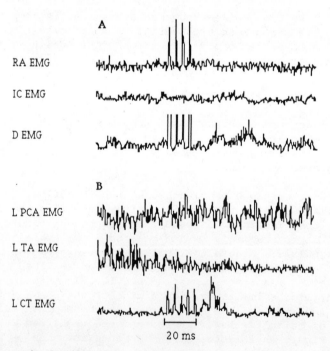

Fig.6. Microstimulation near cells from two monkeys. Trace
      identifications are the same as in other figures. The time
      bar at bottom indicates when the train of pulses was
      delivered. N = 20.

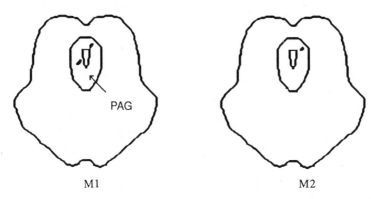

          M1   M2

Fig. 7. Drawings made from coronal sections through midbrains of
    two monkeys (M1 and M2). Marks in PAG indicate locations of
    marking lesions.

location in the PAG, but none was found. Cells related to the
laryngeal muscles were not found in different regions than cells
related to respiratory muscles. Therefore, it does not appear
that PAG cells are topographically organized with respect to
specific muscle groups. Rather, cells primarily of the
dorsolateral and ventrolateral PAG are related to vocalization,
and within these areas, there is an intermingling of cells that
project to motoneurons of different muscle systems. Outside these
areas, cells related to vocalization may be found, but their
density is low compared with the dorsolateral and ventrolateral
PAG.

    After the recording studies were completed, we began a
microstimulation study designed to verify that the dorsolateral
and ventrolateral PAG were related to the laryngeal system and to
determine if there were any other similar areas. In the recording
studies, we had not explored a very large area of the PAG, but
with the microstimulation study it was possible to map a larger
area of the PAG in animals that were not trained to vocalize. By
stimulating at low current levels with short trains of pulses, it
was expected that cell bodies would be excited preferentially. Of
course, it cannot be ruled out that fibers of passage were
stimulated. Moreover, analysis of those EMG changes that occurred
with short latencies would tend to rule out the possibility that
the stimulation excited neural circuits that reached laryngeal
motoneurons over very indirect pathways. As it turned out, we
very rarely observed EMG changes with long latencies.

    In the stimulation studies, 20 to 50 electrode penetrations
were made in each animal into and surrounding the PAG. The
penetrations extended from a position 6 mm anterior of the

interaural line to 3 mm posterior. Since the chamber on the skull
was aimed toward the midline of the dorsal PAG at a 30° angle with
respect to the sagittal plane, the more lateral electrodes passed
from the dorsolateral PAG ventromedially through the ipsilateral
half of the PAG, through the IVth ventricle and then
ventrolaterally through the contralateral half of the PAG. More
medially placed electrodes entered the dorsal PAG near the midline
and passed ventrolaterally through the contralateral half of the
PAG. Therefore, the full mediolateral extent of the PAG, as well
as surrounding areas were stimulated.

Generally, microstimulation elicited EMG changes in the
laryngeal muscles through most of the nine mm A-P extent of the
PAG. However, penetrations more posterior produced EMG changes
less frequently. The most lateral penetrations elicited EMG
changes infrequently since these electrodes passed only through
the most ventrolateral aspect of the ipsilateral PAG, while the
most medial penetrations were unsuccessful since they travelled
dorsal to the dorsal border of the PAG. Between these extremes,
an area of the PAG extending about six mm in the AP direction
yielded EMG changes when stimulated. However, EMG responses
elicited by currents of 60 μA or less were only obtained from A
3.0 to AP 0.

One of the most consistent findings from the
microstimulation study was that the electrical current thresholds
for eliciting EMG changes were lowest in the dorsal PAG,
dorsolateral PAG and tegmental area extending lateral from the
PAG. The area also extended ventrally along the lateral margins
of the PAG into the ventrolateral quadrant. This area was
approximately four mm in width, two to four mm in depth and three
mm in length. Thus, as defined by microstimulation, the PAG area
important in laryngeal control was much larger than that defined
by unit recording.

When the PAG was stimulated, some muscles were excited, some
were suppressed, and sometimes muscles showed a phase of
suppression followed immediately by a phase of excitation.
Computer print-outs of the averaged EMG responses were examined to
note which muscles displayed excitation or suppression. There
were several different patterns of EMG responses. The most typical
muscle responses observed were excitation of the CT and TA
muscles. Sometimes only one of these muscles was excited, in many
cases both were excited, and frequently their excitation was
observed without effects in any other muscle. The latencies for
these effects, as measured from the onset of the stimulus train,
ranged from 12 to 20 ms. The numbers of sites which caused
excitation of these muscles outnumbered sites eliciting their
suppression by about 10 to 1. The sites eliciting excitation of
these muscles were widely distributed within the PGA. Figure 8

illustrates examples of right and left TA excitation from three
different areas in the PAG of one monkey. As may be seen, there
are no remarkable differences in the EMG responses recorded from
these different locations.

A second frequent pattern of EMG change was suppression of
the PCA muscle. Often the PCA suppression was followed
immediately by excitation. In about 25% of the sites eliciting
changes in PCA activity, excitation was observed without
suppression. Although the locations of sites eliciting PCA
suppression were widely distributed, there were more instances of
PCA suppression in the tegmental areas lateral to the PAG than
within the PAG. In most instances where PCA suppression was
observed, excitation of the TA or CT muscles occurred also at the
same location. Figure 9 illustrates an example of PCA
suppression and excitation of the TA muscles from stimulation of a
site within the PAG. Notice in this case that PCA suppression was
followed by PCA excitation.

Figure 9 also shows the effects of varying stimulus current.
As the current was changed from 150 (A) to 80 (B) to 40 (C) to 20
μA (D), the magnitude of the responses declined. In A, B and C
are clear indications of PCA suppression followed by excitation
while the left and right TA muscles only show excitation. Almost
invariably, the excitation in the TA or CT muscles had a shorter
latency (12 - 20 ms) than the suppression in the PCA muscle.

Considering the numbers of muscles studied in each animal (4
to 8), the number of possible combinations of muscle response
patterns was large. "Response pattern" refers to all muscle
responses elicited from a given site. Other than the most typical

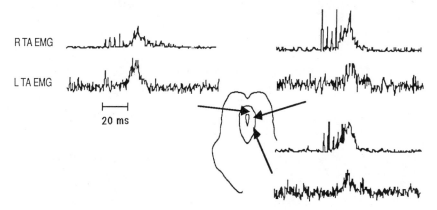

Fig. 8. Results from microstimulation in three different locations
        in PAG of one monkey. Stimulation in widely dispersed areas
        of PAG produced similar effects in thyroarytenoid muscles.

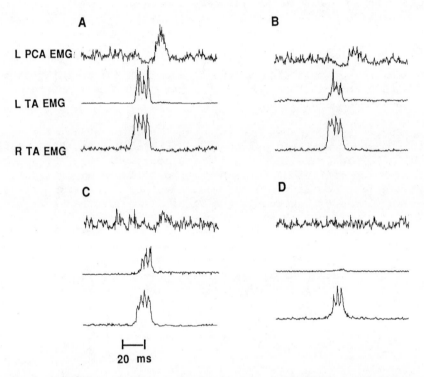

Fig.9. Effects of microstimulation at four different current
intensities: A, 150 μA; B, 80 μA; C, 40 μA; D, 20 μA.

patterns described in the preceding paragraphs, most of the other possible patterns also were observed. However, most other patterns were observed very infrequently. Figure 10 A illustrates an example in one monkey from one of four sites in which the left PCA showed suppression followed by excitation along with left TA excitation. Usually effects such as that in Figure 10 A were observed only from stimulation of a very restricted location. Figure 10 B shows that when the electrode was moved 0.5 mm from the site depicted by the effects in Figure 10 A, the response pattern changed such that only the left TA muscle was excited.

DISCUSSION

The results from unit recording and microstimulation provide different types of data on the function of the PAG with respect to vocalization. These data are consistent inasmuch as the same general conclusions can be drawn from each set. With respect to the anatomical organization of the PAG, the data indicate that the dorsolateral PAG is involved in vocalization and laryngeal control. Unit recordings from one monkey and microstimulation data suggest that ventrolateral areas of the PAG also may be involved in vocalization. Functionally, unit records and results from microstimulation suggest groups of PAG neurons modulate the activity of motoneurons during vocalization. Although most of our data were obtained from the laryngeal system, we have obtained data from one monkey indicating that PAG cells are correlated with the respiratory system. In an earlier study (Larson, 1985) it was shown that PAG stimulation excites respiratory and also facial muscles. In the following discussion, the major points to be made are in reference to the laryngeal system, but preliminary data suggest the same general principles probably apply to other muscles systems involved in vocalization.

Single neurons become active or change their discharge rates with vocalization. These changes usually occur sufficiently far in advance of vocalization, that it seems unlikely they would be responding to sensory activation. The parametric correlations demonstrated that single neurons may be correlated with one or more measures of vocalization or laryngeal muscle activity. The fact that such neurons were not correlated with each and every measure indicates that the cells may be related to rather specific aspects of vocal output. Since anatomical studies have shown that PAG neurons project to the nucleus ambiguus (Jürgens & Pratt 1979a; Yoshida et al., 1985), the site of laryngeal motoneurons and respiratory related neurons (RRNs), it would seem that PAG neurons might influence the activity of the motoneurons and the RRNs, not necessarily directly, but through interneurons, and thereby affect vocalization. The fact that neither the parametric correlations with vocalization or laryngeal EMGs were terribly

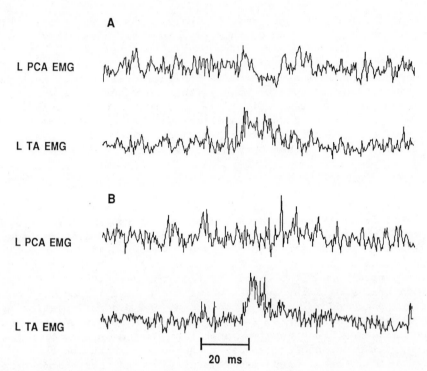

Fig.10. Effects on left posterior cricoarytenoid (L PCA) and left
thyroarytenoid (L TA) muscles from stimulating two points, A
and B, in the PAG.

strong and that weak effects were obtained from spike-triggered
averaging, support the suggestion that the PAG may project to
interneurons rather than motoneurons directly. Regardless of the
directness of these projections, it appears that the influence of
a single PAG neuron on laryngeal motoneurons is weak.

If the effects of a single PAG neuron on laryngeal
motoneurons is weak, it is logical to assume that groups of
similarly discharging units, each projecting to a motoneuron or
groups of motoneurons, would have a stronger effect. In this
sense it is appropriate to assume that groups of PAG neurons are
functionally more important to a motoneuron than a single neuron.
Because we did not simultaneously record from several PAG neurons,
which might constitute a functional group, we cannot verify such a
suggestion, but certainly it is in keeping with most other neural
systems that have been studied. Nevertheless, the results from
microstimulation provide data that are consistent with the above
suggestion as well as other observations from unit recording.

Microstimulation was done throughout the PAG in locations separated by 0.5 to 1 mm. The current levels varied from 150 to 20 µA at locations that yielded effects. It was common in such locations to see very pronounced effects at the higher currents and with each drop in current, the effects became less obvious until at 40 or 20 µA, effects were usually confined to one or two muscles. Follett & Mann (1986) reported that stimulating at a current of 0.5 to 1.0 mA through a monopolar electrode could possibly excite neural elements within a radius of 2 mm. Therefore, in our studies, the strongest stimulating currents probably affected neural elements within a radius of .5 to .75 mm from the electrode, and this would have been reduced to about .25 mm at the lowest currents. We assume, then, that in most cases our microstimulation effects resulted from stimulation of several cells or fibers. However, at the lower current levels, the observed effects were more apt to result from stimulation of cell bodies. It is also clear that at the currents used in this study, microstimulation results would have been confined to relatively small groups of neurons.

At the higher current levels, effects were almost always seen in two or more muscles. Often times, excitation of one or more muscles would be accompanied by suppression of another muscle. The pattern observed most frequently at the lowest current was excitation of the TA and CT muscles. The second most frequently observed pattern was suppression of the PCA muscles. These patterns are similar to those that occur with vocalization. As can be seen in Figure 1, the PCA muscle, which is a vocal fold abductor, usually reduces its activity during vocalization, while the TA and CT muscles, which are vocal fold adductors and tensors, increase their activity. Therefore, microstimulation usually elicited a pattern of muscle excitation similar to that observed in normal vocalization. Moreover, these effects usually were bilateral, confirming the neuroanatomical tracing studies of Jürgens and Pratt (1979a), that showed bilateral PAG projections to the nucleus ambiguus.

An important finding from these studies is that microstimulation leads to patterned responses in functionally related groups of muscles. One way to interpret these data is that relatively small sets of PAG neurons project to certain groups of motoneurons (perhaps through interneurons) and cause excitation of some and suppression of others. The fact that movement of the electrode by 0.5 mm leads to differing EMG patterns is an indication that the sets of PAG neurons are not homogeneous in their projections. Rather, it appears that one set may project predominantly to TA motoneurons, for example, while another will project to PCA motoneurons. There also is anatomical and physiological evidence (Sandner et al, 1986; Gioia et al., 1985) that PAG neurons communicate with one another through axon collaterals, which may indicate that microstimulation, while directly activating only a few cells, could excite and suppress many more distant cells through these interconnections. It would be most interesting to know if the connections between cells in the PAG are made along functional lines.

Although microstimulation in no way mimics the activity of a natural input to a region such as the PAG, it does provide clues as to its function based on analysis of the outputs from the area. Furthermore, knowing the activity of the cells, helps to interpret the effects of microstimulation. Earlier it was suggested that single PAG neurons have a relatively weak effect on laryngeal motoneurons, and that groups of neurons would have a stronger effect.   It should also be considered that the activity of a single cell is representative of a group of similarly discharging cells and that a single group is only one of several that comprise the PAG. Since microstimulation has shown that when groups are activated, coordinated muscle patterns ensue, we may assume further that naturally discharging groups of functionally related groups of PAG neurons would affect functionally related motoneurons. We then suggest that the relative balance of activity in the different PAG groups would determine which laryngeal muscles would contract most strongly and thereby affect specific features of vocalization. It is a well established fact that contraction of laryngeal muscles affects parameters of vocalization such as loudness and fundamental frequency (Hirano & Ohala, 1969). Therefore, vocalizations with different acoustical properties may be determined in part by which groups of PAG neurons are active. This statement also implies that different types of species specific vocalizations are determined by which sets of neurons within the PAG are active. Indeed, we demonstrated (see Fig.) that some cells discharge before one type of vocalization (e.g., bark) but are quiet for another type (e.g., shriek).

On another issue, it was noted that the area within the PAG that appears to be involved in vocalization, based on unit recordings, is smaller than that defined by microstimulation effects. From recording, it appears that an area of about 1 mm^3 of the dorsolateral PAG is involved in vocalization. Although we did not record sufficient numbers of cells from the ventrolateral PAG to make firm statements about the size of this area, our limited observations suggest that it is about the same size as the dorsolateral region. From the microstimulation studies, we noted changes in laryngeal muscles at low current stimulation (20 to 60 μA) in areas exceeding 12 cu mm in size. This discrepancy in size may result from at least two factors. First, microstimulation very likely excited fibers of passage which may travel throughout the PAG. Because of their small size, it would have been very difficult to record from fibers and hence the unit recordings do

not reflect their activity. Second, with unit recording, we
located a few isolated cells outside of the main areas described
above. This observation may indicate that vocalization-related
neurons are widely dispersed in the PAG. Although difficult to
locate for unit recording, the spread of current from
microstimulation of up to 0.5 mm in a radius from the electrode
would likely have activated many of these diffusely located cells.
Hence, microstimulation is more likely to elicit EMG responses
because of the spread of stimulating current to cells hundreds of
microns from the electrode tip.

To summarize, our data show that cells within the midbrain
PAG discharge before and during vocalization. Most vocalization-
related cells are located in the dorsolateral PAG. While
individual cells are weakly related to single muscles or
parameters of vocal output, these relations tend to be somewhat
specific, suggesting that single PAG cells have rather specific
functions. Microstimulation usually caused excitation of
bilateral vocal fold tensor muscles and suppression of vocal fold
abductor muscles. Since these muscle patterns are typical of
those that occur during normal vocalization, the data suggest
microstimulation excites groups of PAG neurons that in turn cause
excitation and suppression of laryngeal motoneurons according to
functional demands. Thus, it may be that groups of PAG neurons are
organized, possibly through intrinsic PAG connections, according
to functional aspects of vocalization. Our data also indicate
that some cells are active only with a specific type of
vocalization but not for another. Therefore, the type of
vocalization emitted may be determined by which sets of PAG
neurons are active. Although this review has not touched on the
projections from higher limbic system structures, those
projections may determine which sets of PAG neurons are excited or
suppressed.   Two important areas for future research are how
limbic projections affect PAG neurons, and how PAG projections
affect various brainstem interneurons and motoneurons.

Acknowledgments: We would like to thank Michael D. Kistler for his
participation on early phases of these studies. This research was
supported by a grant from NINCDS, NS 19290.

REFERENCES

Adametz, J. & O'Leary, J.L. 1959, Experimental mutism resulting
        from periaqueductal lesions in cats. Neurol., 9:636-642·
Beitz, A.J. 1982, The organization of afferent projections to the
        midbrain periaqueductal gray of the rat. Neurosci., 17:133-
        159.

Beitz, A.J. 1985, The Midbrain Periaqueductal Gray in the rat. I.
    Nuclear volume, cell number, density, orientation, and
    regional subdivisions, J. Comp. Neurol., 237:445-459.
Beitz, A.J. & Shepard, R.D. 1985, The midbrain periaqueductal gray
    in the rat. II. A Golgi analysis. J. Comp. Neurol.,237:460-
    475.
Cohen, M.I. 1981, Central determinants of respiratory rhythm, Ann.
    Rev. Physiol., 43:91-104.
Davis, P.J. & Nail, B.S. 1984, On the location and size of
    laryngral motoneurons in the cat and rabbit, J. Comp.
    Neurol.,230:13-32.
Fetz , E.E. & Cheney, P.D. 1980, Postspike facilitation of
    forelimb muscle activity by primate corticomotoneuronal
    cells, J. Neurophysiol., 44:751-772.
Follett, K.A. & Mann, M. D. 1986, Effective stimulation distance
    for current from macroelectrodes, Exp. Neurol., 92:75-91.
Gioia, M., Bianchi, R., & Tredici, G. 1984, Cytoarchitecture of
    the periaqueductal gray matter in the cat: A quantitative
    Nissl study, Acta Anatom., 119:113-117.
Gioia, M., Tredici, & G. Bianchi, R 1984, A Golgi study of the
    periaqueductal gray matter in the cat. Neuronal types and
    their distribution, Exp. Brain Res., 58:318-332.
Hirano, M. & Ohala, J. 1969, Use of hooked-wire electrodes for
    electromyography of the intrinsic laryngeal muscles, J.
    Speech Hear. Res., 12:362-373.
Jürgens, U. 1982, Amygdalar vocalization pathways in the squirrel
    monkey, Brain Res., 241:189-196.
Jürgens, U. & Ploog, D. 1970, Cerebral representation of
    vocalization in the squirrel monkey, Exp. Brain Res., 10:
    532-554.
Jürgens, U. & Pratt, R. 1979a Role of the periaqueductal grey in
    vocal expression of emotion, Brain Res.167:367-378.
Jürgens, U. & Pratt, R. 1979b The cingular vocalization pathway in
    the squirrel monkey, Exp. Brain Res., 34:499-510.
Kalia, M.P. 1981 Anatomical organization of central respiratory
    neuron, Ann. Rev. Physiol., 43:105-120.
Kennedy, M.C. 1975 Vocalization elicited in a lizard by electrical
    stimulation of the midbrain, Brain Res., 91:321-325.
Kirzinger & Jürgens, 1982 Cortical lesion effects and vocalization
    in the squirrel monkey, Brain Res., 233:299-315.
Larson, C. R. & Kistler, M. K. 1984 Periaqueductal gray neuronal
    activity associated with laryngeal EMG and vocalization in
    the awake monkey, Neurosci. Let., 46:261-266.
Larson, C.R. & Kistler, M.K. 1985 Brainsterm neuronal activity
    associated with vocalization in the monkey. In "Vocal Fold
    Physiology: Laryngeal function in phonation and respiration"
    T. Baer, K.S. Harris and C. Sasaki, eds. College-Hill, San
    Diego.
Larson, C.R. & Kistler, M.K. 1986, The relationship of
    periaqueductal gray neurons to vocalization and laryngeal
    EMG in the behaving monkey, Exp. Brain Res., 63:596-606.
Larson, C.R. 1985, The midbrain periaqueductal gray: A brainstem
    structure involved in vocalization. J. Speech Hear. Res.,
    28:241-249.

Magoun, H.W., Atlas, D., Ingersoll, E.H. & Ranson, S.W. 1937, Associated facial, vocal and respiratory components of emotional expression: An experimental study. J. Neurol. Psychopath., 17:241-255.

Mantyh, P. W. 1982, The midbrain periaqueductal gray in the rat, cat and monkey: A Nissl, Weil and Golgi analysis, J. Comp. Neurol., 204: 349-363.

Müller-Preuss, P. & Jürgens, U. 1976, Projections from the cingular vocalization area in the squirrel monkey, Brain Res. 103:29-34.

Ploog, D. 1981, Neurobiology of primate audio-vocal behavior. Brain Res. Rev., 3:35-61.

Robinson, B.W. 1967, Vocalization evoked from forebrain in Macaca Mulatta, Physiol. Beh., 2:345-354.

Sandner, G., Schmitt, P. and Karli, P. 1986, Unit activity alterations induced in the mesencephalic periaqueductal gray by local electrical stimulation, Brain Res, 386:53-63.

Sapir, S., Campbell, C. & Larson, C. 1981, Effect of genoihyoid, cricothyroid and sternothyroid muscle stimulation on voice fundamental frequency of electrically elicited phonation in rhesus macaque. Laryngoscope, 91:457-468.

Suga, N., Schlegel, P. Shimozawa, T. & Simmons, J. 1973, Orientation sounds evoked from echolocating bats by electrical stimulation of the brain., J. Acous. Soc. Am., 54:793-797.

Sutton, D., Larson, C. & Lindeman, R.C. 1974, Neocortical and limbic lesion effects on primate phonation, Brain Res. 71:61-75.

Tredici, G., Bianchi, R., & Gioia, M. 1983, Short intrinsic circuit in the periaqueductal gray matter of the cat. Neurosci. Let., 39:131-136.

Ueda, N., Ohyamna, M., Harvey, J.e., Mogi, G. & Ogura, J.H. 1971, Subglottic pressure and induced live voices of dogs with normal, reinnervated, and paralyzed larynges Laryngoscope, 81:1948-1959.

Winter, P., Ploog, D. & Latta, J. 1966, Vocal repertoire of the Squirrel monkey (Saimiri sciureus), its analysis and significance. Exp. Brain Res., 1:359-384.

Yoshida, Y., Mitsumasu, T., Miyazaki, Tl, Hirano, M. & Kanaseki, T. 1984 Distribution of motoneurons in the brain stem of monkeys, innervating the larynx. Brain Res. Bull., 13:413-419.

Yoshida, Y., Mitsumasu, T., Hirano, M. & Kanaseki, T. 1985, Afferent connections to the nucleus ambiguus in the brain stem of the cat; an HRP study. In "Vocal Fold Physiology: Laryngeal function in phonation and respiration" T. Baer, K.S. Harris and C. Sasaki, eds. College-Hill, San Diego.

Yoshida, Y, Miyazaki, T., Hirano, M, Shin, T. & Kanaseki, T. 1982, Arrangement of motoneurons innervaing the intrinsic laryngeal muscles of cats as demonstrated by horseradish peroxidase. Acta Otolaryngol., 94:329-334.

NEURAL CONTROL OF VOCALIZATION IN BATS AT PERIPHERAL TO
MIDBRAIN LEVELS

Gerd Schuller and Susanne Radtke-Schuller

Zoologisches Institut der Universität München
Luisenstrasse 14, D-8000 München 2, F.R.G.

INTRODUCTION

Vocalizations are important carriers for information
in animal communication and their composition reaches the
most sophisticated level in speech. Besides its role for
interindividual communication, the uttering of vocalizations has gained additional functional significance in
active sonar systems as, e.g., developed by bats and
dolphins. These systems require accurate control of the
spectral composition of the emitted echolocation signals
and auditory feedback is most probably involved in the
control of the motor output.

In active sonar systems the emitted signal serves as
a carrier and reference signal. The information on the
properties of the reflecting target is contained in the
spectral changes superimposed on the emitted reference
signal. Thus the extraction of the spectral differences
between emitted sound and echoes conveys the relevant
information to the echolocating animal. These differences
can be derived by direct comparison of the uttered vocalizations and the returning echoes through the acoustic
channel. In this case the motor control of sound emission
needs only to maintain a roughly standardized spectral
composition of the vocalization as the reference signal
would always be analyzed in parallel to the echoes.
Alternatively, a mechanism in which the structure of the
vocalizations would be accessible by internal neuronal
feedback needs no auditory processing of the emitted call
and thus frees the auditory system for exclusive

processing of echo information. In the latter case a very accurate motor control of echolocation call emission is necessary to guarantee reliable evaluation of the super-imposed echo information.

There are many hints from behavioural studies in bats that the motor programs for echolocation call emission are only partly fixed, and that modulations through auditory feedback can modify the spectral and temporal composition of the sounds (e.g., Pye, 1980). Thus, many bat species adapt the echolocation calls to the currently prevailing demands of orientation or prey capture by altering the temporal and spectral pattern of the vocalizations. Bats have the capability to optimize the structure of the echolocation signals for the specific task within certain limits.

PARAMETERS CONTROLLED IN BAT VOCALIZATIONS

The variety of echolocation calls used by bats is large and here only two major classes of spectral components shall be briefly considered.

The first class is characterized by broadband spectra and by fast frequency transitions, i.e., the calls embody either relatively noisy broadband components or frequency-modulated signals with monotonous frequency changes from high to low frequencies (occasionally viceversa). Both types can have a harmonic structure with one to several harmonics. These echolocation calls generally are short and have durations of no more than a few milliseconds.

In the second class, the main component of the echo-location calls consists of a long constant frequency portion which may be preceded and/or terminated by short frequency modulations. The duration of the constant fre-quency portion is generally long and can reach up to 100 msec. The frequency is kept constant within 50 Hz at its extreme in rhinolophid bats. Also this type of vocaliza-tion can have more or less pronounced harmonic components. Typical representatives of the former class are found in the vespertilionid bats and of the latter class in the rhinolophid bats.

In bats using broadband echolocation calls the time course of the frequency modulations constitutes the most important control parameter, whereas in bats emitting constant frequency pulses the control of the constant

frequency portion is of fundamental importance. The importance of precise frequency control is obvious in rhinolophid bats and Pteronotus p. parnellii, both of which
show a behaviour called Dopplershift compensation
(Schnitzler 1968, 1970). During this behaviour, the
emitted frequency is adjusted in a way that stabilizes the
frequency of the returning echoes within a narrow frequency band (several hundred Hz) of best hearing, despite
the fact that the relative speed between the bat and the
reflecting background creates frequency shifts in the
echoes. In this control circuitry, a feedback mechanism is
active which transfers the information on the frequency
shifts as analyzed in the auditory system to the descending vocal control system.

SUPRALARYNGEAL STRUCTURES

     The supralaryngeal cavities in bats have strong fil-
tering properties and influence the structure of the
emitted vocalizations.

     In bat species emitting the echolocation sounds
through the nostrils (e.g. Rhinolophus and Hipposideros)
little change in the transmission properties can be expected as the dimensions of the nasal cavities are morphologically fixed. Bat species emitting the orientation
sounds through the mouth can modulate the acoustical
transmission properties of the mouth cavity to a greater
extent. The harmonic composition of the echolocation calls
and the relative sound pressure levels of the spectral
components within the call are especially affected by
changes of the supralaryngeal cavities.

     The spectral and temporal composition of the echolo-
cation calls are mainly determined by the source genera-
ting mechanisms in the larynx. But the importance of
modulations of the vocal tract resonances for the fine-
tuning of the spectral composition of sounds in different
species should not be ignored (see also Roberts, 1972).
Consequently, control mechanisms influencing the nose and
mouth cavities should also be investigated.

LARYNX

     The larynx in microchiropterans shows the normal
mammalian morphology but exhibits some hypertrophied
features (Elias, 1908, Fischer and Gerken, 1961). The

cricoid and thyroid cartilages are comparatively strong
and rigid and the cricothyroid muscles are largely hypertrophied, covering the ventral and lateral portions of the
larynx completely. The arytenoid cartilages are rigid and
allow less rotational movements than in other mammals.

Several mechanisms of high frequency sound production
in bats have been proposed. After Fischer and Vömel(1961)
and Fischer and Gerken (1961), the vocal fold is narrowed
at the beginning of sound production through adduction of
the vocal cords, thus forming a whistle-like edge under
the control of the m.vocalis, whereas the arytenoid cartilages should play a minor role because of their rigidity.
Griffin and Novick (Griffin, 1958; Novick and Griffin,
1961) proposed a different mechanism for sound production
involving the laryngeal membranes found in the larynx of
bats formed by the modified vocal and ventricular fold.
These membranes cover small volumes at both sides of the
ventricular lumen which could display resonant properties
in the frequency range which is used by bats. Contraction
of the cricothyroid muscle exerts tension on these membranes and could probably alter the tuning properties of
the system. The rapid succession of short ultrasonic
pulses as emitted by bats requires rapid contraction and
relaxation times of the involved muscles. The cricothyroid
muscle in bats seems to be well adapted for rapid contractions and has very short mean contraction times of around
6.5 msec, which is about one fourth of that in dogs or
rabbits (Suthers and Fattu, 1973). Morphologically these
muscles exhibit an extremely well developed sarcoplasmatic
reticulum   (Revel, 1962).

DENERVATION EXPERIMENTS

In order to investigate the functional significance
of the different muscles in the larynx of bats, several
authors have selectively denervated different muscle
groups by cutting the laryngeal nerves (Griffin, 1958,
Novick and Griffin, 1961, Schuller and Suga, 1976, Suthers
and Fattu, 1982).

The intrinsic laryngeal muscles, except the cricothyroid muscle, receive their innervation through the
recurrent laryngeal nerve (RLN), whereas the cricothyroid
muscle is controlled by the motor branch of the superior
laryngeal nerve (SLN) (e.g. Henson, 1970, Quay, 1970). If
one or both recurrent laryngeal nerves are cut, only minor
changes in the emitted sounds occur. Neither the frequency

or frequency modulation of the emitted calls nor the
timing is profoundly disturbed. Small changes following
surgery (e.g. a small drop in frequency) normally recovered within a short postsurgical period. The denervation of the recurrent nerve led in some bats to light to
severe difficulties in breathing as the internal laryngeal
muscles govern the abduction and adduction of the vocal
cords. Suthers and Fattu (1982) have shown that
sectioning the RLN leads to a 4-5 dB decrease in sound
pressure level of the emitted sounds postsurgically. They
have further demonstrated that variations of the subglottic pressure have little or no influence on the frequency of the emitted sound.
These minor effects of RLN section in bats is in clear
contrast to the effect in humans where lesioning of this
nerve leads to severe deficits in speech production. Evi-
dently, the laryngeal muscles in bats innervated by the
RLN play a subordinate role for the spectral shaping of
the ultrasonic calls.

     Cutting the motor branch of the superior laryngeal
nerve has very prominent consequences on the spectral
composition of the emitted calls. In vespertilionid bats
as well as in bats emitting long constant frequency pulses
the frequency of the echolocation calls drops considerably
(several kHz to more than 10 kHz), and because of the
filtering properties of the vocal tract cavities this can
lead to marked changes in the harmonic composition of the
echolocation calls. In bats emitting FM echolocation
signals, the section of SLN reduces or eliminates most of
the frequency modulation. Only in rare cases could some
recovery be observed. No marked influence of SLN cutting
upon the duration of the echolocation sound could be
observed except in rare cases in which the duration was
lengthened after surgery. Thus, the SLN is obviously the
main laryngeal component involved in the control of frequency of the emitted sound in bats.

RECORDINGS FROM LARYNGEAL MUSCLES AND NERVES

     The functional significance of the different laryn-
geal components is also reflected in the discharges found
during laryngeal activity in laryngeal muscles and nerves.
Recordings of electromuscular potentials have been made
from the cricothyroid muscles by several authors (Novick
and Griffin, 1961, Suthers and Fattu, 1973, Schuller and
Suga, 1976), but no recordings are available from the
other intrinsic laryngeal muscles in bats. The reason for

this is probably the delicacy of the larynx and the
relative inaccessibility of these muscles for recording
without interfering with the laryngeal micromechanics.

The cricothyroid muscle is active prior to the
emission of vocalization, during and beyond the end of the
vocalization. The type of response depends on the recording site in the muscle and different portions of the
muscles which can also be anatomically defined have different functional properties. There is no detailed study
available to clarify these functional differences of the
cricothyroid muscle subunits. During activation of the
cricothyroid muscle prior to pulse emission the tension
of the laryngeal membranes builts up and determines the
frequency at the beginning of the echolocation call. Concurrently the air flow resistance in the larynx is
increased by a coordinated activation of the cricothyroid
muscles together with the other intrinsic laryngeal
muscles controlling the adduction of the vocal fold membranes. The role of intrinsic muscles for the air flow
resistance in the larynx is dramatically demonstrated in
that bats suffocate or show severe breathing difficulties
when both recurrent nerves are cut. The relaxation of the
muscles innervated by the RLN leads to complete adduction
of the vocal fold and subsequent closing of the glottis.

The activity of the laryngeal nerves shows qualitatively similar discharge patterns as the muscles. Quantitative measurements in bats are only available for the
horseshoe bat, Rhinolophus ferrumequinum or Rh. rouxi
(Schuller and Rübsamen, 1981, Rübsamen and Schuller,
1981). Using the Dopplershift compensation behaviour of
these bats, the frequency of the constant frequency
portion of the echolocation sound can be controlled by
appropriate auditory feedback. The nerve activity recorded
from the superior laryngeal nerve under these conditions
shows a clear linear dependence on the emitted CF-
frequency (Fig 1b). The activity of the cricothyroid
muscle shows a similar dependence on the emitted frequency
(Fig 1a) and both recordings directly demonstrate the
importance of the SLN and the cricothyroid muscle for
precise frequency control in the echolocation calls of
rhinolophid bats. In the lower left of the figure (1c)
the dependence of the emitted frequency as a function of
electrical stimulation of the cricothyroid muscle is
shown. The animal has been forced by Dopplershift compensation to emit a 2 kHz lower frequency than its resting
frequency and the electrical stimulation cancels the
decrease progressively with increasing stimulation rate.

The rates of the stimulation correspond roughly to those also found in the recordings from the cricothyroid muscle.

No such frequency dependence of the discharge activity is found for the recurrent laryngeal nerve that shows activity strongly correlated with the start and the end of the vocalizations or the start of the frequency modulated portion. The recordings demonstrate that the RLN activity is controlling the temporal parameters of the echolocation calls.

The function of the SLN and RLN in horseshoe bats is not necessarily specialized for Doppler compensation, but probably characterizes general laryngeal control mechanisms in bats.

THE MOTOR NUCLEUS OF THE LARYNX, THE NCL. AMBIGUUS

As in other mammals, the motoneurons giving rise to the recurrent and superior laryngeal nerves are located in the Ncl. ambiguus (NA) in the lateral portion of the brain stem reticular formation.

Topographic arrangement of motoneurons

From studies in other mammals it is known that the motoneurons for different laryngeal muscles are orderly arranged within this nucleus, creating a topography of functional characteristics of laryngeal muscles. Schweizer et al. (1981) have selectively applied horseradish peroxidase to the cut ends of the superior or the recurrent laryngeal nerves and determined the location of the corresponding motoneurons. The motoneurons of the superior laryngeal nerve axons innervating the cricothyroid muscle are located within the ventrolateral portion of the nucleus and extend over its rostral end until the caudal limit of the Ncl. facialis. The motoneurons of the recurrent laryngeal nerve fibers occupy the dorsocaudal parts of the nucleus. Thus, a distinct segregation of the two main inputs to the laryngeal musculature within the NA is present and differences in neuronal responses can be expected in the different parts of the nucleus.

Response properties of laryngeal motoneurons

Recordings from motoneurons and interneurons within the NA of the bat (Rübsamen et al., 1986) have yielded a

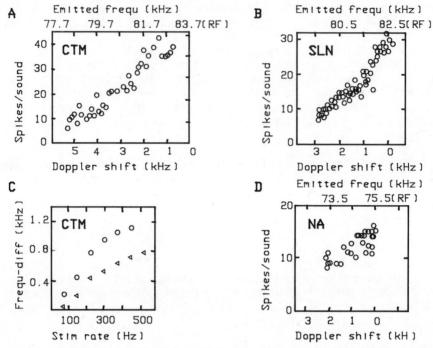

Fig. 1.   Laryngeal control of the emitted frequency in
          horseshoe bats. Activity of the cricothyroid
          muscle (A, CTM, electromygram), the
          supralaryngeal nerve (B, SLN, summated
          activity) and of a motoneuron in the Ncl.
          ambiguus (D, NA, single unit) as a function of
          the frequency of the emitted constant
          frequency portion (CF) of the orientation
          sound. The frequency is indicated as emitted
          frequency in the upper scale (RF = resting fre-
          quency) and as deviation from the RF in the
          lower scale (labeled as Doppler shift). The
          activity is indicated as spikes/sound with typi-
          cal sound durations between 40 and 50 msec.
          Graph C shows how the emitted frequency can be
          increased by electrical stimulation of the
          cricothyroid muscle. (Adapted from Schuller et
          al. (1976, 1981) and Rübsamen et al. (1986))

large variety of response types. A number of neurons were
exclusively active during ongoing vocalization or responded only in correlation with the respiratory cycle. Other
neurons showed activation to both ongoing activities.

The response patterns could be classified after the temporal occurence of maximal spike activity in relation to the onset or termination of the vocalizations or within the respiratory cycle. Based on the response pattern, the neurons could be attributed to distinct laryngeal muscles with specific function during the emission of echolocation calls. One class of neurons showed activity tightly linked to the beginning or end of the vocalization or the frequency-modulated part and the neurons were considered to be responsible for the temporal control of sound emission, whereas in another class of neurons, the neural activity was a function of the frequency of the constant frequency portion of the emitted pulse and thus associated with the frequency control of sound emission. The latter type of neurons has been recorded mainly from rostral portions of the NA and the retrofacial nucleus. These neurons probably were motoneurons sending their fibres via the superior laryngeal nerve to the cricothyroid muscles and displayed a similar dependence of the spike activity as a function of the emitted frequency as superior laryngeal nerve fibers (Fig 1c).

The results of the NA recordings again underline the fact that in bats the main contribution to frequency control comes from the superior laryngeal motoneurons, whereas the temporal parameters are governed by the more caudally situated RLN motoneurons. No further topographical order within the classes could be detected in Rhinolophus.

Anatomical connections of the Ncl. ambiguus

Following neurophysiological recordings from the NA, Rübsamen and Schweizer (1986) used the retro- and anterograde transport of horseradish peroxidase to trace the afferent and efferent projections of this nucleus. The inherent difficulties of this method become obvious, when looking at the size (about 800 um diameter) and anatomical properties of the NA. The NA is located in the reticular formation of the brain stem caudal to the Ncl. facialis. Its anatomical demarcation to surrounding structures is poor and its functional definition is heterogeneous, thus limiting the possibilities for interpreting the projections as areas involved in the efferent vocal system.

These experiments showed that the NA is reciprocally connected with its contralateral counterpart and with parts of the adjacent reticular formation. Reciprocal

links also exist with medial portions of the medulla
oblongata and the parabrachial nuclei, i.e., areas
involved in respiratory control. Afferent pathways to the
injection sites in the NA originate in lateral parts of
the periaqueductal gray and the Ncl. cuneiformis, which
are considered to be part of the descending vocalization
system. Further afferent connections come from the
superior colliculus, pontine nuclei and areas involved in
motor control systems (red nucleus and frontal cortex).

Whether the brain areas marked after HRP injections
into the NA are of functional importance for vocalization
can only be demonstrated by verifying their reciprocal
connection to the NA and by investigating their physiological properties during vocalization.

ELECTRICAL STIMULATION FOR ELICITING OF SPECIES-SPECIFIC
VOCALIZATIONS IN BATS

Electrical stimulation has been widely used as a
method to clarify the involvement of brain areas in
specific pathways controlling different motor programs or
animal behaviour. Although this method cannot distinguish
between different neural elements that are stimulated, it
yields valuable information if the limitations of the
method are taken into account.

The first experiments to elicit echolocation sounds
in bats by electrical brain stimulation were done by Suga
et al. (1973) in various species. At these stimulation
sites the evoked vocalizations corresponded to naturally
uttered echolocation calls and were accompanied by pinna
and mouth movements but not by further gross body movements. Brain sites in which species-specific vocalization
could be electrically elicited were found in the lateral
parts of the central gray at the rostral level of the
auditory midbrain and in dorsolateral parts of the midbrain reticular formation anteroventral to the inferior
colliculus. No further anatomical details on the brain
areas specific for the evocation of vocalizations have
been given in that paper and the detailed correlation of
stimulation sites to morphological brain structures is no
given. No further stimulation studies in midbrain areas o
at lower levels are available for bats.

In higher brain centers, stimulation experiments wer
done by Gooler and O'Neill (1985) who electrically
elicited vocalizations in the anterior cingulate cortex o

the bat Pteronotus p. parnellii. These authors found a topographical correlation between stimulation site and frequency of the constant frequency portion of the emitted orientation sound.

STIMULATION EXPERIMENTS IN THE RUFOUS HORSESHOE BAT, RHINOLOPHUS ROUXI

Our own studies with electrical stimulation were focused on the midbrain of the horseshoe bat, Rhinolophus rouxi. The aim was to accurately define those brain sites where species-specific orientation calls could be elicited, and to correlate them with anatomical structures. Thus, brain areas retrogradely marked by HRP in the same species (Rübsamen and Schweizer 1986) were tested for their involvement into the descending vocal control system and injection of HRP or WGA labeled with HRP was used to verify the anatomical connections within the vocal pathway.

Material and Methods

The electrical stimulation experiments were conducted in 20 rufous bats from Sri Lanka, using a stereotaxic device which allowed a reconstruction of the stimulation sites with high precision (100-200 μm resolution) (Schuller et al., 1987). The electrical stimuli consisted of trains of 0.1 msec long pulses at a rate of 1 kHz. The duration of the trains was 15 msec thus containing 15 pulses. The stimulation bursts were delivered at rates between 3 and 10 Hz and applied through insulated tungsten electrodes with insulation free tips of 2-20 μm diameter. The vocalizations were monitored with a condenser micro-phone and the temporal courses of frequency and amplitude were stored on magnetic tape, together with the electrical stimulus and a signal following the respiratory cycle. The animal was monitored with a video camera system.

The midbrain regions were systematically scanned from the rostral limit of the superior colliculus to the caudal end of the inferior colliculus. The very dorsolateral parts and the areas near the midsagittal plane were less densely scanned or not hit at all.

Strict criteria were applied for considering a stimu-lation site as specific for the evocation of species-specific orientation calls:

a) only stimulation currents below 20 µA (in many cases
10 µA) were considered to yield stimulation of sufficient
spatial resolution;
b) the elicited vocalizations had to be acoustically
indistinguishable from natural echolocation sounds;
c) the stimulation elicited exclusively vocalizations but
no other body movements except some ear or mouth/nose
movements;
d) the elicited vocalizations had a one-to-one relationship to the electrical stimulus at relatively constant
latencies below 100 msec; and, finally,
e) the vocalizations were not a consequence of electrically induced general arousal.

Results of electrical stimulation

At most stimulation sites where vocalization could be
electrically elicited, their spectral composition
corresponded to that of natural echolocation calls. Only
at pontine stimulation sites and in the overlaying fibres,
the elicited vocalizations had extremely short durations
and the CF frequency deviated from that in the natural
calls.

The latencies between electrical stimulus and vocal
response was typically between 20 and 60 msec and
stabilized with increasing stimulation amplitude within
variations of 10 to 20 msec around the mean latency. In
some locations, the latency was consistently longer
(around 80 msec), i.e. considerably longer than at most
locations.

The efficiency of electrical stimulation also
depended on the repetition rate of the stimulus. Repetition rates that interfered with the respiratory cycle most
often led to either a stop of sound emission or to arousal
of the bat. A rate at around 7 Hz, which is about twice
the respiratory rate was often optimum for eliciting
vocalizations.

The spectral parameters of the vocalizations could,
in general, not be influenced by the electrical stimulation, except for the sound pressure level of the emission,
which at some stimulation sites increased systematically
with increasing stimulation amplitude.

The frequency of the constant frequency portion of
the echolocation call could not be systematically
influenced by the stimulation at any stimulation site.

Ear movements could be elicited at many more stimulation sites than vocalization. There were only rare cases
in which the vocalization could be evoked independently of
ear and nose movements and, in these cases, the threshold
for eliciting ear movements was only slightly higher than
that for vocalization. The direction of movement of the
individual ear and the correlation between the ipsi- and
contralateral ear in general were very specific for
distinct stimulation sites. Nose leaf movements could
also be elicited electrically and occurred in conjunction
with vocalizations or ear movements or as isolated
behavioural response.

The correlation of elicited vocalization with
respiration could be twofold. In the first and most common
case, the respiratory cycle was synchronized to the
electrical stimulus and the vocalization occured during
this respiratory cycle. In the second case, the vocalization was electrically elicited and provoked an extra
expiratory pulse during vocalization.

Brain areas specific for eliciting vocalizations

Following the given criteria for electrically evoking
species-specific vocalizations, three areas in the brainstem could be delimited in which the vocalizations
including the accompanying ear and nose-leaf movements
were optimally elicited. The regions are indicated as
shaded areas in the schematic brain sections (Fig. 2) and
are located in
a) intermediate and deep layers of the superior colliculus
(r/c level: 5819-6875 µm),
b) the dorsolateral part of the midbrain reticular formation (Deep mesencephalic nucleus) (r/c level: 6611-7139
µm) and
c) the Ncl. tegmentalis pedunculo-pontinus in the antero-
medial and medial vicinity of the rostral part of the
dorsal nucleus of the lateral lemniscus (r/c level: 7139-
7403µm).

In these areas the spectral parameters of the vocalizations were not influenced by the electrical stimulation
and it can be assumed, therefore, that these stimulation
sites are at a level of the descending vocal motor system
at which vocalization is triggered but not determined in
its acoustical composition.

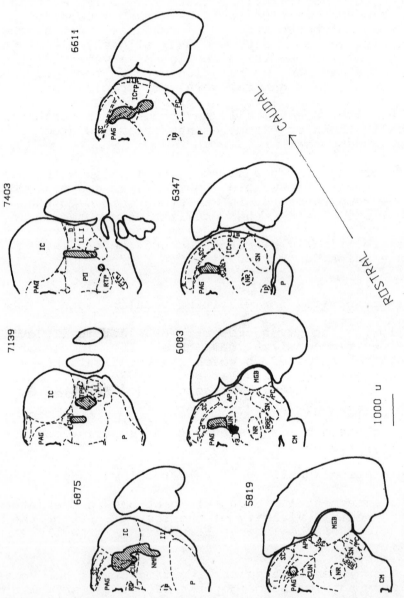

Fig.2. Brain sites for optimal eliciting of vocalizations (shaded areas). Abbreviations see next page. The numbers in the upper right indicate the rostro-caudal level of the sections.

Abbreviations for figure 2: AP area pretectalis, BIC brachium of the colliculus inferior,   CTm medial trapezoid body,   CUN Ncl.cuneiformis, IC(rp) inferior colliculus (rostral pole), LL Ncl. of the lateral lemniscus (d,i,v dorsal, intermediate, ventral), MGB medial geniculate body, NMP deep mesencephalic nucleus, NR Ncl. ruber, NTPP Ncl. tegmentalis pedunculopontinus, P pontine nuclei, PAG periaqueductal gray, PC cerebral peduncle,   PO pontis oralis, RRF retrorubral field, SC superior colliculus (s,i,d superior, intermediate, deep layers), SG suprageniculate nucleus, SN substantia nigra.

Connectivity of areas specific for the eliciting of vocalization

Following the spatial definition of brain sites for specific evocation of vocalizations, horseradish peroxidase (HRP) or wheat germ agglutinin labeled with HRP was injected in order to trace the retro- or anterograde projections of these locations. The connection of these areas presumably involved in the descending motor pathway for the control of vocalization are represented in a schematic way in Fig. 3.

Interestingly, none of these areas showed a direct anatomical connection to the motor nucleus of the larynx, the Ncl. ambiguus, and the link to the output control level could not be established anatomically from these brain areas. Two of these areas (SC and DMN) had anterograde connections to the Ncl. cuneiformis (CUN), which lies ventrolateral to the midbrain periaqueductal gray (PAG). Stimulation in CUN and the very lateral parts of the PAG did not yield vocalizations following our criteria; instead, the vocalizations were elicited with long delays (several hundred ms) after the start of the stimulation and were in almost all cases accompanied by arousal of the animal. Tracer deposits centered in the cuneiform nucleus and slightly overlapping the lateral borders of the PAG showed anterograde transport to the nucleus ambiguus. Thus, the connection between the structures in which stimulation triggers vocalization and the motor control nucleus of the larynx is indirect, while the shortest connection runs via the cuneiform nucleus or lateral border areas of the PAG.

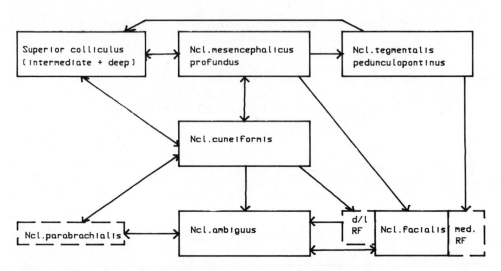

Fig. 3.   Schematic diagram of the anatomical connections
of three midbrain areas where species-specific echolocation calls could be elicited by electrical stimulation.
Only the connections within the descending pathway for
vocal control are represented. Connections to pontine
nuclei, the cerebellum and higher brain levels are
omitted.

        The exact funtional role of these intermediate links
is not readily understood, and must be investigated with
recordings from these structures during vocalization.

        The Nucleus pedunculopontinus has no direct
connection to the above mentioned relay areas, but
projects to the deep SC and the reticular formation
lateral to Ncl. facialis which in turn are linked to the
Ncl. ambiguus.
The connection between the cuneiform nucleus and the
lateral PAG to the Nucleus ambiguus also corroborates the
findings of Rübsamen and Schweizer (1986), who found
retrograde marking in these areas after HRP injections
into the Nucleus ambiguus. All other projections to the NA
as described by these authors can at present not be reciprocally assured as part of the vocal control system.

CONCLUSIONS

        The descending pathway for neural control of vocali-
zation in bats has been systematically traced from the

periphery to the level of the midbrain only in the horseshoe bat (Rhinolophus rouxi or Rhinolophus ferrumequinum).
Physiological recordings during vocalization are available
from the peripheral nerves and the motor nucleus of the
larynx (Ncl. ambiguus), whereas beyond this level, data
stem from electrical stimulation experiments and tracer
experiments revealing the anatomical connections. The
functional involvement of the brain areas sending
information directly or indirectly to the motor nucleus
has to be further investigated by recordings from these
structures. From present knowledge on the descending
vocalization system in bats, it is clear that there is no
simple hierarchical organization as shown in primates
(e.g. Jürgens and Ploog, 1981) but, instead, a complex
system of interconnected areas, the differential function
of which needs further elucidation.

REFERENCES

Elias, H., 1908, Zur Anatomie des Kehlkopfes der
    Microchiropteren., Morph. Jahrb. 37:70.

Fischer, H., Gerken, H., 1961, Le larynx de la chauve-
    souris (Myotis myotis) et le larynx humain.
    Ann.Oto-Laryngol. 78:577.

Fischer, H., Vömel, H.J., 1961, Der Ultraschallapparat
    des Larynx von Myotis myotis. Gegenbaurs
    Jahrb.Morphol.Mikr.Anat.Abt 1. 102:200.

Gooler, D.M., O'Neill W.E., 1985, Central control of
    frequency in biosonar vocaliations of the mustached
    bat, Soc Neurosci. Abstr. 165:5

Griffin, D.R., 1958, Listening in the dark., Yale
    Univ.Press, New Haven

Henson, O.W., The central nervous system, in: "Biology
    of bats II", W. Wimsatt, ed., Academic Press,
    New York

Jürgens, U., Ploog, D., 1981, On the neural control of
    mammalian vocalization, TINS 4(6):135.

Novick, A., Griffin, D.R., 1961, Laryngeal mechanisms in
    bats for the production of orientation sounds.,
    J.Exp.Zool. 148:125.

Pye, J.D., 1980, Echolocation signals and echoes in air, in: "Animal Sonar Systems," R.-G. Busnel, J.F. Fish, eds., Plenum Press, New York and London

Quay, W., 1970, Peripheral nervous system, in "Biology of bats II", Wimsatt, W., ed., Academic Press, New York

Revel, J.P., 1962, The sarcoplasmatic reticulum of the bat cricothyroid muscle, J.Cell Biol. 12:571.

Roberts, L.H., 1972, Variable resonance in constant frequency bats, J.Zool. Lond. 166:337.

Rübsamen, R., Schuller, G., 1981, Laryngeal nerve activity during pulse emission in the CF-FM bat, Rhinolophus ferrumequinum. II. The recurrent laryngeal nerve. J.Comp.Physiol. 143:323.

Rübsamen, R., Betz, M., 1986, Control of echolocation pulses by neurons of the nucleus ambiguus in the rufous horseshoe bat, Rhinolophus rouxi I. Single unit recordings in the ventral motor nucleus of the laryngeal nerves in spontaneously vocalizing bats. J.Comp.Physiol.A 159:675.

Rübsamen, R., Schweizer, R., 1986, Control of echolocation pulses by neurons of the nucleus ambiguus in the rufous horsehoe bat, Rhinolophus rouxi II. Afferent and efferent connections of the motor nucleus of the laryngeal nerves. J.Comp.Physiol.A 159:689.

Schnitzler, H.-U., 1968, Die Ultraschall-Ortungslaute der Hufeisen-Fledermäuse (Chiroptera-Rhinolophidae) in verschiedenen Orientierungssituationen. Z.Vergl.Physiol. 57:376.

Schnitzler, H,-U., 1970, Echoortung bei der Fledermaus Chilonycteris rubiginosa, Z.Vergl.Physiol. 68:25.

Schuller, G., Rübsamen, R., 1981, Laryngeal nerve activity during pulse emission in the CF-FM bat, Rhinolophus ferrumequinum. I. Superior laryngeal nerve (External motor branch), J.Comp.Physiol. 143:317.

Schuller, G., Suga, N., 1976, Laryngeal mechanisms for the emission of CF-FM sounds in the Doppler shift

compensating bat, Rhinolophus ferrumequinum;
J.Comp.Physiol. 107:253.

Schuller, G., Radtke-Schuller, S., Betz, M., 1987, A
stereotaxic method for small animals using
experimentally determined reference profiles.
J.Neurosci.Meth. 18:339.

Schweizer, H., Rübsamen, R., Ruehle, C., 1981,
Localization of brain stem motoneurons innervating
the laryngeal muscles in the rufous horseshoe bat,
Rhinolophus rouxi., Brain Res. 230:41.

Suga, N., Schlegel, P., Shimozawa, T., Simmons, J.,
1973, Orientation sounds evoked from echolocating bats by electrical stimulation of the
brain, J.Acoust.Soc.Amer. 54:793.

Suthers, R.A., Fattu, J.M., 1973, Mechanisms of sound
production by echolocating bats, Amer.Zool.
13:1215.

Suthers, R.A., Fattu, J.M., 1982, Selective laryngeal
neurotomy and the control of phonation by the
echolocating bat, Eptesicus., J.Comp.Physiol.
145:529.

AUDITORY-VOCAL INTEGRATION IN THE MIDBRAIN OF THE

MUSTACHED BAT: PERIAQUEDUCTAL GRAY AND RETICULAR FORMATION

Nobuo Suga and Yukio Yajima[*]

Department of Biology
Washington University
St. Louis, MO 63130
U.S.A.

INTRODUCTION

Acoustic communication and echolocation involve the auditory and vocal systems. In order to understand these systems, research should be performed not only on each system in isolation, but also on auditory-vocal integration. How is the signal processing by the auditory system influenced by vocal activity? How is the activity of the vocal system modified by acoustic stimuli? To date, neurophysiological studies directly related to these questions are very limited, but there are several papers worth mentioning.

In the gray bat _Myotis grisescens_ (Suga and Schlegel, 1972; Suga and Shimozawa, 1974), the squirrel monkey _Saimiri sciureus_ (Jürgens and Ploog, 1981), and canary _Serinus canarius_ (McCasland and Konishi, 1981), auditory responses to self-vocalized sounds are attenuated or inhibited in the central auditory system during vocalization.

In the mustached bat _Pteronotus parnellii_, vocal self-stimulation is used as a referent to process target-velocity and -range information by CF/CF and FM-FM combination-sensitive neurons, respectively (Suga, 1984; Kawasaki et al., 1987). This may also be true in the horseshoe bats, _Rhinolophus ferrumequinum_ and _R. rouni_ (Schuller, 1979; O'Neill et al., 1985).

_____

[*]Present address of Y. Yajima: Lab of Neurophysiology, Hyogo College of Medicine, Mukogawacho, Nishinomiya, Hyogo, Japan.

Neurons in the midbrain periaqueductal gray (PAG) respond to acoustic stimuli in the monkey <u>Macaca</u> <u>fuscicularis</u> (Larson and Kistler, 1984), and neurons in the vocal center (hyperstriatum ventrale pars caudale:HVc) of song birds show auditory responses (McCasland and Konishi, 1981). Since these vocal centers or areas receive auditory information, it has been found that even "vocal" motoneurons and muscles also respond to acoustic stimuli, both in the little brown bat <u>Myotis lucifugus</u> (Jen and Suga, 1976) and in song birds (Williams, 1985; Williams and Nottebohm, 1985).

In this article, we will review our experiments on vocal behavior and single neuron activity related to audio-vocal integration for echolocation in mustached bats. Behavioral experiments, vocal responses to electric and acoustic stimuli, were performed on both unanesthetized mustached bats and a few other species of bats whose species-specific orientation sounds are clearly different from each other (Suga et al, 1973, 1974). Neurophysiological experiments, single unit recording from the midbrain reticular formation (MRF) and PAG were performed only on unanesthetized mustached bats.

VOCAL RESPONSES TO ELECTRIC STIMULI

The orientation sound of the mustached bat always consists of a long constant frequency (CF) component and a short frequency modulated (FM) component. When electric stimuli are applied to the dorsal part of MRF and/or the lateral part of PAG near the boundary between the superior and inferior colliculi (Fig. 1), microchiropterans emit species-specific orientation sounds. For example, in the mustached bat, electric stimulation in MRF elicits emission of a single CF-FM sound which is 20-30 msec long (Fig. 2, A and C). While electric stimulation in PAG elicits emissions of multiple CF-FM sounds which are 10-30 msec long (Fig. 2, B and D). Each of these electrically elicited sounds always contains a 2-3 msec-long terminal FM component, and contains 4 harmonics. The second harmonic is always predominant, and the first harmonic is usually very faint. In the second harmonic, the CF component is about 62 kHz, and the FM component sweeps downward from 62 to 50 kHz. These electrically elicited sounds are indistinguishable from orientation sounds which are spontaneously emitted. While emitting 110-115 dB SPL orientation sounds after the electric stimulation, the bat moves its mouth and pinnae, but shows no other body movements. The latencies of the electrically elicited sounds range between 25 and 60 msec after the beginning of the train of electric stimulus pulses.

In the Myotis bat, electric stimulation in MRF evokes emission of a single FM sound (Fig. 3, B1) which is about 3 msec long and sweeps downward from 100 to 40 kHz (Fig. 3, A and C). Its amplitude is typically 110-115 dB SPL at 10 cm in front of the

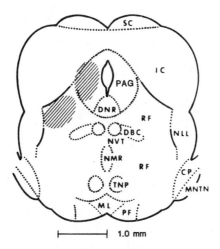

Fig. 1. A frontal section across the midbrain near the boundry
between the inferior and superior colliculi of Myotis
austroriparius. The locations of the tips of the stimulating
electrodes are indicated by the shaded areas. The electric
stimulus used to elicit vocalization was a short train of pulses
delivered at two times per second. The train consisted of six
electric pulses, each of which had a 0.1 msec duration and a 1-15
V amplitude. The estimated amount of current was 1-15 μA. The
interpulse interval was 1.7 msec. CP: cerebellar peduncle. DBC:
decussation of brachium conjunctivum. DNR: dorsal nucleus of
raphe. IC: inferior colliculus. ML: medial lemniscus. MNTN:
mesencephalic nucleus of trigeminal nerve. NLL: nucleus of
lateral lemniscus. NMR: nucleus of medial raphe. NVT: nucleus of
ventral tegmentum. PAG: periaqueductal gray. PF: pyramidal
fibers. RF: reticular formation. SC: superior colliculus. TNP:
tegmental nucleus of pons (Suga et al., 1973).

bat's mouth. The latency of the emitted sound is 40-60 msec after
the beginning of the train of electric pulses. The sound is very
similar to the orientation sound used by the Myotis bat during the
search phase of echolocation. Electric stimulation in PAG evokes
emission of multiple FM sounds (Fig. 3, B2) which each are 1-2
msec long and sweep downward from 40 to 20 kHz (Fig. 3,D). They
are intense, 110-115 dB SPL, and occur in one or more groups (Fig.
3, B2). The repetition rate of the sounds in each group is 80-
140/sec. These sounds are similar to orientation sounds used by
the Myotis bat during the terminal phase of insect-pursuit or
obstacle avoidance. To emit the sounds, the bat moves its mouth
and pinnae. No other body movements are involved.

For echolocation, the mustached bat emits only CF-FM sounds,

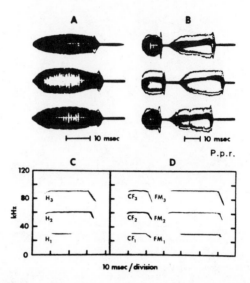

Fig. 2.   CF-FM sounds elicited from a mustached bat $\underline{P}$. $\underline{parnellii}$ $\underline{rubiginosus}$ by electric stimuli applied to the dorsal part of the reticular formation (A) or the lateral part of the periaqueductal gray (B) in the midbrain.   (C) and (D) Sonagrams of some of the sounds in A and B, respectively (Suga et al., 1973).

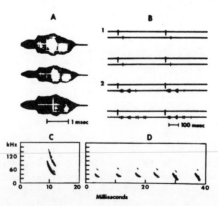

Fig. 3.   FM sounds evoked from $\underline{Myotis}$ $\underline{austroriparius}$ by electric stimuli applied to the midbrain.   (A) FM sounds elicited by the stimulation of the dorsal part of the midbrain reticular formation.   (B) FM sounds elicited by the stimulation of either the dorsal part of the reticular formation (1) or the lateral part of the periaqueductal gray (2) in the midbrain.   The upper and lower traces respectively represent electric stimuli and elicited sounds.   (C) and (D) Sonagrams of some of the sounds shown in B1 and B2, respectively (Suga et al., 1973).

while the Myotis bat emits only FM sounds. The electric
stimulation in MRF and/or PAG elicits only species-specific
orientation sounds. This is also true in other species of bats
tested, such as <u>Pteronotus suapurensis</u>, <u>Eptesicus fuscus,</u> and
<u>Noctilio leporinus</u>. These data imply that the functional
organization of the vocal system differs from species to species
(Suga et al., 1973).

  Some uncertainty exists as to whether the electric stimuli
directly excite the vocal system, rather than evoking an emotional
change, which in turn initiates vocalization. In the above
mentioned areas of the midbrain, electric stimuli apparently
stimulate the vocal system directly, because (1) the latency of
the vocalization is very short, (2) the vocalization is evoked
synchronously with each train of electric stimuli and immediately
stops when the stimulus stops, and (3) no gross body movements are
associated with this vocalization when the electrodes are placed
in a low-threshold area.

  The mammalian vocal system has been best studied in monkeys.
The cingulate cortex is considered to be the highest vocal center,
and the regions of MRF and PAG shown in Fig. 1 are also important
in monkey vocalization (Jürgens and Ploog, 1981). In the
mustached bat, electric stimulation of the anterior cingulate
cortex elicits orientation sounds, and the anterior cingulate
cortex projects to MRF and PAG (Gooler, 1987; Gooler and O'Neill,
1987). In the horseshoe bat, horseradish peroxidase injected into
the nucleus ambiguus labels the lateral part of PAG, cuneiform
nucleus, and several other regions in the brain (Rübsamen and
Schweizer, 1986). The dorsal region of MRF which was electrically
stimulated in our experiments apparently corresponds to the
cuneiform nucleus.

VOCAL RESPONSES TO MASKING SOUNDS

  When the electric stimulus is attenuated, the amplitude of
electrically evoked sounds decreases in amplitude, and the latency
of the vocalization increases and shows large fluctuations. Under
these conditions, a 2 msec-long CF tone (at a repetition rate of
250/sec) or a continuous tone is delivered in addition to the
electric stimulus. Then the electrically evoked sound increases
in amplitude and occurs more regularly. The number of sounds
emitted for each electric stimulus often increases as well. Such
a behavioral response is called a "vocal response to an acoustic
stimulus". The vocal response to an acoustic stimulus varies with
the parameters of the stimulus. An increase in amplitude of the
tone pulse causes an increase in the amplitude of the vocal
response (Fig. 4). In the mustached bat, the frequency-tuning
curve of the vocal response measured with tone pulses is very
sharply tuned to 62-63 kHz (Fig. 5, curve TB). The lowest

threshold of vocal response is 23 dB SPL. When a continuous pure
tone is delivered instead of the tone pulses, the threshold of the
vocal response is 10-25 dB higher than that for the tone pulses,
although the continuous pure tone has energy 3 dB greater than the
repetitive tone pulses (Fig. 5, curve CT).

When a 2 msec-long FM sound is repetitively delivered instead
of the CF tone pulse, the vocal response of the mustached bat is
significantly stronger to the FM sound than to the CF tone, except
around 62 kHz (Fig. 5, arrows). In particular, downward sweeping
FM sounds are most effective in evoking the vocal responses. The
thresholds for downward sweeping FM sounds are 10-20 dB lower than
those for upward sweeping FM sounds at the same frequencies and
about 30 dB lower than those for CF tone pulses, except around 62
kHz.

The very sharp frequency-tuning curve of the vocal response
at about 62 kHz and the low threshold for the downward sweeping FM
sounds suggest that the control of the vocal response is mediated
by particular types of auditory neurons; one type of auditory
neuron with a very sharp frequency-tuning curve at about 62 kHz
and another type more sensitive to downward sweeping FM sounds
than to pure tones (Suga et al., 1974).

The change in the electrically evoked vocalization in the
presence of acoustic stimuli suggests that the bat echolocates
with the electrically evoked sounds, and that the animal increases
the amplitude and the number of orientation sounds to overcome the
masking sound and thereby detect echoes from objects in front of

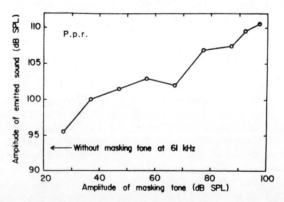

Fig. 4. Vocal response to a masking sound. Electrically elicited
orientation sounds from a mustached bat increased in amplitude
when the amplitude of a 61 kHz tone pulse (masker) was raised.
The tone pulse was 2 msec-long and was delivered at a rate of
250/sec. The arrow indicates the amplitude of the electrically
elicited sounds without the tone pulse (Suga et al., 1974).

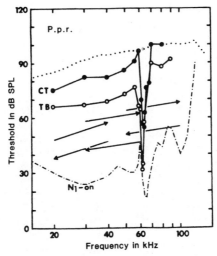

Fig. 5. Thresholds of vocal responses of a mustached bat to acoustic stimuli (maskers). <u>TB</u>: Threshold curve measured with 2 msec CF tone pulses delivered at a rate of 250 pulses/sec. <u>CT</u>: Threshold curve measured with a continuous pure tone. Each arrow indicates the direction of frequency sweep in an FM sound by its head, the range of frequency sweep by its length, and the threshold of the vocal response to the FM sound by its vertical position. A threshold curve for N_1-on response is also presented for a comparison. The uppermost dotted line indicates the frequency response curve of the loudspeaker. The ordinate represents a stimulus amplitude at threshold in dB SPL (decibels in sound pressure level referred to 0.0002 dyne/cm^2 r.m.s.). The abscissa represents the frequencies of the acoustic stimuli in kilohertz (Suga et al., 1974).

the bat. Consistent with this interpretation is the observation that the vocal response to the masking sound is affected by the spectrum of the masking sound, the information-bearing elements or parameters of the orientation sound and echo pair, and also the properties of the auditory neurons used for echolocation. The observed thresholds of vocal responses to acoustic stimuli might be interpreted in the following way: in the CF component of echoes, the second harmonic (about 62 kHz) is much more important than the other harmonics, because the threshold of the vocal response is low only at 62 kHz. The first, second, and third harmonics in the FM component of the orientation sound and echoes are equally important to the bat, because the threshold of the vocal response is lower for downward sweeping FM sounds than the thresholds for upward sweeping FM sounds and for pure tones, except around 62 kHz. [The "resting" frequency of the second harmonic CF component of the orientation sound differs among

individual bats. The mean and standard deviation are 60.87 ± 0.48
kHz for 77 Panamanian mustached bats P. p. rubiginosus (Suga and
Tsuzuki, 1985) and 61.77 ± 0.56 kHz for 116 Jamaican mustached
bats P. p. parnellii (Suga et al., 1987). The resting frequency
of the Panamanian mustached bat, from which the data shown in Fig.
5 were obtained, was probably about 62 kHz.]

SINGLE UNIT ACTIVITIES RECORDED FROM PAG AND MRF

     The behavioral data described above suggest that neurons
responding to acoustic stimuli become active prior to
vocalization, and that the activity prior to vocalization
(hereafter, prevocal activity) is affected by the acoustic
stimuli. To test these hypotheses, tungsten wire electrodes with
5-8 μm tip diameter were inserted into the PAG and MRF in 12
unanesthetized mustached bats (Fig. 6). About 15% of the neurons
recorded showed prevocal activity and/or auditory responses.
These neurons could be classified into 3 types. "V-A" neurons (n
= 37) showed prevocal activity and auditory response. "V-O"
neurons (n = 33) showed prevocal activity, but no auditory
response. "A-O" neurons (n = 87) showed auditory response, but no
prevocal activity.

     The recording sites of these 3 types of neurons were
estimated from the penetration angles and depths of the recording

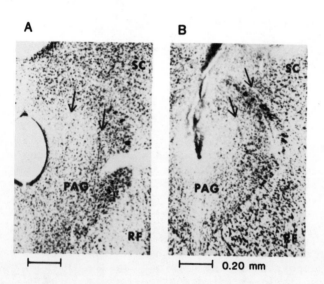

Fig. 6. Frontal sections across the midbrain of a mustached bat.
(A) and (B) Each shows tracts of two parallel electrode
penetrations (arrows). PAG: periaqueductal gray. RE: reticular
formation. SC: superior colliculus. Thionin stain: 30 μm thick.

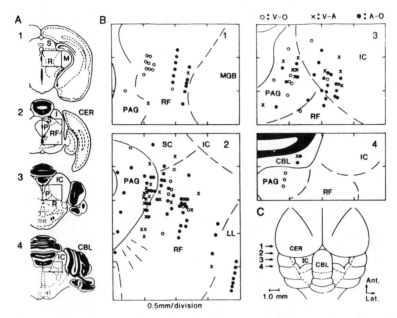

Fig. 7.   Locations of V-O, V-A, and A-O neurons.   (A) Frontal
sections 1-4 across the midbrain of a mustached bat at arrows 1-4
in C.   (B) 1-4 correspond to the rectangular areas shown in A, 1-
4.   Open circles, crosses, and filled circles indicate V-O, V-A,
and A-O neurons, respectively.   The locations of these neurons are
estimated by depths and directions of electrode penetrations. (C)
The dorsal view of the brain.   CBL: cerebellum.   CER: cerebrum.   I
or IC: inferior colliculus.   LL: lateral lemniscus.   M or MGB:
medial geniculate body.   P or PAG: periaqueductal grey.   R or RF:
reticular formation.   S or SC: superior colliculus.

electrodes (Fig. 7).   In our penetrations, 21 of the 87 A-O
neurons were recorded from the medial region of the inferior
colliculus or the lateral lemniscus, and 5 of the 37 V-A neurons
and 2 of the 33 V-O neurons were recorded from the medial region
of the inferior colliculus.   However, the great majority of V-A
and V-O neurons were recorded from the lateral region of PAG and
the dorsomedial region of MRF, as expected from the electric
stimulation experiments.   Most surprising to us were the five V-A
and two V-O neurons recorded from the medial edge of the inferior
colliculus (Fig. 7, B3), and also two V-A neurons recorded from
either the superior colliculus or the region immediately medial to
the lateral lemniscus (Fig. 7, B2).   A horseradish peroxidase
injection into the nucleus ambiguus labels not only PAG and the
cuneiform nucleus, but also other regions in the brain, including
the superior colliculus and fibers running immediately medial to
the lateral lemniscus.   The inferior colliculus is not labelled

(Rübsamen and Schweizer, 1986). Therefore, the V-A neurons recorded from the superior colliculus and the region just medial to the lateral lemniscus are consistent with the anatomical data, but the V-A and V-O neurons recorded from the medial edge of the inferior colliculus are not.

Fig. 8 shows examples of single-unit activity of V-A, V-O, and A-O neurons. The V-A neuron in Fig. 8A showed prevocal activity starting about 132 msec prior to the emission of orientation sound(s). The activity increased toward a peak which occurred within 30 msec before vocalization. Clusters of neural discharges 50 msec after the onset of the emitted sound (time = 0) were associated with multiple vocalizations (Aa). This neuron responded best to a CF tone at 60.27 kHz and 90 dB SPL. The response pattern was phasic-on, and the response latency was 6 msec (Ab). Such a short latency suggests that audio-vocal

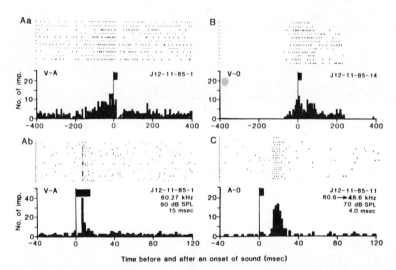

Fig. 8. Prevocal activities and/or auditory responses of V-A, V-O, and A-O neurons. The rasters and histograms display temporal patterns of nerve impulses referenced to the onset of spontaneously emitted orientation sounds (Aa and B) or acoustic stimuli (Ab and C). When a mustached bat emitted short trains of orientation sounds, the onset of the first sound in the trains was used to align nerve impulses in time. The filled rectangles on the zero lines represent the durations of acoustic stimuli or emitted orientation sounds. (Aa) and (B) Orientation sounds emitted by the bat were 15-20 msec long. (Ab) The acoustic stimulus was a 60.27 kHz, 90 dB SPL, 15 msec-long CF. (C) The acoustic stimulus was a 4.0 msec-long, 70 dB SPL FM sound sweeping from 60.6 to 48.6 kHz. These sounds were delivered at a rate of 2/sec.

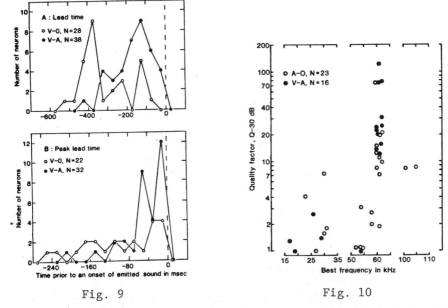

Fig. 9   Fig. 10

Fig. 9. Distributions of lead times (A) and peak lead times (B) of prevocal activities of V-0 and V-A neurons, when mustached bats spontaneously emitted CF-FM orientation sounds.

Fig. 10. Distribution of quality factors of frequency-tuning curves of A-0 and V-A neurons. Best frequencies of these neurons fell within 3 different frequency bands (abscissa). The quality factor, Q-30dB, is calculated as the best frequency divided by the bandwidth of a frequency-tuning curve at 30 dB above minimum threshold.

integration indeed takes place in the midbrain. The V-0 neuron in Fig. 8B showed prevocal activity with a 67 msec lead time. Peak activity appeared within ± 10 msec of the onset of emitted orientation sounds. Clusters of neural activities after the zero time were associated with multiple vocalizations. The A-0 neuron in Fig. 8C responded better to a downward sweeping FM sound than any CF tone tested. The response latency was 13 msec.

The lead time of prevocal activity associated with the emission of orientation sounds varied widely among neurons, ranging from 10 to 550 msec. Interestingly, the lead times of V-0 neurons tended to be longer than those of V-A neurons (Fig. 9A). Prevocal activity was consistent in neurons with a short lead time, but it was inconsistent in those with a long lead time. Since prevocal activity gradually increased toward the onset of vocalization in almost all neurons, "peak" prevocal activity appeared with a lead time between 0 and 260 msec. The "peak" lead time was less than 70 msec in the majority of neurons studied (Fig. 9B).

The emission of orientation sounds is synchronized with expiration (Suthers and Fattu, 1973). In the big brown bat Eptesicus fuscus, the anterior cricothyroid muscle becomes active as early as 100 msec (56 msec on the average) prior to sound emission (Suthers, 1988). In the horseshoe bat, the recurrent laryngeal nerve becomes active about 180 msec prior to .sound emission. The prevocal activity between 30 and 180 msec is associated with respiration and occurs with/without vocalization (Rübsamen and Schuller, 1981). Neurons with extremely long lead time, which were recorded in our experiments, may be related to respiration.

SENSITIVITY OF PAG AND MRF NEURONS TO CF TONES AND FM SOUNDS

Frequency-tuning curves or minimum thresholds of V-A and A-O neurons were measured with CF tones, FM sounds, and/or noise bursts. In the FM sounds, frequency swept downward or upward over a band spanning either 6, 12, or 18 kHz. In the noise bursts, bandwidth was set at either 4, 8, or 16 kHz.

The majority of V-A and A-O neurons recorded were tuned to a sound between 60 and 64 kHz. Their frequency-tuning curves were much sharper than the tuning curves of V-A and V-O neurons tuned to other frequencies (Fig. 10). Among neurons tuned to identical frequencies, there were noticeable differences in responses to CF tones, FM sounds, and noise bursts. For example, both the V-A neurons in Fig. 11 A and B were tuned to 60.0 kHz and responded to both CF tones and FM sounds. But the neuron in A responded better to CF tones than to FM sounds, although the difference between the minimum thresholds for these two types of sounds was only 4 dB. On the other hand, the neuron in B responded better to FM sounds than to CF tones. There was an 8 dB difference between the minimum thresholds. The weaker response and higher threshold to FM sounds shown by the neuron in A may be explained by the fact that, unlike the CF tones, only a fraction of the 4-msec-long FM sounds fell into the tip portion of the frequency-tuning curve. The strong response and low threshold to the FM sounds of the neuron in B may be explained by synaptic summation or facilitation or even by disinhibition which might be evoked by the frequency sweep (Suga, 1965, 1973).

In other neurons, the difference in threshold between responses to CF tones and FM sounds was very large (Fig. 15A). In Fig. 12 A and B, for example, two V-A neurons are tuned to either a 57 or a 54 kHz CF tone. They poorly responded to CF tones, but strongly responded to noise bursts and/or downward sweeping FM sounds. In A, the minimum thresholds of the responses to noise

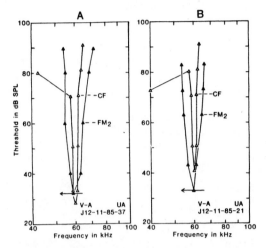

Fig. 11. Excitatory frequency-tuning curves of two V-A neurons (A and B) measured with single 15 msec-long CF tones or single 4 msec-long FM sounds. Threshold for an FM sound is expressed by the stimulus amplitude at the center of its 12 kHz-wide frequency sweep. In each graph, the arrow at the minimum threshold symbolizes the direction and range of frequency sweep.

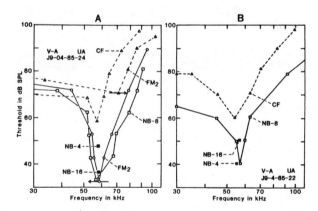

Fig. 12. Excitatory frequency-tuning curves of two V-A neurons (A and B) measured with either single CF tones, FM sounds, or noise bursts. The durations of these sounds were 15, 4 and 15 msec, respectively. The FM sounds swept 12 kHz either upward or downward. The noise bursts had a bandwidth of either 4, 8 or 16 kHz. They are expressed by NB-4, NB-8, and NB-16, respectively. The best frequency bands and minimum thresholds for NB-4 and NB-16 are indicated by the filled squares. In A, each arrow at the minimum threshold symbolizes the direction and range of frequency sweep.

bursts and downward sweeping FM sounds were respectively 22 and 23
dB lower than the minimum threshold for CF tones. Interestingly,
the response to upward sweeping FM sounds was very poor and the
threshold was 34 dB higher than to downward sweeping FM sounds.
In B, the minimum threshold to noise bursts was 20 dB lower than
to CF tones. The neuron did not respond to FM sounds, regardless
of the direction of frequency sweep.

In addition to the variations in responses to CF tones, FM
sounds, and noise bursts, we have found two combination-sensitive
V-A neurons. The response properties of one of these neurons were
extensively studied (Figs. 13 and 14). This neuron showed
prevocal activity with a lead time of about 110 msec. The
prevocal activity stopped within 10 msec after the onset of an
emitted orientation sound (Fig. 13a). The neuron poorly responded
to single CF and FM sounds. Its threshold was low for FM sounds,
but high for CF tones (Fig. 14). This neuron poorly responded to
the second and third harmonics of the CF-FM orientation sound when
separately delivered (Fig. 13, b and c). However, it responded
strongly to the combination of these two harmonics (Fig. 13d).
The essential signal elements in this complex sound were found to
be the FM components, so that the neuron was FM_2-FM_3 combination-
sensitive. Combinations of any two CF tones tested could not
evoke a facilitative response in this neuron (e.g., Fig. 13e).

Fig. 14 shows the excitatory frequency-tuning curves of this
neuron measured with CF tones and FM sounds, and also facilitative
tuning curves measured with pairs of FM sounds. The minimum
thresholds measured with FM_2 or FM_3 were 34 dB lower than
threshold minima at around 51 or 77 kHz measured with CF tones.
The minimum threshold for facilitation was respectively 10 and 5
dB lower for FM_2 and FM_3 than that for excitation evoked by either
FM_2 or FM_3 alone. The neuron was thus FM-sensitive and also FM-FM
combination-sensitive.

The data obtained from PAG and MRF clearly indicate that
there are different types of V-A neurons in terms of auditory
response. Thus the vocal system appears to be coupled with the
auditory system through various types of auditory neurons. What
is interesting in relation to vocal responses to masking sounds is
that some V-A neurons showed lower thresholds to downward-sweeping
FM sounds than to CF tones, while some others were sharply tuned
to CF tones around 61 kHz and responded better to these than to FM
sounds. Thus, differences in minimum threshold between responses
to CF tones and downward sweeping FM sounds were calculated for
individual V-A and A-O neurons and plotted in Fig. 15. "FM-
sensitive" neurons are arbitrarily defined as at least 5 dB more
sensitive to FM sounds than to CF tones, and "CF-sensitive"
neurons are at least 5 dB more sensitive to CF tones than to FM
sounds. Of the 82 V-A and A-O neurons studied, 30 and 32 were
respectively FM- and CF-sensitive (Fig. 15A). FM and CF

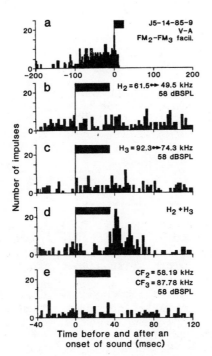

Fig. 13. Prevocal activity and response to a combination of two sounds of a V-A neuron. (a) Peri-event-time histogram displaying prevocal activity associated with the emission of CF-FM orientation sounds. (b)-(e) are peri-stimulus-time histograms displaying responses or no response. (b) Stimulation by a sound similar to the second harmonic of the orientation sound. The stimulus consisted of a 30 msec-long CF component at 61.5 kHz followed by a 4 msec-long FM component sweeping from 61.5 to 49.5 kHz. (c) Stimulation by a sound similar to the third harmonic of the orientation sound. The stimulus consisted of a 30 msec-long CF component at 92.3 kHz followed by a 4 msec-long FM component sweeping from 92.3 to 74.3 kHz. (d) Simultaneous stimulation by the two sounds used in b and c. (e) Simultaneous stimulation by two 34 msec-long CF tones at 58.19 or 87.78 kHz. All the acoustic stimuli were delivered 50 times at 58 dB SPL, and the PST histograms were plotted. The durations of the orientation sounds vocalized and the acoustic stimuli delivered are indicated by the solid rectangles.

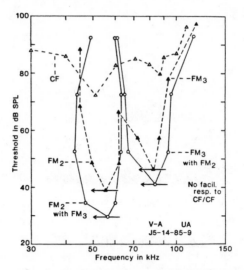

Fig. 14. Excitatory and facilitative frequency-tuning curves of a V-A neuron. The excitatory tuning curves were measured with either 34 msec-long single CF tones (curve CF) or 4 msec-long single FM sounds. The width of frequency sweep in these FM sounds was either 12 kHz (curve FM$_2$) or 18 kHz (curve FM$_3$), which respectively mimicked the FM components in the 2nd and 3rd harmonics of the bat's orientation sound. Threshold for FM sounds is expressed by the stimulus amplitude at the center of their frequency sweeps. The facilitative tuning curves were measured with a pair of FM$_2$ with FM$_3$ sounds, in which either the FM$_2$ (curve FM$_2$ with FM$_3$) or the FM$_3$ (curve FM$_3$ and FM$_2$) was varied in frequency and amplitude to measure thresholds, while the other sound in the pair was fixed. Curve FM$_2$ with FM$_3$ was obtained when the FM$_3$ was fixed at 58 dB SPL and 92.3-to-74.3 kHz sweep. Curve FM$_3$ with FM$_2$ was obtained when the FM$_2$ was fixed at 58 dB SPL and 61.5-to-49.5 kHz sweep.

sensitivities were related to best frequencies of neurons: the ratio of CF- vs FM-sensitive neurons is 81:19 for neurons with best frequencies between 61.0 and 61.9 kHz, while it is 21:79 for neurons with best frequencies between 53.0 and 60.9 kHz (Fig. 15B). That is, neurons tuned to the frequency of the second harmonic CF component (CF$_2$) of Doppler-shifted echoes stabilized by Doppler-shift compensation are mainly CF-sensitive, while neurons tuned to the frequencies swept by the second harmonic FM component (FM$_2$) are mainly FM-sensitive. As shown in Fig. 10, neurons with a best frequency between 60.0 and 62.0 kHz are very sharply tuned. Therefore, our electrophysiological data agree with the behavioral data presented in Fig. 5: (i) the vocal response to a CF tone is very sharply tuned to 61-62 kHz, and (ii)

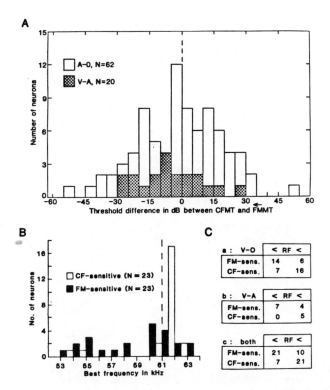

Fig. 15. Differences in sensitivity to CF tones and downward sweeping FM sounds. (A) Differences in minimum threshold between responses to CF tones and FM sounds of A-0 and V-A neurons. (B) Distributions of CF-sensitive and FM-sensitive neurons as a function of their best frequencies. When a neuron is more than 5 dB sensitive to CF tones than to FM sounds, it is called "CF-sensitive". When a neuron is more than 5 dB sensitive to FM sounds than to CF tones, it is called "FM-sensitive". (C) FM-sensitive and CF-sensitive V-0 (a) and V-A (b) neurons are divided into two groups according to whether their best frequencies are within the ranges of the FM components (< RF) or the ranges of the Doppler-shifted CF components (RF <) of the bat's biosonar signals. RF is the resting frequency of either CF_1, CF_2 or CF_3 component of the orientation sound which are either 30.5, 61.0, or 91.5 kHz, respectively.

outside of the 60-63 kHz band, the vocal response is much stronger
to downward sweeping FM sounds than to CF tones.

We do not know how V-A and A-O neurons with these different
auditory responses are spatially arranged in the midbrain vocal
regions. We also do not know how prevocal activity is modified by
acoustic stimuli. The functional organization of the midbrain
vocal regions in terms of audio-vocal integration remains to be
explored.

SUMMARY

1.   In echolocating bats, electric stimulation of the dorsal part
of the reticular formation (MRF) and/or the lateral part of the
periaqueductal gray (PAG) in the midbrain elicits species-specific
orientation sounds. The functional organization of the vocal
system apparently differs among species.

2.   The orientation sound of the mustached bat, <u>Pteronotus</u>
<u>parnellii</u>, consists of four harmonics (H_{1-4}), and each harmonic
consists of a long constant frequency (CF) component followed by a
short frequency modulated (FM) component. Thus, each orientation
sound contains 8 components: CF_{1-4} and FM_{1-4}. In the emitted
sound, H_2 is always predominant. The resting frequency of the CF_2
differs among individual bats within a range of 60 and 63 kHz. It
is 61.0 kHz on the average. FM_2 sweeps downward from 61 to 59
kHz.

3.   Bats respond to acoustic stimuli (maskers) by increasing the
intensity of the electrically-elicited vocalization. In the
mustached bat, this "vocal" response is very sensitive to CF tones
only around 62 kHz, and the frequency-tuning curve of the vocal
response is very sharply tuned to this frequency. The vocal
response is also strong to downward sweeping FM sounds. Its
threshold is much lower for downward sweeping FM sounds than for
upward sweeping FM sounds and CF tones, except for CF tones around
62 kHz. Such vocal responses suggest that when emitting the
orientation sound, the vocal system is strongly coupled with the
auditory system through particular types of auditory neurons:
neurons sharply tuned to the CF_2 component in Doppler-shifted
echoes and also neurons more sensitive to the FM components in the
echoes.

4.   MRF and PAG contain at least three types of neurons:
prevocal-auditory (V-A), prevocal-no auditory (V-O), and no
prevocal-auditory (A-O). Prevocal activity associated with the
emission of CF-FM orientation sounds occurs with a lead time
between 10 and 550 msec and gradually increases toward the onset
of the sound emission. The peak of prevocal activity occurs at 0-
260 msec prior to the emission. The "peak" lead time is less than
70 msec in the majority of neurons.

5. V-A and A-O neurons show various types of auditory responses to CF tones, FM sounds, and noise bursts. Some neurons are very sharply tuned to CF tones around 62 kHz and are much more sensitive to CF tones than the other sounds. Others are sensitive to either FM sounds or noise bursts, and some are sensitive to combinations of two sounds. Thus, the vocal system appears to be coupled with the auditory system through various types of auditory neurons.

6. The great majority of V-A and A-O neurons sensitive to the frequencies of the CF_2 component of a Doppler-shifted echo are very sharply tuned and are CF-sensitive, while V-A and A-O neurons tuned to frequencies swept by the FM components of the echo are FM-sensitive. Therefore, our electrophysiological data agree with the behavioral data for vocal responses to acoustic stimuli.

ACKNOWLEDGEMENTS

This work on mustached bats has been supported by a research grant from the U.S. Public Health Service, R01-NS17333 Javits neuroscience investigator award. We thank W.E. O'Neill and S.J. Gaioni for their helpful comments on this article.

REFERENCES

Gooler, D. M., 1987, Species specific vocalizations elicited by microstimulation of anterior cingulate cortex in the echolocating bat, Pteronotus parnellii parnellii: Characteristics of emissions and topographic representation of vocal frequency. Ph.D. Thesis, Univ. of Rochester, N.Y.

Gooler, D. M. and O'Neill, W. E., 1987, Topographic representation of vocal frequency demonstated by microstimulation of anterior cingulate cortex in the echolocating bat, Pteronotus parnelli parnelli. J. Comp. Physiol, A 160: (in press).

Jen, P. H.-S. and Suga, N., 1976, Coordinated activities of middle-ear and laryngeal muscles in echolocating bats. Science, 191:950-952.

Jürgens, U. and Ploog, D.,1981, On the neural control of mammalian vocalization. TINS, June: 135-137.

Kawasaki, M., Margoliash, D. and Suga, N., 1988, Delay-tuned combination-sensitive neurons in the auditory cortex of the vocalizing mustached bat. J. Neurophysiol. (in press).

Larson, C. R. and Kistler, M. K., 1984, Periaqueductal gray neuronal activity associated with laryngeal EMG and vocalization in the awake monkey. Neurosci. Letters, 42:261-266.

McCasland, J. S. and Konishi, M., 1981, Interaction between auditory and motor activities in an avian song control nucleus. Proc. Natl. Acad. Sci. U.S.A. 78:7815-7819.

O'Neill, W. E., Schuller, G., and Radtke-Schuller, S., 1985, Functional and anatomical similarities in the auditory cortices of the old world horseshoe bat and neotropical mustached bat for processing similar biosonar signals. Winter meeting of Assoc. Res. Otolaryngol. Abst. No.193.

Rübsamen, R. and Schweizer, H., 1986, Control of echolocation pulses by neurons of the nucleus ambiguus in the rufons horseshoe bat, Rhinolophus rouxi. II. Afferent and efferent connections of motor nucleus of the laryngeal nerves. J. Comp. Physiol., A 159:689-699.

Rübsamen, R. and Schuller, G., 1981, Laryngeal nerve activity during pulse emission in the CF-FM bat, Rhinolophus ferrumequinum. II. The recurrent laryngeal nerve. J. Comp. Physiol., A 143:323-327.

Schuller, G., 1979, Vocalization influences auditory processing in collicular neurons of the CF-FM bat, Rhinolophus ferrumequinum. J. Comp. Physiol., 132:39-46.

Suga, N., 1965, Functional properties of auditory neurones in the auditory cortex of echolocating bats. J. Physiol., 181:671-700.

Suga, N., 1973, Feature extraction in the auditory system of bats, in: "Basic Mechanisms in Hearing," Ed. Moller, A.R. Academic Press, N.Y. 675-742.

Suga, N., 1984, The extent to which biosonar information is represented in the bat auditory cortex, in: "Dynamic Aspects of Neocortical Function," Eds. Edelman, G.M., Gall, W.E. and Cowan, W.M., John Wiley & Sons, N.Y. 315-373.

Suga, N., Niwa, H., Taniguchi, I. and Margoliash, D., 1987, The personalized auditory cortex of the mustached bat: adaptation for echolocation. J. Neurophysiol., 58 (in press).

Suga, N. and Schlegel, P., 1972, Neural Attenuation of responses to emitted sounds in echolocating bats. Science, 177:82-84.

Suga, N., Schlegel, P., Schimozawa, T., and Simmons, J. A., 1973, Orientation sounds evoked from echolocating bats by electrical stimulation of the brain. J. Acoust. Soc. Am. 54:793-797.

Suga, N. and Shimozawa, T., 1974, Site of neural attenuation of responses to self-vocalized sounds in echolocating bats. Science 183:1211-1213.

Suga, N., Simmons, J. A., and Shimozawa, T., 1974, Neurophysiological studies on echolocation systems in awake bats producing CF-FM orientation sounds. J. Exp. Biol. 61:379-399.

Suga, N. and Tsuzuki, K., 1985, Inhibition and level-tolerant frequency tuning in the auditory cortex of the mustached bat. J. Neurophysiol., 53:1109-1145.

Suthers, R. A., 1988, The production of echolocation signals by bats and birds, in: "Animal Sonar Systems", Ed: Nachtigall, P.E., Plenum, N.Y. (in press).

Suthers, R. A. and Fattu, J. M., 1973, Mechanisms of sound
    production by echolocating bats. <u>Am. Zool</u>., 13:1215-1226.
Williams, H., 1985, Sexual dimorphism of auditory activity in the
    zebra finch song system. <u>Beh. Neu. Biol</u>., 44:470-484.
Williams, H. and Nottebohm, F., 1985, Auditory responses in avian
    vocal motor neurons: A motor theory for song perception in
    birds. <u>Science</u> 229:279-282.

THE COORDINATION OF INTRINSIC LARYNGEAL
MUSCLE ACTIVATION DURING PHONATORY
AND NON-PHONATORY TASKS

Christy L. Ludlow, Ph.D
Mihoko Fujita, M.D.

Speech Pathology Unit
Human Motor Control Section, MNB
National Institute of Neurological and Communicative
Disorders and Stroke, Bethesda, MD 20892

INTRODUCTION

Lesions at different levels of the central nervous system can
selectively interfere with laryngeal movements during respiration,
vocalization, speech, effort closure and swallow. This suggests
that these actions are controlled by complex programs at different
levels of the nervous system. During respiration, two laryngeal
muscles, the thyroarytenoid (TA) and the cricothyroid (CT) are
activated in a reciprocal pattern with the posterior cricoarytenoid.
Increased CT activity during inspiration and expiration is
phasically related to respiration and most likely driven by the
medullary respiratory center (Sasaki and Buckwalter, 1984). During
inspiration, the CTs contract to lengthen the vocal folds as they
are opened, thus increasing the size of the glottis. The CT is also
active during expiration in relation to the degree of positive
subglottic pressure (Sasaki and Buckwalter, 1984). Others have
observed that the TA activates with the onset of expiration,
increments with expiratory action and drops in activity with
inspiration onset (Wyke and Kirchner, 1976). Human studies however,
have reported that the opposite is true in unanaesthetized subjects
with the greatest amount of TA activity immediately preceding
inspiration onset (Buchthal and Faaborg-Andersen, 1964). Since the
major function of the TA is vocal fold adduction and shortening, it
is difficult to reconcile these observations with the opening and
lengthening of the vocal folds observed during inspiration
(Brancatisano, Collett and Engel, 1983).

During swallow, the larynx elevates and the vocal folds adduct.
This action is the result of a series of reflexes (Wyke and
Kirchner, 1976) and is often disturbed by brain stem lesions
(Morell, 1984). Since respiration and swallow are both life support
mechanisms, these actions can be under involuntary control. On the
other hand, speech production is a learned motor activity disturbed
by lesions to the left hemisphere (Abbs,1986) or the basal ganglia
(Ludlow, Rosenberg, Salazar et al., 1987). Vocalization not
associated with speech, can be disturbed by lesions to other
structures such as the limbic cortex, amygdala, and hypothalamus
(Jurgens and Ploog, 1985). Vocalization may differ from phonation in
its neural control. We distinguish vocalization, an unlearned limbic
system response, from phonation, which is vocalization for speech
and includes extended production of a vowel sound.

Laryngeal muscle actions during speech, phonation, swallow, effort
closure and respiration differ in learning and accuracy
requirements. Effort closure is a less familiar nonphonatory
laryngeal action elicited by the instruction, "deep breath and
hold". This is not easily elicited from naive subjects without
practice and represents a novel non-phonatory laryngeal action.
Speech, a learned action, can have considerable timing variation in
EMG signals between tokens spoken by the same individual (Abbs,
1986). On the other hand, laryngeal muscle activation may be more
tightly coordinated during swallow and respiration, which do not
involve learning, than during phonation, speech and effort closure,
which do. The TA and CT may be independently activated during some
laryngeal tasks. These muscles are innervated by different nerves,
the recurrent laryngeal nerve for the TA and the superior laryngeal
nerve for the CT, and their motoneuron pools are separate in the
nucleus ambiguous.

This paper presents a preliminary investigation of the patterns of
laryngeal muscle activation during phonatory and non-phonatory
tasks. The purpose is to determine whether there are differences in
laryngeal muscle coordination and variance during different
laryngeal actions. Since some of these actions are selectively
impaired in idiopathic speech disorders such as spasmodic dysphonia,
determination of the different characteristics of these actions
might increase our understanding of why some actions are selectively
affected in some disorders.

METHODS

Two adult males (21 and 31 years), naive to the purpose of the
study, agreed to participate after informed consent. Subjects were
in a supine position with Respitrace bands around the chest and
abdomen to measure respiratory movement. A head mounted microphone
recorded vocalization and speech. Four 30 gauge concentric needles
were inserted percutaneously into the TA and CT on each side. For
the TA, phonation was the verifying gesture, while a pitch glide in
the modal voice range, was used for the CT. Head raising was used
to check that the needle was not in strap muscle.

Following needle insertion, the room was darkened and subjects were instructed to "sleep." After 10 minutes, the four EMG signals and respiratory movement were recorded for 5 minutes during quiet respiration on an FM tape recorder. Subsequently, the subjects performed the following actions between three and six times:
- swallow,
- deep breath and hold (effort closure),
- extended phonation of /a/ for 5 to 10 seconds, and
- production of the sentence "A dog dug a new bone" beginning with the same vowel sound as used during extended phonation.

The EMG activity was constantly monitored to assure that there was no needle movement throughout the recording session. The EMG signals were bandpass filtered between 100 and 5000 Hz before recording on FM tape simultaneously with the speech and respiratory signals. Inaccurate movements were documented and deleted from the corpus before off-line digitizing.

The respiratory, phonatory and EMG signals were digitized with anti-aliasing filtering, at different rates: 10KHz for speech, 5KHz for EMG, and 500 Hz for respiration. Two volt peak-to-peak sawtooth calibration tones were also digitized and measured to derive 'm' and 'b' values for linear interpolation of the EMG signals into microvolts. The minimum noise level was detected during 60 seconds of quiet respiration in each of the EMG signals and subtracted before measurement.

A sliding window averaged an EMG signal over 20 milliseconds, prior to automatic measurement of the maximum and minimum values for each inspiration and expiration cycle during 60 seconds of quiet respiration. Further, the total energy was integrated within each inspiration and expiration cycle.

For each of the movement tasks, the time of activation of a muscle was determined by identifying the point where the EMG signal first became 150% greater than the mean of the maximum points during inspiration for that muscle in that subject. The time of inactivation of the muscle was similarly identified using the point where the EMG signal became 150% less than the mean minimum level during inspiration for that muscle for that subject. The automatically detected onset and offset points were reviewed for accuracy by the investigators. The maximum level in the signal and the time at which this occurred between activation and inactivation in each muscle was automatically determined.

RESULTS

Respiration

The maximum and minimum levels and the integrated sum of energy of each of the muscles during inspiration and expiration are presented in Table 1. Maximum and minimum levels did not differ significantly

Table 1. Mean Minimum, Maximum and Total Energy (in microvolts)
         of Each Laryngeal Muscle During Inspiration and
         Expiration

Muscle	Minimum		Maximum		Total Energy	
	Inhal	Exhal	Inhal	Exhal	Inhal	Exhal
Right TA	3.8	3.7	23.4	20.1	947.9	362.2**
Right CT	4.9	4.9	20.6	18.5	864.5	586.9**
Left TA	8.8	9.3	25.1	24.7	1230.6	878.3*
Left CT	1.7	1.6	11.6	10.8	124.0	122.8

* p<.05;   **p <.01

between inspiration and expiration. A significantly greater sum of
EMG energy was found during inspiration than during expiration for
three muscles, the right TA, the right CT and the left TA. When the
ratio of the increase of the maximum level over the minimum level
was computed for the TA and CT muscles, no significant differences
were found (p<.05). Therefore, respiratory activation did not
differ between the TA and CT muscles during either part of the
respiratory cycle.

Pearson Correlation Coefficients between the time of maximum and
minimum levels during inspiration and expiration for the right TA,
the left TA and the right CT were computed to determine the
coordination between muscle activation during respiration. These
are presented in Table 2. Only a few values were statistically
significant (p<.05). Weak relationships were found between the time
of minimum levels of activity during expiration in the right TA, the
left TA and the right CT. A similar relationship was found between
the time of minimum levels between the right and left TAs during
inspiration. When the time of maximum levels during inspiration and
expiration are plotted (Figure 1), the TA and the CT are similar.
However, the time of the maximum level during expiration is somewhat
later in the cycle than during inspiration in both muscles.

Activation During Phonation, Speech, Effort Closure and Swallow

The mean level of activation differed across tasks for each muscle
except the right CT (Table 3). Wilcoxon paired comparisons between
tasks within muscles demonstrated that each of the muscles had
higher activation levels for speech than for phonation (p<.05) and
all but the right CT had higher activation levels during swallow
than phonation.

To examine the pattern of activation across muscles relative to
their level of activation during respiration, the percent increase
over the mean maximum inspiration level was computed for each of the
muscles during the four tasks (Figure 2). The pattern of activation
across the four muscles was similar for phonation, speech and effort

Table 2. Pearson Correlation Coefficients Between Times of Maximum
         and Minimum Levels during Inspiration and Expiration in
         Laryngeal Muscles

Measure	Right TA with Left TA	Right TA with Right CT
Inspiration:		
Maximum Level Time	.03	.09
Minimum Level Time	.36*	.17
Expiration:		
Maximum Level Time	.11	.08
Minimum Level Time	.33*	.42*

* (p<.05)

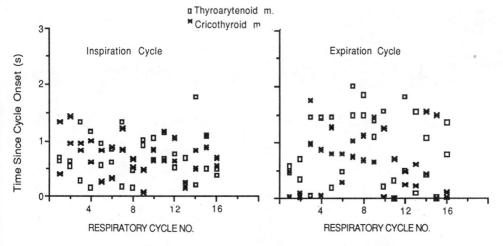

Figure 1. Time of Maximum Activation Levels for the Right TA
(thyroarytenoid) and Right CT (cricothyroid) Laryngeal Muscles
Following the Onset of the Inspiration and Expiration Cycles.

Table 3. Comparisons Between Mean Maximum Levels During Four
         Different Laryngeal Actions (in microvolts)

Muscle	Phonation	Speech	Effort Closure	Swallow
Right TA	24.2	62.7[a]	29.8	96.0[b]
Right CT	58.7	76.8[a]	82.8	49.4
Left TA	34.0	49.5[a]	78.7	141.7[b]
Left CT	36.0	54.9[a]	43.0	55.6

[a] Wilcoxon Test Between Phonation and Speech, p <.05
[b] Wilcoxon Test Between Phonation and Swallow, p <.05

closure. In each, the percent increase over respiration was greatest
for the right CT and less for the other three muscles. On the
Wilcoxon Matched Pairs Test, the right CT was significantly greater
(p<.05) than the right TA during phonation, speech and effort
closure. Within each muscle, the mean percent increase in activation
over respiration ranked the least for phonation, next for speech and
greater for effort closure. Swallow differed from the other three in
that all four muscles were activated to a similar degree, and was
the maximum activation gesture for all of the muscles except the
right CT.

Time of Muscle Action During Phonation, Speech, Effort Closure and
Swallow

The time of muscle activation onset between the TA and CT muscles on
the same side were compared using the Wilcoxon Matched Pairs Signed

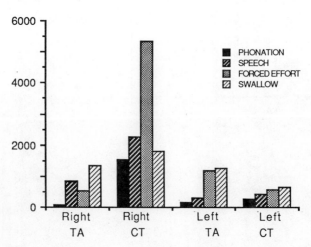

Figure 2. Mean Percent Increase Over Maximum Inspiratory Level for
Each Muscle During Phonation, Speech, Effort Closure and Swallow.

Table 4. Mean Times of Activation Onset for Laryngeal Muscles During Different Tasks (in seconds)

Muscle	Phonation	Speech	Effort Closure	Swallow
right TA	1.07	1.10	2.20	1.90
right CT	1.12	0.97[a]	2.48	1.31[a]
left TA	1.27	1.15	2.04	1.86
left CT	1.20	0.94[b]	1.90	1.90

[a] Wilcoxon Test Between CT and TA, p <.05
[b] Wilcoxon Test Between CT and TA, p <.01

Ranks Test within each task (Table 4). The CTs had their activation onsets significantly earlier than the TAs (p<.05) on Wilcoxon comparisons during speech (the right TA versus the right CT and the left TA versus the left CT). This difference was also found during swallow for the right CT versus the right TA.

The rate of activation to the maximum peak after activation onset was also compared between tasks using the Wilcoxon Test (Table 5), and was faster for phonation than for speech (p<.05).

Coordination of Muscle Action During Phonation, Speech, Effort Closure and Swallow

The relationship between muscle activation onset times within each of the tasks was determined by computing Spearman Rank Correlation Coefficients between the onset times of various muscle pairs (Table 6). The highest correlations were found within speech and swallow,

Table 5. Mean Times of Peak Activation Levels After Activation Onset for Laryngeal Muscles During Different Tasks (in milliseconds).

Muscle	Phonation	Speech	Effort Closure	Swallow
right TA	244	1,320[a]	2,420[b]	263
right CT	224	1,763[a]	2,183[b]	1,230[c]
left TA	179	1,239[a]	4,009[b]	464
left CT	284	1,780[a]	4,820[b]	404

[a] Wilcoxon Test Between Phonation and Speech, p <.05
[b] Wilcoxon Test Between Phonation and Effort Closure, p <.05
[c] Wilcoxon Test Between Phonation and Swallow, p <.05

Table 6.   Spearman Rank Correlation Coefficients Between Muscle
           Activation Onset Times Within Task

Muscle Pair	Phonation	Speech	Effort Closure	Swallow
Right CT with Left CT	.93*	.98*	.19	1.00*
Right TA with Left TA	.73	.97*	.74	.93*
Right TA with Right CT	.82*	.90*	.43	.93*

* p <.01

with all four muscles related. During phonation, significant
relationships were found between the two CT muscles and between the
TA and CT muscles on the right side, but not between the two TAs.
Effort closure was the only task where the onset times of all four
muscles were unrelated.

CONCLUSIONS

These preliminary results indicated that both muscles were similarly
activated during quiet respiration. The TA and CT muscles were both
more active during inspiration than during expiration. Therefore,
the evidence did not support the conclusion that the CTs were
primarily active during expiration. Although the times of maximum
peak levels of the TA and CTs were not coordinated, they did not
demonstrate distinct differences in their activation patterns during
respiration. No differences were seen in the times of maximum peak
levels of the CT and TA muscles during the respiratory cycle. The
observed motion of the vocal folds during inspiration is an
increased glottic opening due to posterior cricoarytenoid action.
The increase in CT activity during inspiration may be active
lengthening of the vocal folds to increase the airway while
increased inspiratory activity in the TA muscles may be the result
muscle stretch feedback to the motoneuron pools. However, no
differences were found in the maximum activation times of these two
muscles during inspiration that would substantiate different
mechanisms for their activation.

Distinct differences were found in the activation levels, timing and
coordination of the laryngeal muscles during the different phonatory
and non-phonatory tasks studied. During effort closure, the only
non-learned task, there was no coordination between muscle onset
times. In contrast, during each of the other tasks, there was
considerable coordination between all four muscles. Further, the
percent increase in muscle activation during effort closure was more
variable and differed between muscles to a greater degree than the

percent increase during the other tasks. However, the pattern of increase across muscles found during this task was similar to that seen during phonation and speech, the two other adduction tasks.

Muscle activation timing during phonation, speech and swallow differed. During both phonation and swallow, muscle activation was quick and ballistic in that the maximum peak activation level was reached quickly after activation onset. All of the muscles except the right CT, were most active and to a similar degree during swallow, making this task the best task for measuring maximum recruitment in laryngeal muscles. Phonation showed the least amount of activation for all of the muscles studied and can be characterized as a small and rapid activation pattern with activation greatest prior to phonation onset.

Speech was the only task where distinct differences in activation onset times were found between the CT and TA muscles, with the CT muscles preceding the TA muscles in activation. This pattern was highly coordinated and consistent with as high a correlation between muscle activation times as was found for swallow. However, the muscle recruitment pattern was not as fast for speech as it was for phonation or swallow, with the peak activation times occurring on the most stressed syllable, "dog," in all four muscles. Therefore, it was only during speech onset that the activation onset times of the two sets of muscles differed. Further, during this task activation was not an immediate burst but increased later with speech stress. Therefore, during speech both the timing of muscle activation onset and the rate of recruitment seems to be distinctive. The potential for pathophysiology of the laryngeal musculature to disturb the normal activation pattern during speech, therefore, seems greatest, while phonation and swallow have simpler patterns and may require less precise control.

In conclusion, different recruitment patterns were found between the laryngeal tasks studied. Highly learned and reflexive tasks had coordinated muscle actions while the less familiar task, effort closure, was more variable with incoordinated muscle actions. Only speech had distinct time differences between TA and CT muscle activation with the maximum activation point independent from vocal fold movement onset. This suggests that since muscle activation and recruitment patterns in the larynx are most precise for speech, these would be most sensitive to laryngeal muscle pathophysiology.

REFERENCES

Abbs, J.H., 1986. Invariance and variability in speech production , in:"Invariance and Variability in Speech Processes," Joseph S. Perkell and Dennis H. Klatt, eds., Lawrence Erlbaum Associates, Inc., Hillsdale, N.J.

Brancatisano, T., Collett, P.W. and Engel, L.A., 1983, Respiratory movements of the vocal folds, J.Appl. Physiol., 54:1269.

Buchthal, F. and Faaborg-Anderson, K., 1964, Electromyography of laryngeal and respiratory muscles, Ann. Otorhinolaryngol. 73:118.

Jurgens, U. and Ploog, D., 1985, On the neural control of mammalian vocalization, in: "The Motor System in Neurobiology," Edward V. Evarts, Steven P. Wise and David Bousfield, eds., Elsevier Biomedical Press, Amsterdam.

Ludlow, C.L., Rosenberg, J., Salazar, A., Grafman, J. and Smutok, M., 1987, Site of penetrating brain lesions causing chronic acquired stuttering, Ann. Neurol. 22: 60-66.

Morell, R.M., 1984, The neurology of swallowing, in: "Dysphagia: Diagnosis and Management," M.E. Grober, ed., Butterworth Publishers, Stoneham, M.A.

Sasaki, C.T. and Buckwalter, J., 1984, Laryngeal function, Am. J. Otolaryngol. 5:281.

Wyke, B.D. and Kirchner, J.A., 1976, Neurology of the larynx, in: "Scientific Foundations of Otolaryngology," R. Hinchcliffe and D. Harrison, D., ed., W. Hennemann, London.

THE FELINE ISOLATION CALL

J.S. Buchwald, C. Shipley, I. Altafullah,
C. Hinman, J. Harrison and L. Dickerson

Department of Physiology
Brain Research Institute and
Mental Retardation Research Center
UCLA School of Medicine
Los Angeles, CA 90024

I. INTRODUCTION

The vocalization of the human neonate has been called an 'acoustical umbilical cord' insofar as it serves as a primary survival mechanism in obtaining food, warmth, and comfort for the otherwise helpless infant. Through these vocalizations, which utilize only variations in pitch, duration and intensity for differences in meaning, the infant signals different emotional and affective messages to caregivers. For the first six to nine months of life, this form of communication comprises a universal language common to all infants and independent of cultural bias (Olney and Scholnick, 1975). Subsequently, phoneme imitation and word production begin to obscure this prelinguistic form of communication and, with the development of a vocabulary, a grammar, and a syntax, a qualitatively different, culturally-bound linguistic communication system emerges.

We have been interested in the prelinguistic communication of the human infant because of its obvious ontogenetic importance to the sensori-motor integration required for the production of more complex intonations and phonemic sounds, and because of its fundamental importance as a universal human behavior. This form of graded, or non-linguistic, communication, however, is not restricted to human infant behavior and similar vocal repertoires have been described for a number of other mammalian species including, in our own work, the kitten and cat. Thus we have attempted to develop an animal model of human infant vocalization in which the behavioral significance and neurophysiological substrates of particular vocal response types can be characterized and systematically investigated.

II. CAT VOCAL REPERTOIRE

        The cat has a vocal repertoire which we have defined in
terms of 1) auditory properties (how it sounds), 2) behavioral
correlates (the behavioral context in which the call is emitted),
and 3) acoustic characteristics (quantitative data resulting from
both sonographic and digital-statistical analyses of the call).
Calls which showed similarities were found to occur across sessions
for a given subject as well as across subjects. Different call
types occurred in such behavioral contexts as isolation, food
deprivation, pain, defensive threat or aggresive threat, and were
notable for their graded, non-syllabic structure (Brown et al.,
1978).

        Of particular interest to us has been the call emitted by
the socially isolated kitten or adult cat, a voiced call very
similar in harmonic form to the hunger call emitted by the food
deprived animal. The feline isolation call is also acoustically
and sonographically very similar to the human infant's isolation
call (Newman, 1985).

III. CALL ANALYSIS

        Cat isolation cries are characterized by a sustained
fundamental frequency and several harmonics of this fundamental,
some of which can be resonated by the vocal tract so that they
contain more energy than the fundamental throughout parts of the
call. Calls were initially analysed with a storage oscilloscope and
spectrograph to determine fundamental frequency, duration and peak
intensity. More complex acoustic analyses were carried out by the
methods described in Carterette et al., (1979, 1983). Calls were
first filtered by a Krohn-Hite filter set to the range 100-9000 Hz
(to prevent aliasing), then sampled by a 12-bit analog to digital
converter at 20 kHz, and stored on the magnetic disc of a PDP 11/10
minicomputer. Analysis programs used a combination of the discrete
fast Fourier transform, autocorrelation and linear prediction
techniques to determine a number of statistical measures of
acoustic parameters, such as the fundamental frequency of the call
and its harmonic structure (Fig. 1).

IV. BEHAVIORAL STUDIES. SIGNIFICANCE OF THE ISOLATION CALL

        The isolation calls of individual kittens or cats vary
considerably.   Although these cries are all emitted under similar
conditions of social isolation, a wide range of modulation in the
general cry pattern occurs both within and across animals.

        In order to define significant acoustic parameters within the
highly variable isolation cries of the kitten, a behavioral assay
was developed that utilized the adult cat's maternal retrieval

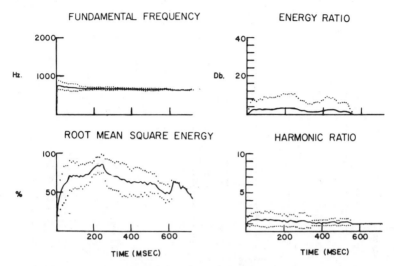

Fig. 1.   Graphs obtained from the analysis of the average of five
          spontaneous isolation calls using a combination of fast
          Fourier transform, autocorrelation and linear prediction
          techniques. Mean values are indicated by solid lines,
          standard deviations by dotted lines. The Fundamental
          Frequency (FF) in this example shows little variation.
          The Root Mean Square Energy reflects the total loudness
          of the call, the Energy Ratio indicates the ratio of the
          energy in the harmonic with maximum energy to that in the
          FF, and the Harmonic Ratio indicates the ratio of the
          frequency of the harmonic with maximum energy to that of
          the FF.

response (Harrison, et al., 1979; Buchwald, 1981).   During the 4
weeks before and 4 weeks after delivery, females were found to
retrieve kittens emitting the isolation call at virtually a 100%
level whether or not the kittens were seen.   Males and non-pregnant
or non-lactating females showed no retrieval, thus indicating that
the response was hormonally-bound.   In the experimental situation,
a   curtain   separated   the   adult   cat   from   the   kitten.   A
tape-recorded series of naturally varying kitten cries and a
tape-loop recording of a single kitten cry were subsequently found
to trigger the same maternal retrieval response, although somewhat
less reliably than the actual crying kitten (Figure 2).   The
naturally varying cries were more effective than the single
repeated cry.   Presentations of synthesized stimuli that temporally
reversed the call to a backward presentation or that contained only
isolated   components   of   the   total   call   structure,   e.g.,   the
fundamental frequency, first formant, initial segment or terminal
segment, were clearly less salient than either the varying or
invariant total call, and little or no retrieval was elicited by
these component stimuli.

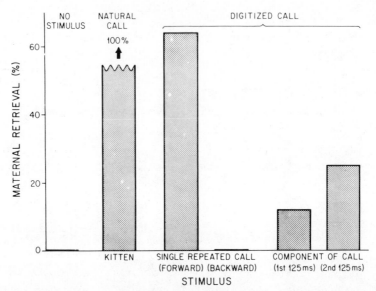

Fig. 2.   Summary of retrieval responses of 6 female cats over 11
test sessions during the month immediately before and
after parturition. Experimental sessions consisted of
12 2 min stimulus trials separated by 5 min intertrial
intervals with no more than two sessions per week per
subject.   In the 6 different test conditions illustrated,
no stimulus was delivered, the living kitten called
(from behind a curtain), a digitized call was repeated
in a forward or backward direction, and the 1st or 2nd
125 ms component of the call (as shown in figure 3)
was presented.

From these experiments several conclusions are suggested: 1)
in the absence of visual, olfactory, or thermal cues, the kitten
isolation cry can trigger maternal retrieval, which indicates that
the acoustic signal per se has behavioral significance, i.e., it
produces a maternal response essential for the kitten's survival;
2) vocal communication with the mother is enhanced by cry
variability along the dimensions of pitch, duration, and intensity
and is diminished by decomposition of total call structure into
isolated acoustic parameters; and 3) as a corollary, brain
mechanisms have evolved which provide for highly sensitive maternal
reception of kitten isolation call production.

V.   CALL RECEPTION STUDIES

Participation of different auditory pathways for different
aspects of auditory information processing is suggested by a
variety of behavioral and anatomical data.   Behavioral testing
procedures indicate that bilateral lesions of the primary auditory

cortex cause no loss in discrimination of temporal sequencing of auditory stimuli (Colavita, 1979) or in discriminations between complex vocal stimuli (cat: Dewson, 1964; dog: Heffner, 1977), whereas bilateral lesions of the insular and temporal cortical areas produce marked disruption in these functions (cat: Goldberg et al., 1957; Cornwall, 1967; Kelly, 1973; Colavita et al., 1974; Dewson, 1964).   Insular and temporal cortical regions have been further separated from each other insofar as bilateral lesions confined to insular cortex produce loss of temporal pattern discrimination, not produced by temporal cortex lesions (cat: Colavita et al., 1979), while lesions largely confined to temporal cortex result in loss of harmonic discriminations (e.g., vowel sounds "u" versus "i", cat: Dewson, 1964).

Such functional differentiation is supported by anatomical data which indicate that, while the major thalamic projections to areas AI, II and EP originate in the principal division of the medial geniculate body (MGB), the major projection to temporal cortex originates in the caudal division of the MGB, and the major projection to insular cortex originates in the medial division of the posterior nuclear group of the thalamus (Winer et al., 1977; Diamond, 1978).   Furthermore, brainstem input to each of these thalamic subdivisions appears to originate differentially so that the parallel but separate anatomical identity of the forebrain pathways is an extension of more caudal separation in the region of the lateral lemniscus and inferior colliculus (Diamond, 1978).

We have been interested in further testing the hypothesis that a particular class of stimuli is preferentially processed by a particular thalamo-cortical subsystem. To this end we have carried out electrophysiological recordings in the MGB of single unit responses to the kitten isolation call, as well as to neutral click and tone stimuli (Hinman et al., 1979).

METHODS

Pilot experiments indicated marked changes in evoked potential and unit responses for some of the MGB regions of interest when the animal was anesthetized with pentobarbital. Thus, all recordings were made from awake unanesthetized adult cats restrained by head-cap fittings which secured the head in the stereotaxic plane but induced no discomfort.   Recordings were carried out in a sound isolation chamber. Stimuli were delivered through a speaker at a constant location 15 cm in front of the head and all stimuli were 70 dB+/-6 dB SPL, measured at the external auditory meatus.

Single unit recordings were carried out with a stimulus protocol which included a set of isolation call stimuli, pure tones and clicks.   An estimate of best frequency was provided by 125 ms

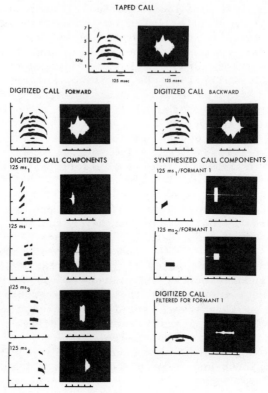

Fig. 3   Some of the test stimuli prepared from a single kitten
          isolation call. Sonogram and oscillogram tracings are
          shown for each stimulus. Both temporal and harmonic
          aspects of call structure have been emphasized. A tape
          recorded call is compared with a digitized version of the
          same call played forward and backward. Successive 125 ms
          chunks of the 500 ms call were also used as stimuli, as
          were narrow-band filtered calls and synthesized format
          components, examples of which are shown.

duration pure tones delivered with a 5 ms rise-fall time over a
0.4 to 10 kHz range. Click responsiveness was tested with a 0.1 ms
square wave stimulus. The isolation call stimuli consisted of
digitized presentations of the entire call as well as of call
components similar to those used in the maternal retrieval
experiment (Figure 3). The entire stimulus protocol had a duration
of approximately 20 min during which 15 trials of each stimulus
were presented at a rate of 1/2 sec, with a series of the complete
isolation call presented both at the beginning and at the end of
the protocol.

        Confirmation of recording locations was carried out by
terminally marking sites along the electrode tracks, subsequently

identifying these sites on the relevant brain sections, and reconstructing the electrode tracks and unit recording sites on brain atlas diagrams of the MGB.

RESULTS
        Of the 555 units studied in the MGB, approximately one-third was in each of the three major MGB subdivisions studied i.e., the principal, the posterior dorsal and the magnocellular (nomenclature after Morest, 1964 and Winer, 1985). A variety of response patterns characterized units throughout the MGB, none of which appeared to be regionally restricted. Responses of sustained increase or decrease in discharge, with or without rebound, were found in all MGB divisions, as were "on", "off", and "on-off" responses and a number of other complex patterns. Moreover, a unit response pattern to the complete isolation call stimulus was not necessarily predictable from the responses elicited by the various call component and tone stimuli.

        With regard to the isolation call, the 'principal' MGB sudivision showed no selectivity i.e., none of the units responded only to this stimulus; moreover, all of the units were highly responsive to clicks and/or tones. In the 'magnocellular' subdivision less than 10% of the units responded only to the isolation call, and many units were responsive to clicks and tones. In contrast, in the 'posterior dorsal' subdivision virtually none of the units responded to clicks. On the other hand, approximately 30% of these units responded only to the isolation call (Figure 4). Thus, the 'posterior dorsal' caudal MGB differentially showed a high degree of receptive field selectivity biased toward the isolation call and call components.

        As noted previously, the 'posterior dorsal' MGB provides the major input to temporal cortex (Winer et al., 1977; Diamond, 1978), and lesions in this thalamo-cortical subsystem result in a loss of discrimination of harmonic, i.e., vowel sounds (Dewson, 1964). Consistent with these data is our electrophysiological result showing that only in the 'posterior dorsal' division did a large proportion of the units, approximately 30%, respond selectively to the isolation call.

        In summary, the 'posterior dorsal' MGB-temporal cortex system is suggested as particularly important for processing such complex stimuli as vocalizations. Moreover, the temporal cortex is known to project to entorhinal cortex which, in turn, projects heavily to limbic centers and to the hypothalamus. Insofar as the hypothalamus is believed to be the primary regulator of hormonally bound maternal behavior, we postulate that MGB-temporal cortex relays to the hypothalamus may provide the necessary circuitry for call reception whereby the kitten isolation call induces the maternal retrieval response.

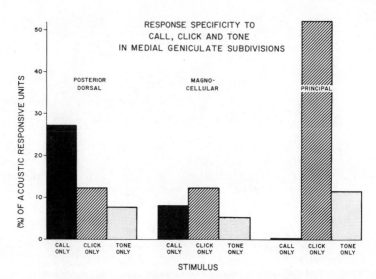

Fig. 4.   A comparison of unit response specificity to isolation
          call, tone and click stimuli in each of the three MGB
          subdivisions tested. The largest proportion of units
          which responded only to the call stimuli were recorded
          in the posterior dorsal MGB; essentially none of the
          cells in the principal division of the MGB showed this
          characteristic. (From Hinman et al., 1979).

VI. CALL PRODUCTION STUDIES

A. ROLE OF AUDITORY FEEDBACK

     Modulation of vocal behavior by mechanisms of auditory
feedback exemplifies one level of "vocal learning". If vocal
learning plays any role in the development of kitten cries, then
calls of deaf animals should differ from those of hearing
littermates.

     In order to assess the importance of auditory feedback to the
isolation call, cochlear function was eliminated in a series of
kittens at two weeks of age postnatally, before the ear canals were
completely opened and while hearing thresholds to peripheral sounds
are still very high (Shipley et al., 1981; Shipley et al.,
submitted).   Vocal recordings from the deaf kittens and their
normal littermates were continued through the first year of life
and two deaf animals with their littermates were studied over a
period of three years. Persistent and marked effects of deafening
on the vocalizations were evident at all ages. These were: 1) a
significant increase in call loudness (consistently at least twice
as loud as the controls) and 2) a significant decrease   in
variability of the harmonic structure, i.e., the call of the deaf

animals was more monotonous. The fundamental frequency did not change significantly in initial or peak frequencies.

These results were supported by another series of experiments in which the 4 week old deaf and hearing kittens were fitted with earphones through which varying levels of white noise were presented. As the level of noise was increased from 0-80 dB SPL, the calls of the normal animals increased approximately 10 dB in loudness, while there was no effect upon calls of the deaf animals. In normal hearing humans, a similar response (the Lombard reflex) functions to adjust the level of vocal output so that the speaker can hear his/her own voice in varying levels of background noise. Lack of auditory feedback prevents such a reflex from functioning in deaf kittens.

Thus, abnormal loudness and, particularly, loss of normal variability, all characterize the call structure of deaf animals and indicate a significant role for auditory feedback. Moreover, the active vocal modulation carried out through mechanisms of auditory feedback by the hearing animals, which are absent in the deaf animals, suggest that a type of vocal learning is normally present in the developing kitten and cat.

B. ROLE OF HYPOTHALAMUS

We have also recently carried out a stimulation study of the hypothalamus in order to compare evoked calls with spontaneous isolation calls in the adult cat, to analyze quantitatively the calls evoked by electrical stimulation of the hypothalamus, and to study the effects of changes in stimulus parameters upon the evoked calls (Altafullah et al., 1983; Altafullah et al., submitted).

METHODS

Six adult cats were used in the study. Under Nembutal anesthesia a well was placed over the hypothalamus, and a head mount was cemented to the skull to permit painless immobilization of the animal. Animals were allowed to recover from the effects of surgery for at least one week before the next phase of the experiment.

Calls were recorded with the cat comfortably restrained and isolated in a sound attenuating chamber. Stainless steel concentric electrodes were used for stimulation of areas which extended from the pre-optic region (A+16) to the zona incerta (A+8) antero-posteriorly, and across the full medio-lateral extent of the hypothalamus (L 1-4).

Stimuli consisted of trains of biphasic rectangular pulses. Various parametric combinations were tested early in the investigation and, based upon the relative ease with which calls could be evoked, the following were adopted as standard: pulse duration 5 ms, frequency 70 Hz, train duration 1-1.5 sec, and measured current intensity 100-400μA. For each track studied, the electrode was lowered in 0.5 mm steps through the hypothalamus, and each site was initially stimulated with a current intensity of 100 μA. Stimulus intensity then increased until either the animal vocalized or the upper limit of 400μA was reached. In the latter event the site was considered unresponsive for vocalization.

If the animal vocalized, the threshold intensity for evoked vocalization was determined, and at least five vocalizations evoked at supra-threshold intensity were recorded without altering the parameters of stimulation between trials. The entire track was explored in this manner. Effects of manipulating stimulus parameters were studied by varying only one parameter in a set of trials while other parameters were held constant.

Vocalizations were recorded on a tape recorder through a microphone placed 8 inches in front of the cat's head. The frequency response of this system was +/- 3dB in the range of 50-12,000 Hz. At the end of each session a 2 kHz 80 dB (SPL) calibration signal, played at the position of the cat's head, was recorded as a reference for determinations of peak intensity of the vocalizations. The spontaneous and evoked calls of each animal were analysed in an identical manner.

At the termination of the experiment, small lesions were made at the bottom of several of the stimulation tracks for post-mortem histological verification of the accuracy of stereotaxic placement. Stimulation sites for each electrode track were plotted onto appropriate brain atlas diagrams.

RESULTS

VOICED CALL PRODUCING AREAS IN THE HYPOTHALAMUS

Stimulation was carried out at 320 sites in the hypothalamus. For purposes of this study, a stimulation site was considered responsive only if the evoked vocalization was: 1) a voiced call, i.e., 'hisses' and 'growls' were not studied), 2) replicable over at least five trials of stimulation, and 3) had a stable latency from stimulus onset across successive stimulation trials. Applying these criteria, 64 sites were found in the hypothalamus that produced 470 voiced calls upon electrical stimulation.

SPONTANEOUS CALLS

To establish some standard for judging the acoustic properties of evoked calls, groups of from 5-10 spontaneous vocalizations were recorded from each cat in the study (Figure 5).

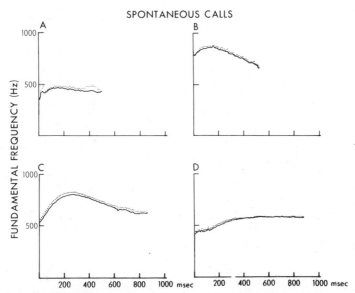

Fig. 5. Average fundamental frequency profiles for 10
spontaneous calls from each of four cats. The
standard deviation of the fundamental is indicated
by dots above the solid line. (From Altafullah
et al., submitted).

In general, the spontaneous calls displayed a structure consistent
for each animal, as evidenced by the small standard deviations in
average pitch. However, there was considerable variation in call
structure across different animals. Average fundamental frequency,
for example, varied from 452 to 818 Hz across the six animals
studied.   Four of the cats had spontaneous calls that were
characterized by a relatively flat and smooth pitch profile, while
the other two cats had pitch contours that were slightly convex
upward.   Such call differences may be due to variations in
laryngeal or vocal tract morphology, physical characteristics of
the animal such as sex and body weight, or pattern of jaw and
tongue movement during vocalization.

EVOKED CALLS

     Threshold intensity for stimulation at 70 Hz, with a duration
of 1 to 1.5 sec ranged from 90 to 259 A, with typical values
between 120-160 A.   Acoustic analysis of the calls evoked by
hypothalamic stimulation showed a variety of call patterns, most of
which were similar to spontaneous vocalizations.   The vocal
response elicited from a specific electode location was
reproducible in repeated trials and, with few exceptions, had a
highly consistent acoustic structure.   The most common pattern
elicited by hypothalamic stimulation had a relatively flat and

smooth pitch profile with little modulation of the pitch through
the duration of the call.

At sites from which voiced calls were evoked, there was not
consistently any accompanying behavior, such as pupillary dilation
salivation and lip retraction. Such rage like behavior was
however, elicited from other sites of hypothalamic stimulation from
which hisses and growls were evoked.

The distribution of representative responsive and
non-responsive sites at six levels of the hypothalamus is shown in
Figure 6. Responsive sites were scattered over a diffuse area
with the largest number in the preoptic region, the ventromedial
area, the perifornical region, the lateral and the dorso-medial
hypothalamus. There appeared to be a general tendency for more
rostral stimulation points to evoke calls with longer latencies.

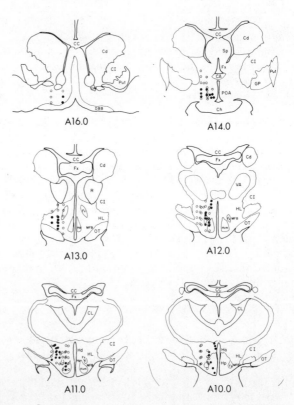

Fig. 6.   Summary of representative responsive (filled
          circles) and non-responsive (open circles)
          stimulation sites at 6 levels of the hypothalamus.
          Data from 6 cats. (From Altafullah et al., submitted).

The pre-optic region with an average latency of 4.4 sec, and the zona incerta, with an average latency of 0.4 sec from stimulus onset, marked the upper and lower limits of the range of latencies seen. All three stimulation sites that produced calls of average latency greater than 4 sec were at levels of A14 to A16.

The majority of cases, responsive sites were confined to a 1-2 mm range and raising or lowering the electrode abolished the response, even when stimulus intensity was raised. The number of responsive sites varied across animals; for two cats, relatively few calls were evoked, while for the other four cats large numbers (e.g., up to 149 calls per individual) were evoked. These differences were not due to differences in the number or position of points stimulated, which were similar across animals but, rather, appeared to be correlated most clearly with the tendency of the individual cat to vocalize spontaneously.

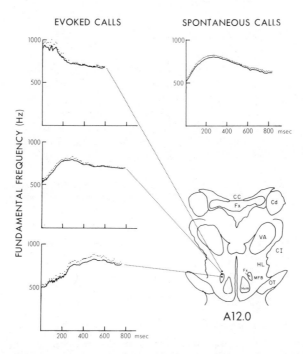

Fig. 7   Average fundamental frequency profiles for 5-10 evoked
          calls from each of three stimulation sites along the same
          electrode track in the perifornical region of the
          hypothalamus. Average fundamental frequency profile for
          ·10 spontaneous calls from the same cat are shown at the
          upper right. (From Altafullah et al., submitted).

While calls evoked from the hypothalamus generally showed small variability across groups of 5-10 calls, considerable variability was seen across recording sites. Figure 7 shows calls elicited by stimulation of the perifornical region in which extensive variation in call structure was seen across three sites with 0.5 mm separation. The first stimulation site produced vocalizations characterized by an unusually high starting pitch (average 916 Hz) which declined thereafter to a lue approximately equal to average values found in spontaneous calls for this animal (average pitch for the evoked call=764 Hz vs. 730 Hz for the spontaneous call). Stimulation at the second electrode site, 0.5 mm below, produced calls that resembled in almost every detail the spontaneous call (average evoked pitch = 721 Hz). Stimulation 0.5 mm deeper produced calls that were, in some respects, the opposite of those seen at the first site. These calls began at a normal pitch but reached their maximum in the second half of the call rather than in the first half, as seen in the spontaneous calls of this animal. The average value of the pitch was, however, similar to that in the spontaneous calls (average evoked pitch = 725 Hz).

EFECTS OF STIMULUS PARAMETERS ON EVOKED VOCALIZATIONS

Effects on call loudness, latency and duration caused by manipulation of stimulus frequency (i.e., the pulses per sec delivered within a pulse train), intensity, and duration were tested with analyses of variance on the correlations between stimulus and call parameters. As the frequency of stimulation was increased from 30 to 120 Hz, the loudness of the evoked call increased (n=50, p<.0001), the latency decreased (p<.0001), and call duration increased (p<.0001). Increases in stimulation intensity from 120 to 420 μA and in stimulus duration from .3 to 2 sec did not have significant effects on any of these call parameters.

Frequency of stimulation also caused consistent changes in the energy relationships between harmonics of the call, which did not occur as a function of either intensity or duration of stimulation. As stimulus frequency increased, higher harmonics of the fundamental tended to be resonated by the vocal tract (N=34, p<.0028).

In summary, voiced calls with a harmonic structure were evoked at a number of sites in the hypothalamus which appeared to be independent of rage vocalizations or other components of a general rage response. The structure of these voiced calls, e.g., call latency, duration, intensity, was not significantly affected by stimulus intensity or duration but all three call parameters were significantly affected by changes in stimulus frequency. In general, call latency was longest at sites in the rostral hypothalamus and shortest at sites in the caudal hypothalamus. In all cats, the voiced calls evoked from some hypothalamic sites were identical to spontaneously occurring isolation calls.

C. EFFECTS OF CINGULATE STIMULATION

In only one cat thus far have we attempted to evoke calls from the cingulate gyrus. In this animal the anterior cingulate gyrus was stimulated on four different occasions, and 15-20 calls were recorded which sounded like spontaneous isolation calls and showed similar pitch profiles. The latencies of these calls were very long, i.e., 7-10 sec, so that they commenced after stimulation had ceased. However, because the latencies were so long and the calls were not consistently evoked, we could not be certain that they were indeed the result of cingulate stimulation rather than random, spontaneous calls. We hope to extend these observations in the future.

D. EFFECTS OF MIDBRAIN STIMULATION

In four cats the midbrain area of the periaqueductal gray and the area immediately ventral and lateral to it were stimulated. At most of these stimulation sites calls were consistently elicited. While these data have not yet been analyzed, there appears to be a wide range of call types, as indicated by a variety of pitch profiles, which can be evoked at this level. Included in the vocalizations evoked at this level was the typical isolation call, with the calls at any one site showing a relatively short and constant latency.

VII. SUMMARY AND CONCLUSIONS

1. These studies have described the vocal repertoire of the cat, which utilizes gradations of pitch, intensity and duration to communicate in a manner similar to that of the human infant.

2. The isolation call of the kitten triggers maternal retrieval, a response essential for the kitten's survival. Thus, brain mechanisms for both production and reception of the isolation call appear to be adaptively significant to the species.

3. The isolation call selectively activates neurons in the posterior dorsal MGB, a subdivision with direct terminal projections to temporal cortex, but not to primary auditory cortex. From this MGB-temporal cortex system, relays to the hypothalamus may provide the necessary circuitry for reception of the isolation call by the hypothalamus during hormonally primed periods resulting in the triggering of the maternal retrieval response.

4. Active modulation of vocalization through mechanisms of auditory feedback has been demonstrated by comparing the vocalizations of normal and deaf animals. Such data suggest that a rudimentary type of vocal learning, e.g., that associated with the self-monitoring and modulation provided by auditory feedback, is normally present in the developing kitten and cat.

5. The isolation call, a call of fundamental importance to the animal's survival, can be evoked by hypothalamic stimulation. Responsive sites extend from the pre-optic region to the zona incerta, with latencies decreasing from more than 4 sec to less than 1 sec along a rostro-caudal gradient.

6. The restricted radius of sites at which calls could be evoked, and the lack of effect of increasing stimulus intensity upon the evoked call, support the concept of specific low threshold nodes within the hypothalamus which serve to trigger the isolation call.

7. As a system which is functionally ancient in phylogenetic terms and functionally precocious in ontogenetic terms, the hypothalamus is proposed as the primary locus for integrating the thermal, chemical, and affective stimuli resulting from social isolation and for triggering the vocal effector system of the isolation call.

8. The feline isolation call appears to be both behaviorally and acoustically similar to the isolation cry of the human infant. Thus, the hypothalamus may also be an important integrating center in the human for vital pre-linguistic expressions of isolation and hunger.

REFERENCES

Altafullah, I., Shipley, C. and Buchwald, J.S., 1983, A quantitative study of the vocalization elicited by hypothalamic stimulation in the cat, Neurosci. Abst., 9: 365.

Altafullah, I., Shipley, C. and Buchwald, J.S., Voiced calls evoked by hypothalamic stimulation in the cat, Submitted.

Brown, K.A., Buchwald, J.S., Johnson, J.R, and Mikolich, D.J., 1978, Vocalization in the cat and kitten, Dev. Psychobiol., 11:559.

Buchwald, J.S., 1981, Development of acoustic communication processes in an experimental model, in: "Pre-term Birth and Psychological Development," S.L. Friedman and M. Sigman, eds., Academic Press, New York.

Carterette, E.C., Shipley, C., and Buchwald, J.S., 1979, Linear prediction theory of vocalization in cat and kitten, in: "Frontiers of Speech Communication Research," B. Lundbloom and S. Ohman, eds., Academic Press, London.

Carterette, E., Shipley, C. and Buchwald, J.S., 1983, On synthesizing animal speech: the case of the cat, in: "Electronic Speech Synthesis," G. Bristam, ed., McGraw-Hill, New York.

Colavita, F.B. and Weisberg, D.H., 1979, Insular cortex and perception of temporal patterns, Physiol. and Behav., 22:827.

Colavita, F.B., Szeliga, F.V. and Zimmer, S.D., 1974, Temporal pattern discrimination in cats with insular-temporal lesions, Brain Res., 79:153.

Cornwall, P., 1967, Loss of auditory pattern discrimination following insular-temporal lesions in cats, J. Comp. Physiol. Psychol., 63:165.

Dewson, J.H., 1964, Speech sound discrimination by cats, Science, 144:555.

Diamond, I.T., 1978, The auditory cortex, in: "Evoked Electrical Activity in the Auditory Nervous System," Academic Press, New York.

Goldberg, J.M., Diamond, I.T. and Neff, W.D., 1957, Auditory discrimination after ablation of temporal and insular cortex in the cat. Fed. Proc., 16:47.

Harrison, J.B., Buchwald, J.S., Norman, R.J. and Hinman, C., 1979, Acoustic analysis of maternal retrieval to kitten stress call, Neurosci. Abst., 5:22.

Heffner, H.H., 1977, Effect of auditory cortex ablation on the perception of meaningful sounds, Soc. Neurosci. Abst., 3:6.

Hinman, C., Buchwald, J., Harrison, J. and Norman, R., 1979, Neuronal response to the kitten stress call in cat medial geniculate nucleus, Neurosci. Abst., 5:22.

Kelly, J.B., 1973, The effects of insular and temporal lesions in cats on two types of auditory pattern discrimination, Brain Res., 62:71.

Morest, D.K., 1964, The neuronal architecture of the medial geniculate body of the cat, J. Anat., 98:611.

Newman, J.D., 1985, The infant cry of primates. An evolutionary perspective, in: "Infant Crying," B.M. Lester and C.F.Z. Boukydis, eds., Plenum Press, New York.

Olney, R.L. and Scholnick, E.K., 1975, Adult judgments of age and linguistic differences in infant vocalizations, J. of Child Language, 3:145.

Shipley, C., Buchwald, J.S., Carterette, E.C. and Strecker, J., 1981, Differences in the cries of deaf and hearing kittens, Neurosci. Abst., 7:774.

Shipley, C., Buchwald, J.S. and Carterette, E.C., 1987 The role of auditory feedback in the vocalizations of cats, Exp. Brain Res. 101:1.

Winer, J.A., 1985, The medial geniculate body of the cat, "Advances in Anatomy, Embryology and Cell Biology," 86:1.

Winer, J.A., Diamond, I.T. and Raczkowski, D., 1977, Subdivisions of the auditory cortex of the cat: The retrograde transport of horseradish peroxidase to the medial geniculate body and posterior thalamic nuclei, J. Comp. Neurol., 176:387.

AMYGDALOID ELECTRICAL ACTIVITY IN RESPONSE TO CONSPECIFIC CALLS
IN SQUIRREL MONKEY (S. SCIUREUS):   INFLUENCE OF ENVIRONMENTAL
SETTING, CORTICAL INPUTS, AND RECORDING SITE

Robert L. Lloyd and Arthur S. Kling

Psychiatry Service, Veterans Administration Medical
Center, Sepulveda, CA and Department of Psychiatry
UCLA School of Medicine, Los Angeles, CA

INTRODUCTION

Experimental evidence from primates and other species,
suggests that a major function of the amygdala is in the control
of social/affective behavior (Kling, 1972). Behavioral and
electrophysiological studies also indicate that responses of the
amygdala to sensory stimulation are, themselves, governed by the
ethological/social milieu in which the animal finds itself. The
first aspect of the amygdala is demonstrated by the fact that
electrical stimulation of various regions of the amygdala will
induce distinct forms of somato-motor and autonomic responses, as
well as aggressive and defensive behaviors (Kaada, 1972;
Koikegami, 1963; MacLean and Delgado, 1953). In turn,
stimulation of the various efferent targets of these amygdaloid
nuclei will also induce the corresponding distinct behavioral and
affective responses.

The second aspect is demonstrated by the fact that the
Kluver-Bucy syndrome can be reproduced by bilateral lesions which
are restricted to the amygdaloid nuclei (Schreiner and Kling,
1956). However, if the same animals which are displaying this
syndrome while in confined cages are observed in semi-free or
free-ranging situations, an entirely distinct constellation of
behavioral symptoms emerges (Dicks, Myers, and Kling, 1969;
Kling, Lancaster, and Benitone, 1970). Rather than the loss of
fear and the excessive approach behavior, orality, and sexuality,
which is observed in the laboratory, these animals become
fearful, isolated, and reject appropriate positive communications
and may become hypophagic. It is clear, therefore, that the
environment, and especially the social context, is critical in

137

assessing the response of the amygdala to sensory stimuli and in
evaluating the contribution which this structure makes in
determining the behavior of the animal.

One interpretation of these findings is that this structure
serves as a filter which extracts motivationally meaningful
information form sensory traffic (Gloor, 1975). In this respect,
the amygdala is thought of as a channel conveying information
from the cortex, which is involved in feature analysis and memory
processes, to the hypothalamus and brainstem areas which are
responsible for survival functions of the animal. Others,
however, have concluded that the actions of the amygdala are
biased by visual information. This interpretation is derived
from ablation studies conducted with old world primates who's
behavior appears to be dominated by visual information (Barrett,
1969). The amygdala is, however, a structure which receives
information from all sensory modalities (Turner, 1981), and these
sensory projections overlap to an appreciable degree within the
various nuclei of the amygdala. In addition, within the
amygdala, those nuclei which do not receive direct input from a
given sensory projection quite often are relayed this information
by other amygdaloid nuclei (Aggleton, 1985). This sensory input
arrives indirectly, via temporal cortex, as well as directly from
the thalamus.

In previous studies, we have examined the
electrophysiological response of the amygdala to various social
and visual stimuli using the African green monkey, C. aethiops.
The EEG recorded from the amygdala manifests distinct
quantitative responses, in terms of total power within the
frequency spectrum, depending upon the saliency of the stimulus
evoking these responses (Kling, 1981). The most potent stimuli,
in terms of their association with increases in total power, were
those associated with sexual inspection or threat, followed by
those which may have been considered ambiguous, such that a
number of different consequences could have followed these
postural or visual signals. Conversely, reductions in these
measures were associated with tension-reducing behavior or
stimuli, such as mutual grooming or sitting with conspecifics.
Another index of stimulus saliency is the percentage of total
power in the EEG of the amygdala which exists in the delta band.
More salient stimuli evoke electrical responses which have a
greater proportion of power in the delta range. Hence, in the
amygdala, there is a strong positive correlation between the
amount of power in the EEG spectrum and the proportion of power
in the delta band.

In order to assess the physiological and behavioral
contributions of discrete temporal lobe projections to the
amygdala, several studies were conducted in which the saliency of

a number of visual and social stimuli was first assessed,
vis-a-vis the electrical response of the amygdala, and the
stimuli re-presented following ablation of one of the
subdivisions of the temporal lobe. These studies indicate that
the the region comprising the pole has a marked facilitatory
influence on the response of the amygdala to sensory and social
stimulation. The electrical activity of the amygdala to a number
of situations in a social setting was assessed. Following
ablation, the electrographic response of the amygdala to both
visual and social stimuli was markedly reduced vis-a-vis total
power. Correspondingly, these animals became socially isolated,
and were unwilling to interact with their conspecifics (Kling,
1981).

Lesions of the temporal neocortex produced a more complex
picture. No overt effects upon social/affective behavior were
observed. However, the electrical responses of the amygdala to
individual sensory stimuli were differentially, yet consistently,
affected. The magnitude of the response to some stimuli was
diminished while, in other cases, the response was augmented.
These data led to the conclusion that the inferior and middle
portions of the temporal lobe have both facilitatory and
inhibitory influences upon the amygdala, and, by extension, upon
social behavior (Kling, 1981; Kling et al., 1984).

As indicated above, little work has been done concerning the
influence of auditory stimuli upon amygdaloid functioning. The
new world monkey, S. sciureus or squirrel monkey, is a species
whose behavior appears to be directed, to a much greater extent,
by auditory information. Accordingly, a more recent series of
studies was undertaken in which this species was used to assess
the effects of acoustical stimuli upon amygdaloid functioning, in
addition to those produced by visual and social stimuli, and to
extend the work done on the differential influences within the
temporal lobe upon this structure. In an unpublished study we
have reproduced many aspects of the Kluver-Bucy syndrome
following bilateral ablation of the amygdala in squirrel monkeys.
These included a fall in rank, decreases in social affiliation
and fear, and increases in orality and tameness, and loss of fear
toward a live snake. the characteristic autoerotic and
hypersexual behavior noted in old world species, when in
confinement, was absent.

Having determined that elements of the Kluver-Bucy could be
established in the squirrel monkey, with lesions restricted to
the amygdala, we proceeded to examine the consequences of partial
amygdaloid deafferentation, through lesions of temporal lobe
areas which project to this structure. In the first phase, we
ablated the temporal poles of two squirrel monkeys after having
made detailed assessments of their responses to visual and social

stimuli.   Both animals became less social, lost rank, showed
transient hyperorality, and did not flee from threatening
stimuli.   In addition, the was a substantial reduction in the
electrical response of the amygdala to all social and visual
stimuli, and often there was no response at all.   These findings
are consistent with the observations made on old world primates
which suggested that the temporal pole supplies a major
facilitatory input to the amygdala.

PRESENT EXPERIMENT

        In the present study, a set of conspecific vocalizations was
added in order to determine the response of normal and lesioned
subjects to auditory stimuli, a procedure which had not been done
in any previous experiments.   This procedure was of considerable
interest due to this species richer auditory repertoire and the
fact that the behavior of the squirrel monkey, unlike its old
world counterparts, is mediated to a far lesser extent by visual
stimuli.   In addition, previous observations of the behavioral
changes seen following amygdalectomy were interpreted as
reflecting disruptions of visual perception.   In this regard, we
were particularly interested in the influence of the inferior
temporal cortex upon amygdaloid functioning, since, in at least
old world species, this area has been shown to subserve
visual-perceptual functions.   Reports concerning deficits in
visual discrimination following ablations of inferior temporal
cortex are numerous.   Thus we undertook to examine the responses
of the amygdala to various conspecific vocalizations and to
determine if there is a hierarchy of response, based upon
emotional significance.   In addition, we sought to examine
whether lesions of inferior temporal cortex would affect these
auditory responses, and whether such lesions would affect social
interactions.   One further concern was the assessment of
amygdaloid responses to auditory stimuli under diverse
environmental conditions.   We were interested to see whether the
response of the amygdala to the same stimuli would be different
during a state of social isolation as opposed to when the animal
was free to interact with a group of conspecifics.   As indicated
before, the greater the degree of social-environmental
complexity, the less manifest are the various aspects of the
Kluver-Bucy syndrome, such that in a totally free-ranging
situation such individuals demonstrate a totally distinct
constellation of behaviors.

METHODOLOGY

        Bipolar electrodes implanted in one or both amygdala were
connected to radiotransmitters which broadcast the electrical

activity of the amygdala on an FM band. This approach allowed
the animal completely unrestricted movement and interaction with
conspecifics in a group cage. Four second epochs of electrical
activity were recorded while the animal was engaged in a variety
of social activities with a group of conspecifics in a large
lexan cage (Kling et al., 1987). While in this setting,
recordings of various conspecific vocalizations, the meanings of
which are thought to be well understood, were broadcast. These
test stimuli consisted of: isolation peep, snake call, alarm
peep, trill, twitter, and errchuck. The response of the amygdala
to these vocalizations was compared to the electrical activity of
the amygdala during spontaneous social interaction, and to the
response of the amygdala when these same stimuli were broadcast
to the monkey when it is in isolation. The response of the
amygdala to these stimuli is also contrasted with its response to
400Hz tones. Along with this control stimulus, a short musical
passage was presented to the monkey in order to determine if the
amygdala was merely responding to stimulus complexity. In
addition, 35mm color slides of both ethologically relevant and
complex control stimuli were presented to the animal while it was
in isolation (sitting in a restraining chair), and the electrical
activity of the amygdala sampled. The test stimuli consisted of:
snakes, monkey facial threat, conspecific in benign pose,
alligator, butterfly, crawling insect, and human face. The
control stimuli consisted of histology slides, and were chosen
because of their pattern and color complexity.

   The electrical activity of the amygdala was picked up by a
radioreceiver and recorded on FM modulated magnetic tape.
Simultaneous with the recording of amygdala electrical activity,
a voice channel recorded a description of the behavior of the
animal, that of the conspecifics, and any stimuli which were
presented. Four second epochs of electrical activity, time
locked to behavior or stimulus onset, were digitized by a MINC
computer and stored on disk. The digitized waveforms underwent a
discrete Fourier transform (using the Fast Fourier Transform
algorithm, FFT), and the real and imaginary components combined
to produce the power spectral density function of the time domain
signal. These frequency domain spectra were then parsed into the
various EEG frequency bands, and the percentage of the total
power of the signal contained within each frequency band was
computed.

   These subjects were also used in a parallel study (Perryman
et al., 1987) to assess the effects of inferior temporal cortex
lesions upon visual and auditory evoked potential recorded from
the amygdala. The purpose of procedure was to assess whether
these lesions were depriving the amygdala of the basic sensory
information, or whether these lesions were preventing the
amygdala from appropriately processing the sensory information

which had arrived through more direct routs. To accomplish this, a series of 500 clicks or flashes was presented to the subject while it was seated in a restraining chair.

RESULTS

Several findings emerged from this study. First, the total amount of power contained in the EEG signal increased when stimuli were presented, as compared to the amount present when the animal was engaged in spontaneous social behavior (Fig. 1). Second, the collections of ethologically relevant stimuli, in both sensory domains, produced a greater increase in power than did their associated control stimuli. Within the set of auditory test stimuli (conspecific vocalizations), the increase in power in the signal generated by the amygdala was in proportion to the "affective content" of the vocalization. The "isolation peep", which MacLean (1985) considers to be the most potent vocalization, was consistently associated with the greatest increase in power. In the two presentation conditions, these auditory test stimuli produced strikingly similar response hierarchies. For each animal, the test stimuli were assigned rank scores according to the percentage of power which occurred in the delta band subsequent to their presentation. The rank scores were summed across monkeys, for each stimulus, with a lower rank sum reflecting a greater response. Using this criterion, the isolation peep was again the most potent stimulus in each of the two presentation conditions. The snake call ranked second or third, in the two conditions, while music was last or next to last in potency (Table 1). The third major finding was that the auditory stimuli produced a greater increase in total power when they were presented in the social setting, with the ethologically relevant stimuli again producing a greater response than the control stimuli.

The same regimen of sensory and social stimuli were presented to the monkey following lesion of inferior temporal cortex. Total power in the various conditions was again compared to that recorded during spontaneous social interaction, but the baseline used was one taken following the lesion. Following the cortical lesion, baseline electrical activity increased, but, strikingly, the response of the amygdala to presentations of the same stimuli was now in the opposite direction. All combinations of sensory stimulation produced a decrease in power from baseline.

Interestingly, the relationship between test and control stimuli remained, as did the influence of the social setting. Test stimuli were associated with more power than were control stimuli, the latter producing a greater decrease in power.

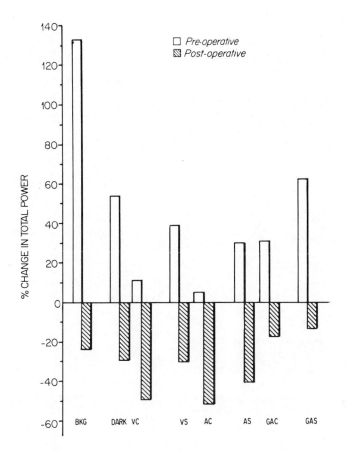

Fig. 1. Percent change in total power for all stimulus and
         control conditions compared to spontaneous group
         behavior. Open bars represent preoperative comparisons,
         hatched bars represent comparisons after the lesion to
         post-lesion spontaneous group behavior.
         VC & VS = visual control and test stimulation;
         AC & AS = auditory control and test stimulation;
         GAC & GAS = group auditory control and test stimulation.

Table 1. Sum of Rank Ordering of Percent of Total Power
in the Delta Band Evoked by Conspecific Calls

Group Auditory Condition

Pre-Op		Post-Op	
Iso Peep	21	Alarm Peep	23
Errchuck	23	Trill	25
Snake Call	24	Twitter	27
Twitter	29	Iso Peep	28
Alarm Peep	30	Snake Call	28
Trill	34	Errchuck	28
Music	35	Music	37

Chaired Condition

Pre-Op		Post-Op	
Iso Peep	25	Trill	26
Snake Call	27	Music	29
Twitter	27	Twitter	33
Alarm Peep	30	Snake Call	33
Trill	36	Errchuck	34
Music	39	Alarm Peep	34
Errchuck	40	Iso Peep	35

Again, the auditory stimuli presented in a social setting were
associated with more power (less of a decrease), and the
relationship between vocalizations and control stimuli was still
preserved; the lowest decrease in power occurred when test
stimuli were presented in the social setting. Even with impaired
input from a major pathway, the social context influences the
response of the amygdala to sensory stimuli, and this social
influence still preserves the relationship, in terms of the power
output of the amygdala, between ethologically relevant
vocalizations and irrelevant control stimuli. However, within
the set of vocalizations, the "affective hierarchy", in terms of
power output originally observed in the pre-lesion recording
sessions, was disrupted (Table 1). The isolation peep, which
previously displayed such primacy, falls to mid-rank in the
social condition and to lowest rank in the isolated condition.
The second most potent stimulus, the snake call, also suffers a
similar reduction in rank. Another striking feature of this
hierarchy is the contraction in the spread of summed ranks for
the various vocalizations. The difference between the highest
and lowest summed rank (excluding music) is 160% greater before
lesion in the social setting. Similarly, the range in ranks is
88% greater before lesion in the isolated condition.

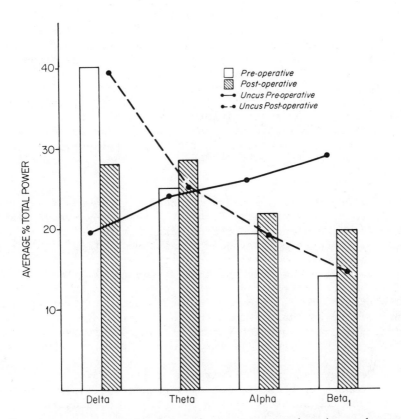

Fig. 2. Average percent of total power occurring in each
frequency band from recordings taken from the amygdala
and uncus. Preoperative pattern of the amygdala
consisted of highest power in the delta band, gradually
diminishing to the beta band. Postoperatively, there is
a flattening out of this difference between bands. An
opposite pattern is seen in the uncal recordings, with
delta having the lowest percent power and beta the
highest. Following inferior temporal cortex lesion, the
pattern is reversed, becoming similar to the
preoperative amygdala recordings.

The relationships described above are also observed in the frequency profile of the EEG. Meaningful stimuli, and stimuli presented in the social setting, produce EEG epochs with a greater proportion of the total power in the delta band than in any other frequency band. Progressively higher frequency bands contain progressively lower proportions of total power. Less relevant stimuli do not produce records with such a large percentage of power in the delta range. Following lesion of the inferior temporal cortex, records taken in these same situations (high meaning or affect) show a much more even distribution of power (Fig. 2). It would appear that lesions of this input structure impedes the animal's ability to interpret, or place affective tone, upon sensory information which, according to Perryman et al. (1987), is still available to the amygdala. These frequency relationships, in the intact subject, are consistent with earlier work (Kling, 1981) done on old world primates.

The nature of these sensory responses, vis-a-vis frequency, also appears to be regionally distinct. Recordings taken nearby, from the uncus, manifest a quite different response topography. Affectively laden stimuli produce a response profile with the greatest percentage of total power in the beta range, with progressively less power in the lower frequencies. Lesions of inferior temporal cortex reverse this ordering, such that the response of the uncus following lesion is quite similar to the response of the amygdala before the identical lesion (Fig. 2). This indicates that both the nature of the sensory response, and the effect of this type of lesion, are specific to the amygdala.

Finally, as reported by Perryman et al. (1987), lesions of inferior temporal cortex did not disrupt the earlier, sensory, components of the auditory evoked potential recorded from the amygdala. In addition, these early components of the auditory evoked potential preceded in time the same components recorded from the inferior temporal cortex. This latter finding reinforces the notion that inferior temporal cortex lesions do not disrupt sensory input into the amygdala because the information reaches the amygdala before it arrives at the overlying cortex. The later components of the auditory evoked potential, conversely, are profoundly attenuated by this lesion. This would suggest that inputs from inferior temporal cortex are necessary for appropriate assessment by the amygdala. The early components of the visual evoked potentials are, however, influenced by this lesion, suggesting that the information concerning the stimulus itself may be degraded.

DISCUSSION

The findings from this study confirm that, as in old world species, the electrical activity of the amygdala, as measured by the power of discrete frequency bands, is sensitive to the conspecific saliency of the stimulus. For conspecific calls, the isolation peep appeared to be the most potent, with a progressively decreasing response to snake call, twitter, alarm peep, and trill. Only the errchuck appeared to evoke an inconsistent response, the magnitude of which depending upon the environmental setting in which the stimulus was presented. Thus, in the intact subject, auditory information appears to produce a ranking of response magnitude which is dependent upon the relevance of the stimuli. This is similar in nature to the response hierarchies produced by visual and social stimuli. These data are consistent with MacLean proposal that the isolation peep is the most primitive and potent of all mammalian vocalizations and are also consistent with the interpretations which have been made of the other squirrel monkey vocalizations. In addition to lending electrophysiological confirmation to the interpretation of these various vocalizations, these data also suggest a locus for the primacy of the isolation peep and for the magnitude of the responses engendered by these vocalizations.

The second major finding to this study is that the responses of the amygdala to the same auditory stimuli are greater when the subject is in an unrestrained setting, with conspecifics, than when isolated in a chair. This is the first direct comparison of the influence of environmental setting upon the magnitude of the response of the amygdala to sensory stimuli. The third major finding was that the marked attenuation in power from the same electrode placement, following ablation of the inferior temporal cortex, seems to be most noticeable in the lateral nuclei. This is in contradistinction to the medial nuclei, which, in some circumstances, demonstrates an increase in power following the same lesion.

Our working model of amygdaloid functioning divides this structure into two major subunits. The lateral aspect of the amygdala receives cortical inputs which convey information from all sensory modalities (Van Hoesen, 1981). Thus, this aspect of the amygdala is in a position to integrate all the various sensory aspects of a stimulus event into a perceptual gestalt. This compilation of the information from cortical "feature detectors" may also be integrated with information from the organisms memory. Apoplexies involving cortical areas associated with the amygdala have been associated with agnosias in which the patient could describe all the features of a picture without understanding what the picture represented. The medial aspect of the amygdala, on the other hand, does not receive direct sensory projections from inferior temporal cortex, but, instead, is relayed information from the lateral amygdala. We suggest that it is at this stage that the medial amygdala places an emotional interpretation upon an integrated sensory experience. In this regard, damage to the amygdala produces not only a prosopoagnosia, in which patients have difficulty recognizing familiar faces, but, in the case of bilateral damage, may also produce a prosop-affective agnosia, in which the patient can not discern emotional expressions on the faces of others.

We interpret the third finding, in which there is a greater lesion-induced attenuation of power in the lateral nuclei, as resulting from the loss of neocortical facilitatory inputs to the lateral amygdala, which, in turn, may have a tonic inhibitory effect upon the medial nuclei. Although direct neocortical inputs to the lateral amygdala, which have been demonstrated in macaques, are yet to be examined in new world species, these data would be consistent with a parallel evolutionary expansion of the temporal neocortex and development of the lateral amygdala. As the social behaviors of the organism became more complex, a greater analysis of social stimuli would be required of the lateral amygdala, which, in turn, would require a more elaborated input from peri-cortical areas.

The more wide-spread representation in the amygdala of auditory, as opposed to visual, evoked potentials (Perryman et al., 1987) is surprising in view of the suggested bias, at least in old world species, of the amygdala toward the visual system. However, the greater distribution of auditory evoked potentials in the squirrel monkey is consistent with the more dominant role of auditory communication in this species. The fact that lesions of inferior temporal cortex can affect the auditory FFT can be interpreted either as a non-specific reduction of facilitatory inputs to the lateral amygdala, with all sensory modalities being affected equally, or as indicating a more specific role for the inferior temporal cortex in the processing and transmission of auditory information.

The reduction in power brought about by these lesions is not, however, uniformly extended to the medial nuclei. It is possible that preservation of the function of the medial nuclei is the reason why the subjects did not show observable disruptions of affective behavior, social rank, or conspecific bonding. It would be necessary to observe these preparations in a more natural free-ranging, or semi-free ranging, condition in order to get a clearer assessment of this hypothesis.

With regard to these qualitative and quantitative shifts, it should be emphasized that the amygdala does not appear to be "blind" to the sensory stimulation. First, the same response was not just reduced in magnitude, and, in addition, the magnitude of sensory evoked potentials recorded from the amygdalas of these same subjects, following lesion, was not reduced (Perryman et al., 1987). It would appear, therefore, that the amygdala was receiving the sensory information but, perhaps, not the memorial information that had come to be associated with these stimuli. According to Gloor's formulation, the amygdala would then be more greatly biased toward filtering these stimuli out, as the amygdala has been associated with affect, and the magnitude of the electrical response of the amygdala has been associated with the affective content of the stimulus. The affective content of the stimuli and the presence of the social milieu would then tend to offset this lesion-induced negative bias.

The fact that the nature of the response was qualitatively altered following the lesion (a change in the direction of the response to below baseline) suggests a modification to Gloor's model of how the amygdala functions. Rather than just acting as a filter which allows some information to pass to various drive centers, the amygdala may be sending a tonic influence to these centers which is modulated up or down, depending upon the saliency of the stimulus. In this way, the amygdala may bias the response of these areas to information, particularly sensory information, which they may be getting from other centers. The role of the amygdala may be to determine "saliency", analogous to the way cortical areas detect "features", and to place affective tone or "bias" upon this sensory information in a manner analogous to the way in which the reticular formation generates arousal commensurate with incoming sensory stimulation.

A partial deafferentation of the amygdala would deny it the necessary feature analysis and memorial referents to adequately assess the incoming information and, thus, cause the amygdala to under-assess it or reject the saliency of the stimulus. This could account for both the change in direction of the electrical response of the amygdala and the contraction in range of its response hierarchy vis-a-vis the conspecific vocalization. This may also be reflected behaviorally in the blunted affect manifested by animals with amygdaloid lesions; a phenomenon which we have just now begun to observe with lesions restricted to insular cortex, a structure with substantial projections to the amygdala.

REFERENCES

1. Aggleton, J. P., A description of intra-amygdaloid connections in old world monkeys, Experimental Brain Research, 57:390 (1985).
2. Barrett T. W., Studies of the function of the amygdaloid complex in M. mulatta, Neuropsychologia, 7:1 (1969).
3. Dicks, D., R. E. Myers, and A. Kling, Uncus and amygdala lesions: Effects on social behavior in the free-ranging rhesus monkey, Science, 165:69 (1969).

4. Gloor, P., Electrophysiological studies of the amygdala
    (stimulation and recording): Their possible contributions
    to the understanding of neural mechanisms of aggression,
    in: "Neural Basis of Violence and Aggression," W. S.
    Fields and W. H. Sweet, eds., Warren H. Green, St. Louis,
    (1975).
5. Kaada, B. R., Stimulation and regional ablation of the
    amygdaloid complex with reference to functional
    representations, in: "The Neurobiology of the Amygdala,"
    B. E. Eleftheriou, ed., Plenum Press, New York (1972).
6. Kling, A., Influence of temporal lobe lesions in
    radio-telemetered electrical activity of amygdala to
    social stimuli in monkey, in: "The Amygdaloid Complex," Y.
    Ben-Ari, ed., Elsevier /North Holland Biomedical Press,
    Amsterdam (1981).
7. Kling, A., Effects of amygdalectomy on social-affective
    behavior in nonhuman primates, in: "The Neurobiology of
    the Amygdala," B. E. Eleftheriou, ed., Plenum Press, New
    York (1972).
8. Kling, A., J. Lancaster, and J. Benitone, Amygdalectomy in
    the free-ranging vervet (Cercopithecus aethiops), J.
    Psychiat. Res., 7:191 (1970).
9. Kling, A., K. M. Perryman, and T. Parks, A telemetry system
    for the study of cortical-amygdala relationships in the
    squirrel monkey (S. sciureus), in: Modulation of
    sensorimotor activity during alterations in behavioral
    states," R. Bandler, ed., Alan R. Liss, New York (1984).
10. Kling, A., R. L. Lloyd, and K. M. Perryman, Slow wave
    changes in amygdala to visual, auditory, and social
    stimuli following lesions of the inferior temporal cortex
    in squirrel monkey (S. sciureus), Behavioral and Neural
    Biology, In Press (1987).
11. Koikegami, H., Amygdala and other related limbic structures;
    experimental studies on the anatomy and function. I.
    Anatomical researches with some neurophysiological
    observations, Acta Medica Biologica (Niigata), 10:161
    (1963).
12. MacLean, P. D., Brain evolution relating to family, play and
    the separation call, Archives of General Psychiatry,
    42:405 (1985).
13. MacLean, P. D. and J. M. R. Delgado, Electrical and chemical
    stimulation of fronto-temporal portion of limbic system in
    the waking animal, Electroencephalography and Clinical
    Neurophysiology, 5:91 (1953).
14. Perryman, K. M., A. Kling, and R. L. Lloyd, Differential
    effects of inferior temporal cortex lesions upon visual
    and auditory evoked potentials in the amygdala of the
    squirrel monkey (S. sciureus), Behavioral and Neural
    Biology, In Press (1987).

15. Schreiner, L. and A. Kling, Rhinencephalon and behavior,
     Amer. J. Physiol., 184:468 (1956).
16. Turner, B.H., The cortical sequence and terminal
     distribution of sensory related afferents to the
     amygdaloid complex of the rat and monkey, in: "The
     Amygdaloid Complex," Y. Ben-Ari, ed., Elsevier/North
     Holland Biomedical Press, Amsterdam (1981).
17. Van Hoesen, G.W., The differential distribution, diversity
     and sprouting of cortical projections to the amygdala in
     the rhesus monkey, in: "The Amygdaloid Complex," Y.
     Ben-Ari, ed., Elsevier/North Holland Biomedical Press,
     Amsterdam (1981).

THE CENTRAL CONTROL OF BIOSONAR SIGNAL PRODUCTION IN BATS
DEMONSTRATED BY MICROSTIMULATION OF ANTERIOR CINGULATE CORTEX
IN THE ECHOLOCATING BAT, PTERONOTUS PARNELLI PARNELLI

David M. Gooler[*1] and William E. O'Neill[*]

Center for Brain Research[*] and Department of
Physiology
University of Rochester
Rochester, N.Y. 14642

INTRODUCTION

Overview

One of the ultimate goals of sensory neurobiology is to
understand how sensory feedback controls subsequent motor behavior.
For both auditory and speech scientists, it is of particular
interest to know how auditory information influences vocalizations,
and conversely how vocalization affects auditory processing. Such
questions have an important bearing on both the vocal behavior of
the mature organism, and the acquisition of vocal repertoires in the
young during development. In many vertebrate species, communication
sounds are learned from a combination of exposure to the sounds
produced by adults, listening to self-vocalized sounds, and
laryngeal and orofacial motor feedback. Thus there is a feedback
loop established which involves learning a model of the signal via
auditory stimulation, subsequent attempts to duplicate the model
vocally, and comparison of the resulting vocalization with the
internalized model again via auditory analysis. This process has
been well documented for the learning of species-specific song
patterns in many songbirds (Konishi and Nottebohm 1969; Marler and
Peters 1977), and is thought to guide the development of human
speech patterns (Marler 1976).

To clarify the role of auditory feedback in the regulation of
vocal behavior, it is important to use an animal model whose

[1]Current address: Department of Physiology and Biophysics,
University of Illinois, Urbana, Illinois

153

behavior emphasizes the interaction of acoustic information
processing and vocal control. Echolocating bats are especially
suited to this research.

Orientation Sounds

    The structure of the vocalized orientation pulses that bats
emit for echolocation can vary significantly among species.
Echolocation signals often contain a broadband frequency-modulate
sweep or a group of harmonically related sweeps, and in some spec
can be produced in combination with a sustained constant frequenc
(pure tone) portion. In particular, the biosonar system of the
mustached bat, Pteronotus p. parnelli provides an excellent mode
for investigating the sensory-motor complements of echolocation.
The mustached bat emits stereotyped orientation sounds consistin
of a sustained constant frequency (CF) component followed by a sh
downward sweeping frequency modulated (FM) sound, and is thus
grouped with the so-called "CF/FM" bats; a short, low intensity
upward sweeping FM sound (1-2 kHz) occurs prior to the CF portion
(Novick and Vaisnys 1964; Grinnell 1970; Schnitzler 1970; pers.
obs.). The biosonar signal of the mustached bat is comprised of
four harmonics (H_{1-4}) each of which contains a CF and FM componen
the second harmonic (H_2) is usually dominant (emitted with the
greatest energy). The actual frequencies of the CF components
depend on the individual bat, but are around 30, 60, 90, 120 kHz
H_1-H_4, respectively. Each harmonic in an FM sweep decreases by
about 6, 12, 18 and 24 kHz for H_1-H_4, respectively. Total pulse
duration varies from 3-30 ms for the CF component and 2-4 ms for
FM sweep. Pulse repetition rate ranges from 4 to 100 per second
depending on the behavioral phase of flight.

Doppler-Shift Compensation

    Throughout all phases of echolocation, the long CF/FM bat ma
experience a frequency shift in the returning echo (Doppler-shift
produced by the difference in the bat's velocity with respect to
surroundings. In a behavior known as "Doppler-shift compensation
(DSC), long CF/FM bats actively compensate for Doppler-shifts in
echo by changing the frequency of the orientation sound (Schnitzl
1968,1970; Trappe and Schnitzler 1982). The new frequency of the
emitted sound is proportional to the magnitude of the frequency
shift in the echo. In P. parnelli, neurons in the cochlear nucle
can respond to sinusoidal frequency modulations as small as 0.01%
the frequency of the CF_2 component (Suga and Jen 1977).

    While compensating, long CF/FM bats such as the mustached ba
and the European horseshoe bat, Rhinolophus ferrumequinum, stabil
the echo frequency in a preferred, very narrow band called the
"reference frequency" (Schnitzler 1968, 1970). The reference
frequency is about 100-150 Hz higher than the "resting frequency"

(frequency emitted when the bat detects no Doppler-shifts) for P. parnelli (Schnitzler 1970) and 50-300 Hz higher for R. ferrumequinum (Schuller et al. 1974). The variability in the CF frequency emitted during DSC (and therefore the echo frequency) as observed during obstacle avoidance tests is typically ±10 to ±100 Hz for P. parnelli (Jen and Kamada 1982); in R. ferrumequinum the frequency of the echo is maintained within 50-200 Hz, i.e., as small as 0.06% of the reference frequency (Schuller et al. 1974). Under most conditions, the bat's relative flight velocity is positive with respect to its surroundings and it therefore receives echoes that are shifted to higher frequencies, i.e., a positive Doppler-shift; both P. parnelli (Kobler et al. 1985) and R. ferrumequinum (Schuller et al. 1974; Schuller et al. 1975) do not compensate negative frequency shifts.

The auditory system of P. parnelli is extremely sharply tuned peripherally (Pollak et al. 1972; Suga et al. 1975; Suga and Jen 1977) and centrally (Suga and Jen 1976; Pollak and Bodenhamer 1981) to the mustached bat's reference frequency. In addition, a region of auditory cortex (DSCF; Suga and Jen 1976) and a portion of the central nucleus of the inferior colliculus (IC; Pollak et al. 1983) constitute disproportionately large areas consisting of neurons tuned to these frequencies.

Doppler-shift compensation has been compared functionally to retinal foveation (Schuller and Pollak 1979; Neuweiler et al. 1980). The acoustic foveation process depends on the feedback between auditory and vocalization systems which show distinct interactions for high resolution analysis and subsequent precise stabilization of the emitted pulse (and thereby the returning echo) frequency (Schuller et al. 1975; Schuller and Suga 1976a; Schuller 1977). Neurons in the inferior colliculus, tuned to the CF component at the "foveal" (reference) frequencies, are particularly sensitive to small Doppler-shifts induced in the echo (e.g. insect wing beats) (Schuller 1979). Such echoes can provide the bat with information on the angular orientation of insect prey based on spectral and temporal components of the echo (Schnitzler et al. 1983). In addition, neurons in the inferior colliculus (Schuller 1984) and auditory cortex (Ostwald 1980) of R. ferrumequinum can encode modulation at rates equal to the fundamental frequency of the insect wing beat as well as more subtle frequency and amplitude modulations. In CF/FM bats such as R. rouxi, R. ferrumequinum and P.parnelli behavioral studies have shown that the bat will only pursue fluttering insects and that bats can discriminate different wing beat frequencies produced by Doppler-shifts in the echo (Goldman and Henson 1977; Schnitzler and Flieger 1983; Schnitzler et al. 1985). It is strongly suggested that selection of prey may be determined by information from wing beats. Thus, the stabilized echo frequency acts as a carrier for the more subtle Doppler-shifts which can provide information about the insect prey. The precision with which mustached bats control the frequency of their emitted sounds, and consequently maintain the echo at reference frequency, is regulated directly by feedback of information from echoes.

Laryngeal Mechanisms and Nucleus Ambiguus

While aspects of auditory physiology and behavior have been explored for their roles in DSC, the investigation of the control of vocal parameters has centered on laryngeal mechanisms. Novick and Griffin (1961) found that denervating the cricothyroid muscles by severing the superior laryngeal nerve (SLN) bilaterally in FM bats lowered the frequency and disrupted the organization of vocalization. Suthers and Fattu (1973) showed further evidence of SLN control of ultrasonic frequencies in FM bats via modulation of tension of cricothyroid muscles controlling vocal and ventricular membranes; release of tension may produce the downward sweeping FM They suggested that the vocal folds regulate pulse duration by acting as a glottal stop. Vocal folds are shown to be under the control of the recurrent laryngeal nerve (RLN) in CF/FM bats (Schuller and Suga 1976b; Rübsamen and Schuller 1981).

In the bat, R. rouxi, Schweizer et al. (1981) traced the SLN and RLN to their origins in the nucleus ambiguus (NA). The affere and efferent connections of NA in R. rouxi have been traced recent (Rübsamen and Schweizer 1986). Similar to other mammals, the NA i R. rouxi receives inputs from the midbrain periaqueductal gray (PAG), a nucleus important in the production of vocalization. The NA has reciprocal connections with parabrachial nuclei and lateral reticular formation (RF), nuclei involved in modulating the respir atory rhythm and vocal motor pattern. In bats, auditory input fro the inferior colliculus may influence the NA indirectly via efferents from PAG (Frisina, O'Neill and Zettel in prep.), the superior colliculus and lateral pontine nuclei (Schweizer 1981). The lateral pontine nuclei in particular project to the anterior part of the NA from which SLN fibers originate. Rübsamen and Betz (1986) found that in this portion of NA changes in neural activity were associated with changes in the frequency of emissions during DSC. The most rostral inputs to NA in the bat originated in front (motor) cortex (Rübsamen and Schweizer 1986).

Midbrain Control of Vocalization

In various mammals from rodents (Wetzel et al. 1980; Yajima e al. 1980) to primates (Jürgens and Ploog 1970; Jürgens and Pratt 1979a,b) to bats (Rübsamen and Schweizer 1986), anatomical and electrophysiological studies show strong similarities in the vocal control system descending from the midbrain: the midbrain PAG projects to NA which in turn sends efferents in the SLN and RLN. The midbrain PAG occupies an important position in the vocal contr system. All areas in the squirrel monkey brain from which vocaliz

ation could be elicited by electrical stimulation project to PAG
(Jürgens and Pratt 1979b; Müller-Preuss and Jürgens 1976; Jürgens
and Müller-Preuss 1977). As a corollary, lesions of the PAG
abolished all species-specific vocalizations which were elicited
from these regions (Jürgens and Pratt 1979b). Direct stimulation of
caudal PAG elicits the greatest number of different species-specific
vocalizations (Jürgens and Ploog 1970). This suggests that the role
of the PAG is one of integration of inputs from areas where species-
specific vocalizations could be elicited, but that it is above the
level of motor-coordination.

It is less clear what role the PAG plays in the control of
vocalization in bats. The use of electrical stimulation to study
the importance of the midbrain for vocalization in bats has been
pursued by Suga et al. (1973). The regions stimulated are anteroventral to the IC. Electrical stimulation of the dorsal RF in
Myotis (FM bat) evoked vocalizations similar to search phase orientation sounds. Stimulation of the lateral PAG produced orientation
pulses similar to those emitted during terminal phase. In both
cases, vocalization was elicited by summation from repetitive,
subthreshold electrical stimuli. Latencies for vocalization, once
stable responses were evoked, were 25-60 ms and vocalizations were
locked to the stimulus pulse train on a one-to-one basis. Only
movements of the pinnae and mouth were observed.

Emitted sounds evoked in a similar manner from P. parnelli were
indistinguishable from CF/FM pulses produced by the bat during
target pursuit. Further studies (Suga et al. 1974) of P. parnelli
suggested a strong influence of auditory input on vocalization.
Acoustic stimuli enhanced the amplitude of the vocal response and
the number of sounds elicited by subthreshold electrical stimulation. Increasing the amplitude of auditory stimuli increased the
amplitude of the vocalization.

Control of Vocalization and Auditory Influences Rostral to Midbrain

Besides acoustic influence via direct input from auditory
nuclei to PAG, another mechanism for regulating vocalization at PAG
would be by afferent input from other regions known to be important
for vocalization (Jürgens and Pratt 1979b). Electrical stimulation
of a number of brain regions leads to vocalization in the monkey,
but most vocalizations are thought to be secondary to a stimulus
induced change in emotional or motivational state (Jürgens 1976b).

The anterior cingulate cortex (ACg) is thought to play a
prominent role in the descending vocalization system. Single units
in the ACg have been shown to change activity 200-800 ms prior to
vocalization in rhesus monkeys; latencies in this range suggest that
the ACg plays a more integrative role in phonation than one of
direct motor control (Sutton et al. 1978). Electrical stimulation

of the ACg has been shown to elicit vocalization in the squirrel
monkey, as well as in other mammals (Jürgens and Ploog 1970; Jürgen
1976b). While stimulation of a number of anterior limbic regions
leads to "primary" vocalization (i.e., not secondary to specific
stimulus-induced motivational changes) in the squirrel monkey
(Jürgens and Pratt 1979a; Jürgens 1976b), the ACg projects directly
to PAG (Jürgens and Pratt 1979a) and is the only region which
receives direct input from laryngeal motor cortex (Jürgens 1976a).
In addition, most regions of the brain from which vocalizations can
be elicited by electrical stimulation receive direct projections
from the ACg.

An important aspect of vocal control is the reciprocal
interaction of sensory and motor processing. The cingulate cortex
has been shown to have a significant number of connections with
sensory areas in the monkey brain (Jones and Powell 1970). The ACg
has reciprocal connections with the secondary auditory cortex in the
monkey (Pandya and Kuypers 1969; Jones and Powell 1970; Müller-
Preuss et al. 1980; Jürgens 1983). Müller-Preuss et al. (1980)
found that twenty percent of units studied in part of the superior
temporal gyrus (STG) show predominately inhibitory changes in
spontaneous activity coincident with, and lasting 100-300 ms beyond
electrical stimulation (subthreshold for vocal response) of ACg.
Neural response to recorded vocalizations following electrical
stimulation of ACg showed suppressed activity in 4 of 28 STG units.
Neural activity in the ACg in rabbits was shown to be differentiall
affected during positive and negative avoidance conditioning tasks
where the conditional stimulus was a tone (Gabriel et al. 1977).
Thus there is some evidence that the auditory-ACg connections are
functional. These studies suggest that the ACg may be performing a
integrative function above the level of motor coordination involvir
the selection and initiation of specific vocal patterns (Jürgens an
Pratt 1979a; Sutton et al. 1981).

Greater emphasis in studies of the biosonar system of bats has
been placed on acoustic signal processing in auditory nuclei. The
relationship between brain structures and regulation of orientation
sounds has focused on the neural connections of brainstem nuclei an
manipulation of emissions elicited from the midbrain PAG-RF.
Considering the similarity of the auditory system in bats to other
mammals, the disproportionately large area of the brain devoted to
processing of acoustic information, and the variety of information
that can be extracted from biosonar signals, an equally complex and
parallel hierarchical arrangement was expected for motor control of
sound production for echolocation in bats. The aim of this study
was to explore higher centers in the mustached bat brain involved i
the regulation of biosonar vocalization to begin to reveal a level
of motor control complementary to the level of complexity
established in the auditory system.

MATERIALS AND METHODS

Preparation

Nine mustached bats (Pteronotus p. parnelli) were prepared for microstimulation under methoxyflurane anesthesia. The muscles overlying the skull were reflected and a 1.8 cm brad was cemented to the skull over the cerebellum to stabilize the animal's head during the experiments. Animals were allowed to recover for at least two days prior to the experiment. Experiments were performed in an acoustic chamber modified to be anechoic for ultrasound. Spontaneous vocalizations were recorded from bats roosting individually in a small, open-mesh cage, because mustached bats do not vocalize readily while restrained.

Experimental Procedures

Electrical Stimulation.For stimulation, glass-insulated platinum-iridium (70%/30%) electrodes were produced. Stimuli consisted of 350 μs negative monophasic pulses presented in trains of 10 pulses at a rate of 100 pulses per second. Pulse train repetition rate was typically 2 per second. Stimuli were presented every 50-100 μm along a penetration. The current amplitude was typically 10-30 μA although stimulus currents as high as 70 μA were used.

Horseradish Peroxidase Injections.Horseradish peroxidase (10% HRP, Sigma Type VI) or horseradish peroxidase wheatgerm-agglutinin (2% HRP-WGA) was deposited electrophoretically following the last penetration in most preparations in order to mark stimulation sites in the ACg and to trace neural connections. The central core regions of the injection sites for tetramethylbenzidine (TMB) reacted tissue were 400 to 600 μm in diameter and those for the diaminobenzidine (DAB) reaction were 100-300 μm in diameter. HRP histochemistry was performed to visualize the marker and trace neuroanatomical pathways (modified from Mesulam 1982; Frisina and O'Neill 1985).

Recording and Analysis of Vocalizations.Vocalizations were captured from 9 bats by a 1/4 inch condenser microphone (Brüel & Kjaer 4135) positioned 10 cm in front of the bat and were recorded on 1/4 inch magnetic tape on a Nagra TI instrumentation recorder at 30 ips. The amplitude spectra of 829 elicited and 291 spontaneous vocal pulses were generated by a real-time spectrum analyzer (Scientific Atlanta SD380-1).

Topographic Organization.Contour plots (isofrequency contours) were derived from the frequency of biosonar emissions produced by microstimulation and the location of the stimulation sites in the brain. Contours were produced by a computer program (subroutines produced by the Scientific Computing Division of the National Center for Atmospheric Research (Boulder, Co.) which calculates the emitted frequency along a regular grid (100 μm intervals in this case) by a

Gaussian interpolation between data points in 3 dimensions.   Slice
were then made through the grid of interpolated points and
isofrequency contours were plotted in the sagittal plane.

RESULTS

Location of cortical region subjected to microstimulation

        The region from which vocalizations could be elicited by
electrical microstimulation was located anterior and dorsal to the
corpus callosum. The dimensions of the area from which
vocalizations were elicited by near-threshold stimuli were typical
no more than 300 μm wide, and spanned about 900-1300 μm in the
rostro-caudal and 500-1000 μm in the dorso-ventral directions. An
artist's drawing of the brain reconstructed from a sagittal sectio
(Fig. 1a) shows the region (arrow) from which echolocation sounds
were elicited in one bat on the left side of the brain. The
vertical lines connect points within penetrations from which
vocalizations were elicited by microstimulation. The electrode
penetrations ran roughly parallel to the cortical layers in this
region of ACg. The drawing of a frontal section in Fig. 1b shows
the center of an HRP deposit located at one stimulation site about
midway along the rostro-caudal extent of the area from which
biosonar emissions could be elicited on the right side of the brai
The HRP was visualized using the DAB method and the dark center an
the gray corona represent the dense core and the halo regions of t
injection site respectively. There was no apparent morphological
asymmetry or lateralization of function to either side of the brai
observed in the present study.

Characteristics of electrically-elicited and spontaneous
vocalizations

        Stimulation subthreshold for eliciting vocalization.The use o
repeated subthreshold stimuli (5-10 μA below the threshold for
eliciting vocalization) enabled visual examination of the stimulus
synchronized oro-facial movements leading to the vocalization. A
video camcorder with macro lens was used to view and record the
electrically-elicited movements. The threshold for elicited oro-
facial behavior was always lower than for the associated vocal
emission. Initially, synchronized low amplitude movements of the
pinnae occurred, followed in turn by flapping movements of the
mandible, strong pulse-like exhalations, and finally vocalization.
Prominent contralateral deviations within the range of movements o
the pinnae and to some degree the mouth were produced at stimulus
levels near the threshold for eliciting oro-facial behavior.
Increasing stimulus current yielded more bilaterally symmetrical
deflections of the pinnae and mouth, and increased the amplitude o
pulse-like exhalations, as well as oro-facial movements. In

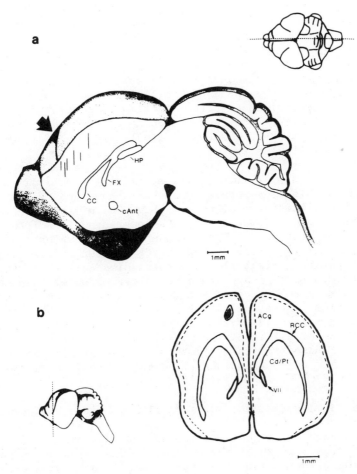

Fig. 1. Sites in the mustached bat brain from which biosonar
        vocalizations were elicited by electrical microstimulation
        in this study. The horizontal and lateral views of the
        brain (insets) indicate the levels of the respective
        sections. a The ranges of penetrations containing only
        vocalization-evoking stimulation sites are shown in this
        sagittal section by vertical lines (arrow). b A frontal
        section containing an HRP deposit (dark spot) midway along
        the rostrocaudal extent of the stimulation site. anterior
        cingulate cortex (ACg); anterior commissure (cAnt); corpus
        callosum (CC); caudate/putamen (CdPt); fornix (Fx);
        hippocampus (HP); radiations of the corpus callosum (RCC);
        lateral ventricle (VII) (a bat P8-18-85; b bat P2-13-86;
        modified from Gooler and O'Neill 1987).

contrast to elicited emissions which are synchronized to the
stimulus train rate, the movements associated with spontaneous vo
behavior are smoother and more continuous. In no case were gross
inappropriate body movements observed during vocalization elicite
by microstimulation of the ACg.

Suprathreshold stimulation. Electrical microstimulation of th
ACg at 10 μA above threshold typically elicited a burst of 2 to 8
vocal pulses per stimulus train. At stimulus levels of 30 μA (10-
μA above threshold), latency to response at different stimulation
sites ranged from 50-275 ms (typically 150-200 ms) following the
onset of each stimulus train.

Vocal pulses elicited by microstimulation were virtually
indistinguishable from spontaneously-emitted sounds. The
electrically-elicited vocal pulses (Fig. 2c) mimicked the pattern
and the shape of the envelope of the spontaneously-emitted
vocalizations (Fig. 2a). The envelope of the waveform generally
shows a rise in intensity during the CF portion until just prior
the FM component. Similarly to natural biosonar cries, the termi
FM portion can rise in amplitude to a level greater than that
produced during the CF component ("sweep peak pulse") or decay
smoothly ("sweep decay pulse") from the CF (Pye 1980). Both type
of FM sweeps were evident in elicited and spontaneous emissions.
The durations of all electrically-elicited vocalizations ranged f
8-32 ms per pulse (typically 12-24 ms), well within the range of
naturally emitted vocal pulses (7-40 ms; Novick and Vaisnys 1964;
Schnitzler 1970; Henson et al. 1987).

Electrical microstimulation of ACg at a rate of 2 trains per
second elicited rates of biosonar vocalization within the realm
typical of natural bat behavior. The rate of emission for elicite
sounds, yields a range of about 33-45 pulses per second (pps) with
peak in the distribution at 42 pps. Similar to natural vocalizatic
emitted at these rates, durations of pulses were typically 8-18 ms

Amplitude spectra of the harmonics of biosonar emissions. In
naturally-occurring vocalizations at least four harmonics have bee
recognized with a fundamental frequency of about 30 kHz. In our
data there is also evidence in both the natural and elicited
vocalizations for a fifth harmonic, about 30 dB less intense than
CF_2. This can be seen in the spontaneously-emitted pulses in Fig.
2a,b. Five harmonically related frequencies identified in an
elicited vocalization (Fig. 2c,d) are similar to those in the
spontaneous emission (Fig. 2a,b). The frequencies of the CF_2
component emitted by the bat during stimulation of ACg were most
often in the range from 57-62 kHz, typical of natural biosonar
vocalizations (Fig. 2b,d).

The relative amplitudes of the harmonics (re CF_2) of

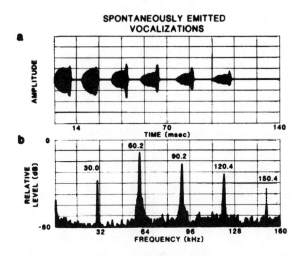

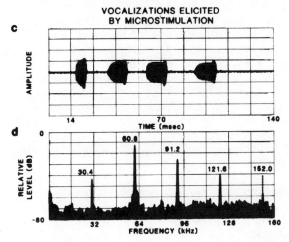

Fig. 2. Waveform analysis of mustached bat vocalizations. a and b
Spontaneously emitted vocalizations. c and d Vocalizations
elicited by microstimulation. As shown in a and c the
envelopes of the vocal pulses have similar characteristics.
b and d Frequency analysis of the CF component (FFT; 200 Hz
resolution). Analysis of one of the spontaneously emitted
pulses in a and one of the elicited pulses in c demonstrates
5 prominent harmonics typically found in each type of
emission. The dotted line which extends above the CF_5
corrects the relative intensity level for attenuation (14
dB) in the recording instrumentation. (from bat P9-9-85;
modified from Gooler and O'Neill 1987).

Table 1.   Range of relative amplitudes (dB <u>re</u> CF_2) of CF
components of spontaneous and electrically-elicited
vocalizations from the ACg in <u>P</u>. <u>p</u>. <u>parnelli</u>

	Elicited[a]	Spontaneous[b]	Spontaneous[c]
CF_1	-28.4 to -40.1	-23.1 to -36.1	-18 to -36
CF_3	- 7.1 to -17.6	- 6.1 to - 8.2	- 6 to -12
CF_4	-18.6 to -33.5	-16.5 to -29.0	-12 to -24
CF_5	-23.3 to -33.8	-23.8 to -33.3	NA

[a] Range of means from 5 bats (P4-7-85, P8-7-85,
P8-18-85, P9-9-85, P2-13-86; total vocal pulses = 829)
[b] Range of means from 4 bats (P9-9-85, P2-13-86,
P2-3-87, P2-10-87; total vocal pulses = 291)
[c] Range from Suga (1984)

electrically-elicited vocalizations are similar to those observed
for spontaneous vocalizations. The range of mean relative
amplitudes for elicited (for each of 5 bats) and spontaneous (for
each of 4 bats) vocalizations are summarized in Table 1 along with
amplitude ranges recorded by Suga (1984) from bats flying in a
hallway. No one group of the minimum or maximum values in Table 1
are from any particular bat in this study. The relative levels fo
each CF harmonic covered similar ranges for both elicited and
spontaneous vocalizations (Table 1). Based on the amplitude range
the harmonic components in order of decreasing amplitude relative
CF_2 are CF_3, CF_4 followed by CF_5 and CF_1. The FFTs in Fig. 2b and
show a similar pattern of relative intensities for typical
spontaneous and elicited vocal pulses.

The variability in the pattern of relative amplitudes was
generally predicted by the distributions in Table 1, but in about
of spontaneous and elicited emissions in all bats the CF_3 and the
CF_4 of elicited sounds were as intense as the CF_2. This variation
in the relative amplitude of the harmonics might alternatively be
interpreted as a selective attenuation of CF_2.

<u>Elicited sounds with complex amplitude spectra</u>. Besides the
biosonar signal, spectrally-complex sounds with a prominent audibl
component can be elicited by microstimulation of the ACg. The sou
is similar to that produced by bats in social interactions as they
scramble about the roost. When these sounds are elicited by micro
stimulation the oro-facial and pinnae movements are diminished in
amplitude compared to those seen with elicited biosonar signals.
Also, the spectrally-complex sounds are of shorter duration and ar
emitted at a higher rate in very tight bursts (Fig. 3). The laten
to emission of the audible sounds is much shorter, occurring 20-50
ms after stimulus onset. The fundamental frequency is about 6-8.5

kHz and 8 or more harmonics are evident in the spectrum.   While
there is always a predominant component in the amplitude spectra
near 12-17 kHz (second harmonic), ultrasonic frequencies are also
evident. The spectrum shown in Fig. 4 from an elicited audible sound
has a peak in the audible frequency range (16.4 kHz).   However, much
of the energy in the spectrum is distributed across the harmonically
related frequencies in the ultrasonic range.   The expression of the
ultrasonic harmonics in spectrally-complex emissions varied to the
degree that they were often buried within the noise, 40 dB down from
the peak in the audible range.   Whether the spectral differences
define functionally different sounds or are stimulus dependent is
uncertain.   Also, it is unclear whether the different emissions are
represented in an organized fashion in the brain.

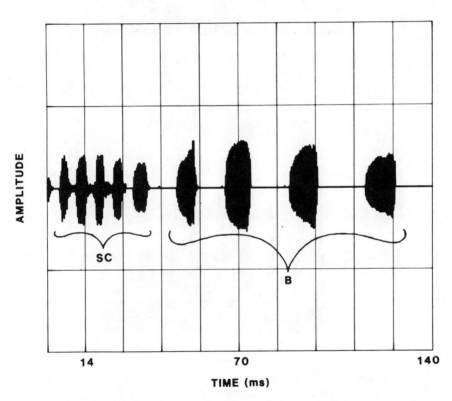

Fig. 3. The envelopes of spectrally complex and biosonar pulses
        elicited by a single stimulus train.   The burst of
        spectrally complex pulses (SC) begins about 50 ms prior
        to the burst of biosonar emissions (B).   The spectrally
        complex pulses were shorter in duration and emitted at
        a higher rate than the biosonar emissions. (from bat
        P8-18-85).

BIOSONAR SOUND

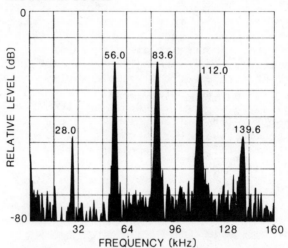

SPECTRALLY COMPLEX SOUND

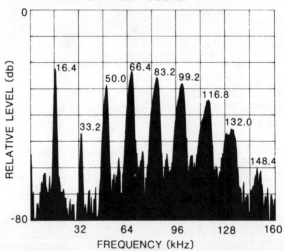

Fig. 4. Amplitude spectra of an elicited spectrally complex sound
and the CF component of an elicited biosonar sound. The
amplitude spectra cover a similar frequency range for both
sounds (FFT; 400 Hz resolution). The peaks of each spectrum
are harmonically related, but the fundamental frequency is
different for each type of sound. The spectrally complex
sound has a typically prominent peak in the audible
frequencies (16.4 kHz). (from bat P8-18-85).

In some cases both biosonar and spectrally-complex sounds can be elicited by an individual stimulus train. The burst of audible sounds always preceded the biosonar emissions (Fig. 3) and the paired bursts containing both types of sounds often occurred repeatedly in response to multiple stimulus trains. The spectra in Fig. 4 are from the last pulse in a burst of spectrally-complex sounds and the first pulse in a subsequent burst of biosonar sounds. While the ultrasonic components in the spectrally-complex sounds cover the same range of frequencies as the biosonar sounds the harmonic relationships were different.

Functional organization of the anterior cingulate cortex for vocalization

Studies were performed to explore the organization of the ACg for vocalization, and to examine its neural connections via injections of HRP. For these complete mapping studies, all penetrations were made in one continuous experiment in order to maintain accuracy in the relative positions of stimulation sites in each bat.

The results of the mapping studies show that a functional organization based on the type of vocalization produced by microstimulation exists in ACg. The anterior portion is associated with echolocation sounds, and the posterior section with audible, spectrally-complex sounds. The two areas are continuous, and in the transition zone both types of vocalization can be elicited by an individual stimulus train, the burst of spectrally complex sounds occurring prior to the biosonar emissions as previously discussed (Fig. 3). Previous work had also shown that in the midbrain PAG-RF the two areas are also adjacent, but the biosonar region is posterior to the area from which audible sounds were elicited (unpubl. obs.) Most interestingly, in contrast to the midbrain PAG-RF where electrically-elicited biosonar vocalizations are always emitted near the resting frequency (Suga et al. 1974), the vocal frequencies elicited by microstimulation of anterior ACg increase along a rostro-caudal axis. There is little variation in the isofrequency contours in the medio-lateral direction.

An example of the resulting tonotopic organization is demonstrated in Figs. 5 and 6 by isofrequency contours derived from a computer-reconstructed slice through the penetration space. The contours viewed in the sagittal plane (Fig. 6) were derived from the CF_2 frequencies of elicited vocalizations and the associated map of stimulation sites (Fig. 5). In Figs. 5 and 6 the vocalizations were elicited from stimulation sites made on the right side of the brain, but no laterality of function was observed in this study. The position of the stimulation sites and the respective frequency of vocal pulses are shown in the sagittal and horizontal planes (Fig. 5a and b). The order in which penetrations were made proceeded in a

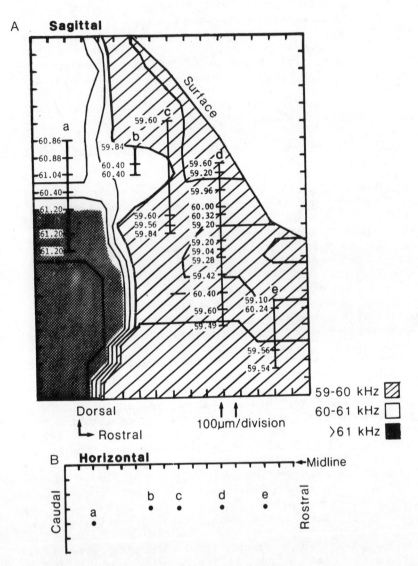

Fig. 5. Map of CF_2 frequencies of biosonar emissions elicited at
stimulation sites in the ACg of one bat and associated
isofrequency contours. The positions of the 5 electrode
penetrations (a-e) relative to the antero-dorsal "surface"
of the brain are shown from a sagittal perspective in A.
The horizontal view in B shows the positions of the penetrations with respect to the midline. (from bat P8-7-85).

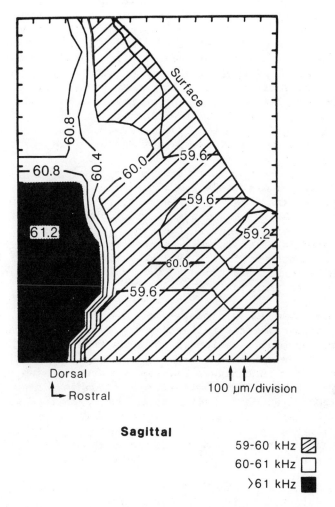

Fig. 6. Isofrequency contours representing the CF$_2$ component of
biosonar vocalizations elicited from the ACg in one bat.
The isofrequency contours were derived from the frequency
data in Fig. 5. The sagittal slice is located 300 μm
lateral to the midline (plane of penetrations b-e in Fig.
5). The interval between isofrequency contours is 0.4 kHz.
The shading emphasizes 1 kHz contour intervals (see key).
Increasing frequency is represented along a ventro-anterior
to dorso-posterior axis. (from bat P8-7-85).

rostro-caudal direction from **e** to **a**. The area spanned 1200 μm in
the rostro-caudal direction and 100 μm in the medio-lateral
direction. Penetrations where vocalizations could not be elicited
were located at the anterior and posterior borders of the area from
which vocal pulses were elicited; one penetration was made 300 μm
anterior to and before **e**, and one was made 300 μm posterior to and
after **a**. The isofrequency contours in Fig. 6 represent a slice mad
in the sagittal plane that is 300 μm from the midline and includes
in the plane of section 4 of the 5 penetrations. The pattern of
contours in the plane containing penetration **a** was 100 μm lateral t
the one shown and essentially identical to it. The isofrequency
contours span CF_2 frequencies from 59.10-61.20 kHz; however
frequencies between the 59.2-60.4 kHz contours are overrepresented.

    The isofrequency contours show an increasing frequency of
elicited pulses from stimulation sites along an anteroventral-to-
dorsoposterior axis (Fig. 6). The contours are a good prediction o
the pattern of the tonotopic organization, but there are limitation
based on the interpolations of frequency information to create a
frequency grid at all points in space. For example, in Fig. 5 ther
are no data points within the 59.2 kHz contour. It is likely that
the 59.2 kHz contour was produced from the intersection of
information from penetrations **e** (59.10 kHz) and **d** (59.04 kHz).

    In this example, it appears that the samples may have been
deficient in covering the full range of frequencies. An estimate
of the rostro-caudal location of the area from which vocal pulses
were elicited, relative to a reference site on the skull of the bat
supports the idea that higher frequencies are represented more
caudally in the ACg. This bat emitted sounds in a range skewed
towards higher frequencies (Fig. 5) and the area from which pulses
were elicited was displaced more caudally from the reference site
(1900-3100 μm re reference site). In contrast, the area in anothe
bat whose frequency range emphasized more low frequencies was
located more rostrally (1300-2600 μm re reference site).

    It is important to note other possible explanations of the
tonotopic pattern that is described in Fig. 5 and 6. There are two
ways in which the frequency of the elicited vocal pulses may appea
to depend on a different type of map and secondarily the level of
stimulus current. The first proposal is that a gradient of
thresholds exists for eliciting the range of frequencies in biosona
emissions such that equivalent levels of stimulus current yield a
frequency axis. However, the frequency is proportional to neither
absolute nor relative stimulus current; if this were not the case
then any frequency within the limits of the system could be elicite
from any part of the ACg in question. The current required to
reflect the true frequency approaches an asymptote beyond which
there is little change in the frequency or pattern of the
vocalizations.

A second proposal is that the different frequencies were elicited from a "locus of high-frequency vocalization" such that for a given stimulus current at a distance from the site, particular lower frequencies would be elicited. This suggests that at a point distant from the "locus", the "locus frequency" could be elicited by increasing the stimulus current. This second possibility is unlikely since the frequency of elicited pulses is not dependent on stimulus level and because the frequency axis would be expected to be symmetrical about the "locus" whereas the axis is linear. Thus, the ACg appears to be tonotopically organized for the frequencies normally emitted during Doppler-shift compensation.

Neural connections of the anterior cingulate cortex determined with HRP histochemistry

Studies in primates using microstimulation and behavioral tasks have suggested an important role for the ACg in initiating vocalization which is dependent on integration of sensory information and motivational factors (Jürgens 1976b; Sutton et al. 1978; Kirzinger and Jürgens 1982). The ACg in primates has reciprocal connections with secondary auditory cortex (Pandya and Kuypers 1969; Müller-Preuss et al. 1980; Jürgens 1983) suggesting a possible route for auditory-vocal interaction. Since it was found in the present study that vocalizations can also be elicited from the ACg in the mustached bat a study of its neural connections was undertaken to see if a pattern of connections similar to those in other mammals is present. It was of particular interest to determine if a potential source of auditory feedback is available, since microstimulation elicits biosonar emissions identical to those used by the bat in DSC.

The location of the stimulation sites injected with HRP was recovered in 6 bats and significant transport was achieved in 4 of these bats. Moderately- and lightly-labeled cells were found in dorsal frontal cortex on the contralateral side of the brain at the level of the injection site and extending 150 μm caudally. A few cells were found in lateral frontal cortex on both sides of the brain at the level of the injection site. Cells were labeled in layer II of the contralateral ACg. Moderately- and lightly-labeled cells were found predominantly in layers II and III of ipsilateral auditory cortex. In the most rostral portion of auditory cortex labeled cells were located just lateral to the temporal sulcus. Labeled cells were also found in deeper layers located in more caudal portions of auditory cortex.

In the ipsilateral thalamus, many cells in the ventral anterior (VA) and the medial lateral (ML) nuclei were consistently and heavily-labeled. The ipsilateral medial geniculate body of the thalamus contained only one labeled cell in the dorsal division in each of two bats.

In one bat, additional areas containing labeled cells ipsilateral to the injection site were found in the following areas: motor cortex; diagonal band of Broca; claustrum; amygdala; the anterior medial nucleus, n. rhomboidalis and n. reuniens of the thalamus; and n. interpeduncularis of the midbrain. The only terminals labeled by anterograde transport were found bilaterally in the medial pontine nuclei, also in this same bat. The difference between this case and the others examined is that this bat received two deposits of HRP 300 μm apart along the rostral-caudal axis of the ACg. While the extent of the injection sites were restricted to the ACg the cumulative large volume filled by the injection may have contributed to the inclusion of the additional regions described.

DISCUSSION

The present study has focused on vocalizations elicited by electrical microstimulation of a supracallosal region (anterior cingulate cortex) in the brain of the mustached bat, P. parnelli. The characteristics of vocalizations elicited by microstimulation and the organization of stimulation sites in the ACg for emission o biosonar-like vocal pulses were examined. Elicited vocalizations consisted of one of two forms: spectrally-complex sounds with prominent audible components and ultrasonic biosonar pulses. The latter are of great interest because they were essentially indistinguishable from spontaneous biosonar vocalizations and covered the frequency range used by this species for Doppler-shift compensation. In addition, the ACg is tonotopically organized for the frequency of emissions elicited by microstimulation. This is the first demonstration of a functional organization in the mammalian ACg for the control of a specific parameter of a vocal signal. Microstimulation of the ACg produced orofacial and respiratory movements appropriate to the emission of biosonar sounds. Afferents to the ACg were typical of most found in primates. The projections included sources of auditory input via the auditory cortex and medial geniculate body which are potential available for the acoustic feedback necessary for proper DSC. It strongly suggested that the ACg in the mustached bat is vocalization-specific, as indicated for the ACg of primates (Jürge 1976a,b; Jürgens and Müller-Preuss 1977).

Elicited vocal pulses and Doppler-shift compensation

The spectral and temporal characteristics of the elicited vocalizations were similar to natural vocal emissions. The CF_2 component was normally dominant and fell within a band from 57-62 kHz, but was most often elicited at frequencies between 59-61 kHz. The reference frequency of P. parnelli is at the top of this range near 61 kHz (Pollak et al. 1972; Suga et al. 1975; personal obs.). Since the bat emits pulses at frequencies lower than the reference frequency during flight the frequency range of elicited pulses is functionally relevant to DSC behavior. During typical non-target oriented flight P. parnelli attains a velocity of about 4.5 m/s (Novick and Vaisnys 1964). If velocities are small relative to the speed of sound, an estimate of the frequency shift detected by the bat (Schnitzler 1973) is:

$$f_e - f_p = f_p \ (2v/c)$$

where f_p is the frequency of the emitted pulse, f_e is the frequency of the echo, $f_e - f_p$ is the Doppler shift, v is the bat's velocity and c is the speed of sound in air (345 m/s at 23° C). At such velocities, a mustached bat emitting at 60.6 kHz would receive a frequency shift in the echo of about 1.6 kHz. The bat would compensate the frequency shift by emitting subsequent sounds at approximately 1.6 kHz lower (about 59 kHz) than the reference frequency. The lower end of the frequency range of the CF_2 component in elicited biosonar pulses was 57 kHz suggesting that the bat can compensate for even larger Doppler-shifts. Such emissions would occur during pursuit of prey especially during rapid flight maneuvers. Thus, microstimulation of the ACg can elicit biosonar vocalizations in the frequency range used by the bat in typical DSC situations.

The connections of the anterior cingulate cortex

All areas that sent afferents to the ACg in this study have also been reported to project to the ACg (area 24 according to Brodmann, 1909) in the rhesus monkey (Baleydier and Mauguiere 1980), squirrel monkey (Jürgens 1983), and in the rat (Finch et al. 1984).

Because an atlas does not exist for the mustached bat brain the thalamic nuclei were defined primarily from drawings of thalamic nuclei in the horseshoe bat (Henson 1970). The ML as well as the intralaminar nuclei are ill-defined in microchiroptera and the ML may represent a transitional zone within the surrounding nuclei according to Henson (1970). It may be that the ventromedial and lateral clusters of label in the ML are equivalent to labeling in the medial part of the ventral lateral nucleus, and/or the nucleus limitans, central lateral, paracentral and central superior lateral nuclei of the intralaminar group. The medial part of the ventral lateral nucleus (Jürgens 1983) and the intralaminar group (Jürgens 1983; Baleydier and Mauguiere 1980) are typically labeled following injections of HRP into the ACg in monkeys. The projections from the auditory cortex and the medial geniculate body of the thalamus provide two levels of possible input from areas that process acoustic information. The ACg has been reported to have reciprocal connections with secondary auditory cortex in the monkey (Pandya and Kuypers 1969; Jones and Powell 1970; Müller-Preuss and Jürgens 1976; Müller-Preuss et al. 1980; Jürgens 1983). Despite the dense

reciprocal connections between the ACg and the thalamus, there are
no reports in the literature of connections with the medial
geniculate body as were found here. Further study of connections t
ACg is needed in the mustached bat to assess the ascending and
determine the descending pathways.

Elicited vocal pulses with complex spectra

The other type of emission elicited by microstimulation of the
ACg appears similar to calls associated with social behavior. In
contrast to the biosonar emissions, these calls contain a significant amount of energy in the audible frequency range, but have
harmonically-related ultrasonic components as well. There is a
consistent prominence of the audible portion in the spectrally-
complex sounds, however the dominant frequency recorded for
different audible sounds covers a 5 kHz bandwidth. A more dramatic
contrast in the amplitude spectra is the wide variation in the
energy devoted to ultrasonic components of the spectrally-complex
pulses. There does not seem to be any relationship between the
fundamental frequency and the energy devoted to the ultrasonic
portion of the sounds. It is unclear whether changes in the
particular dominant frequency of the audible portion, and the amoun
of energy devoted to the ultrasonic components reflect functional
differences in the communication sounds or modifications of the san
sound. A complete study of the types of social cries elicited fron
this part of the ACg is needed. It will also be important to
determine the effect of electrode location and stimulus parameters
on the amplitude spectra of the complex sounds, and to consider to
what degree individual differences influence the emissions.

Jürgens and Ploog (1970) found that the types of call elicite
by electrical stimulation were dependent on the stimulus strength
well as the site of stimulation in the brain of the squirrel monke
In the mustached bat, the stimulation sites of elicited biosonar
pulses are organized tonotopically in the ACg and the frequency of
the emission is not a function of stimulus intensity. However, th
spectrally-complex sounds elicited from the ACg may be more
analogous to the communication calls elicited from monkeys. The
mustached bat emits about 6 different calls attributed to differen
behavioral situations (Suga pers. comm.; unpubl. obs.), but furthe
studies of the types of sounds elicited from the ACg and other bra
regions are needed to better understand control of vocalization i
the bat and assess the relevance of different sounds in the
behavioral context. For example, it would be interesting if
vocalizations associated with aggressive behavior in the bat could
be elicited from nuclei similar to those homologous systems in the
monkey (growling) and the cat (growling and hissing) which subserv
aggressive vocalizations (amygdala, stria terminalis, ventral
amygdalofugal system, perifornical hypothalamus, periaqueductal gr
a..d mesencephalic tegmentum; Jürgens and Ploog 1970).

A theoretical model for the control of Doppler-shift compensation: a role for the auditory cortex and the anterior cingulate cortex in the control of emitted frequency

The source and functional aspects of auditory feedback for control of biosonar emissions are yet to be fully determined. Kobler et al. (1983) have shown a possible indirect pathway to ACg from auditory cortex via frontal cortex in P. parnelli. Schweizer and Radtke (1980) have found connections between auditory cortex and the cingular area in the CF/FM bat, R. ferrumequinum, and preliminary evidence suggested that the auditory cortex could provide acoustic information to the ACg in P. parnelli (Gooler and O'Neill 1985). The current study confirms the consistently large number of cells labeled in the auditory cortex following HRP injections in the ACg and adds the finding that the dorsal division of the MGB also projects to the ACg.

The proposed model is based on both empirical information derived from microstimulation of the ACg in the mustached bat, experiments by Suga, O'Neill and colleagues on the combination-sensitive neurons in the auditory cortex of the mustached bat, and a theoretical mechanism which explains a possible functional relationship between acoustic input and control of vocal frequency in the ACg. The two initial assumptions of the model are that 1) the ACg subserves control of vocal frequency during DSC, and 2) that information on the magnitude of Doppler-shifts is provided to the ACg by CF/CF neurons of the auditory cortex.

In the auditory cortex of P. parnelli, "CF/CF" combination-sensitive neurons (Suga et al. 1978; Suga et al. 1983) that respond to pairs of CF components are excellent candidates for providing Doppler-shift information. CF_1/CF_2 and CF_1/CF_3 neurons could encode the frequency of the PCF_1 (= CF_1 in the vocal pulse) and either the ECF_2 or ECF_3 (= CF_2 or CF_3 in the echo) respectively. The frequency tuning curves of CF/CF neurons are very sharp suggesting that these neurons are sensitive to precise CF/CF combinations. The magnitude of Doppler-shift could be represented by the degree to which the frequency of the ECF_2 or ECF_3 component differs from a precise harmonic relation with the PCF_1 frequency. While different CF/CF neurons are sensitive to different combinations of frequencies, they could encode the same frequency-shift.

We propose that PCF/ECF pairs coding for equal Doppler-shifts of various magnitude would send information to the locus in the ACg which specifies the frequency of the subsequent vocal pulse needed to produce the appropriate DSC (maintain the echo at the reference frequency = RF). For example, assume the RF is 60 kHz. In this model, the locus in ACg corresponding to a PCF_1 emission at 29 kHz (i.e., PCF_2 = 58 kHz) should receive inputs from CF_1/CF_2 neurons tuned to the following combinations: 28.5/59, 29/60, 29.5/61, 30/62, etc. This sequence should be appropriate for adjusting the emitted frequency in response to any 2 kHz (CF_2) Doppler-shift when the reference frequency is 60 kHz. The model works equally well for either adjusting or maintaining the frequency of the emission to keep the echo at reference frequency. As an example, if a bat is flying at a constant velocity such that emitting a pulse with a CF_1 of 29 kHz provides the compensation needed to maintain the echo at reference frequency (60 kHz), inputs from CF_1/CF_2 neurons activated by a frequency combination of 29/60 kHz will continue to activate the same locus in the ACg and subsequent pulses will remain at 29 kHz (58 kHz).

However, the input from the CF/CF area of auditory cortex coding the Doppler-shift information is probably not sufficient itself to trigger vocalization since mustached bats do not vocalize in response to such acoustic stimuli, however much they resemble the pulse/echo pair. It is likely that the ACg acts to integrate a number of inputs in order to initiate vocalization. A trigger or "enable" input is suggested as a mechanism for influencing the probability of vocalization. The input from the CF/CF area combined with the enable command could summate to exceed the threshold for initiating vocalization. Also, lateral inhibitory circuits ("disable") could function to suppress other elements in ACg from influencing the emission during a particular vocalization.

The source of the putative "enable" command may be the thalamic nuclei VA and ML found in this study to be densely labeled as a result of HRP injections into the ACg. As discussed previously, the ML of microchiropteran bats may be homologous to the intralaminar nuclei or the medial portion of the ventral lateral nucleus, all of which show projections to ACg in primates (Baleydier and Mauguiere 1980; Jürgens 1983). These ventral thalamic nuclei are generally associated with efferent control mechanisms (Poggio and Mountcastle 1980). More specifically, VA is thought to be functionally related to the intralaminar nuclei and it is thought that VA sends synchronous discharges to a broad array of cortical and thalamic regions (Carpenter 1976). The connections of the intralaminar nuclei and VA with the ACg were cited by Baleydier and Mauguiere (1980) as strong suggestions that the ACg is involved in "control the arousal reaction and the programming of kinetic response to sensory stimulation". The functional aspects of efferent motor control, attention and arousal from these thalamic inputs to ACg are at least suggestive of the role of an "enable" command.

In conclusion, the cingulate cortex, as a limbic structure, is thought to take the somewhat segregated functions of sensory integration and motor programing a step further by combining attentional, emotional and motivational factors. Referring to the contrast between the roles of the limbic system and midbrain in primate communication Ploog et al. (1975) stated that "...the limbic system sets the stage for the motivational aspects of communication by evaluating the external world and the internal state of the individual, whereas the midbrain executes the appropriate motor expression of the evaluation process.".

For the echolocating bat the regulation of vocalization via DSC involves not only motor programming of biosonar emissions, but processing of acoustic stimuli which represent a highly biologically significant behavior. Vocalization, whether for purposes of social communication in primates (and for that matter bats) or for foraging and navigation in echolocating bats, is a highly motivated behavior and requires a similar level of attention to sensory cues for success.

REFERENCES

Baleydier, C., and Mauguiere, F., 1980, The duality of the cingulate gyrus in monkey: Neuroanatomical study and functional hypotheses, Brain, 103:525.

Brodmann, K., 1909, Vergleichende Lokalisationslehre Der Grosshirnrinde in ihren Prinzipien dargestellt auf Grund des Zellenbaues, J.A. Barth, Leipzig.

Carpenter, M.B., 1976, The diencephalon, in: "Human Neuroanatomy," M.B. Carpenter, ed., Williams and Wilkins Co., Baltimore.

Finch, D.N., Derian, E.L., and Babb, T.L., 1983, Afferent fibers to rat cingulate cortex. Exp. Neurol., 93:468.

Frisina, R.D., and O'Neill, W.E., 1985, Functional organization of mustached bat inferior colliculus: connections of the FM_2 region, Soc. Neurosci. Abstr., 11:733.

Gabriel, M., Miller, J.D., and Saltwick, S.E., 1977, Unit activity in cingulate cortex and anteroventral thalamus of the rabbit during differential conditioning and reversal, J. Comp. Physiol. Psychol., 91:423.

Goldman, L.J., and Henson, O.W., 1977, Prey recognition and selection by the constant frequency bat, Pteronotus p. parnellii, Behav. Biol. Sociobiol., 2:411.

Gooler, D.M., and O'Neill, W.E., 1985, Central control of frequency in biosonar vocalizations of the mustached bat, Soc. Neurosci. Abstr., 11:547.

Gooler, D.M., and O'Neill, W.E., 1987, Topographic representation of vocal frequency demonstrated by microstimulation of anterior cingulate cortex in the echolocating bat, Pteronotus parnelli parnelli, J. Comp. Physiol., 161:283.

Grinnell, A.D., 1970, Comparative neurophysiology of neotropical
    bats employing different echolocation signals, Z. vergl.
    Physiol., 68:117.

Henson, O.W., 1970, The central nervous system of Chiroptera, in:
    "Biology of Bats," W.A. Wimsatt, ed., Academic Press, New
    York.

Henson, O.W. Jr., Bishop, A., Keating, A., Kobler, J., Henson, M.,
    Wilson, B., and Hansen, R., 1987, Biosonar imaging of insects
    by Pteronotus p. parnellii, the mustached bat, National
    Geographic Res., 3:82.

Jen, P.H-S., and Kamada, T., 1982, Analysis of orientation signals
    emitted by the CF-FM bat, Pteronotus p. parnellii and the FM
    bat, Eptesicus fuscus during avoidance of moving and
    stationary obstacles, J. Comp. Physiol. A, 148:389.

Jones, E.G., and Powell, T.P.S., 1970, An anatomical study of
    converging sensory pathways within the cerebral cortex of the
    monkey, Brain, 93:793.

Jürgens, U., 1976a, Projections from the cortical larynx area in th
    squirrel monkey, Exp. Brain Res., 25:401.

Jürgens, U., 1976b, Reinforcing concomitants of electrically
    elicited vocalizations, Exp. Brain Res., 26:203.

Jürgens, U., 1983, Afferent fibers to the cingulate vocalization
    region in the squirrel monkey, Exp. Neurol., 80:395.

Jürgens, U., and Müller-Preuss, P., 1977, Convergent projections o
    different limbic vocalization areas in the squirrel monkey,
    Exp. Brain Res., 29:75.

Jürgens, U., and Ploog, D., 1970, Cerebral representation of
    vocalization in the squirrel monkey, Exp. Brain Res., 10:532

Jürgens, U., and Pratt, R., 1979a, The cingular vocalization pathw
    in the squirrel monkey, Exp. Brain Res., 34:499.

Jürgens, U., and Pratt, R., 1979b, Role of the periaqueductal grey
    in vocal expression of emotion, Brain Res., 166:367.

Kirzinger, A., and Jürgens, U., 1982, Cortical lesion effects and
    vocalization in the squirrel monkey, Brain Res., 233:299.

Kobler, J.B., Isbey, S.F., and Casseday, J.H., 1983, Evidence for
    connections between auditory cortex and frontal cortex of th
    bat, Pteronotus parnellii, Soc. Neurosci. Abstr., 9:956.

Kobler, J.B., Wilson, B.S., Henson, O.W. Jr., Bishop, A.L., 1985, Echo intensity compensation by echolocating bats, Hearing Res., 20:99.

Konishi, M., Nottebohm, F., 1969, Experimental studies in the ontogeny of avian vocalizations, in: "Bird Song," R. Hinde, ed., Cambridge University Press, London.

Marler, P., 1976, Sensory templates in species-specific behavior, in: "Simpler Networks and Behavior," J.C. Fentress, ed., Sinauer Associates, Sunderland.

Marler, P., and Peters, S., 1977, Selective vocal learning in a sparrow, Science, 198:519.

Mesulam, M.M., 1982, Principles of horseradish peroxidase neurochemistry and their applications for tracing neural pathways - axonal transport, enzyme histochemistry and light microscopic analysis, in: "Tracing Neural Connections with Horseradish Peroxidase," M.M. Mesulam, ed., John Wiley & Sons, Chichester.

Müller-Preuss, P., and Jürgens, U., 1976, Projections from the "cingular" vocalization area in the squirrel monkey, Brain Res., 103:29.

Müller-Preuss, P., Newman, J.D., and Jürgens, U., 1980, Anatomical and physiological evidence for a relationship between 'cingular' vocalization area and the auditory cortex in the squirrel monkey, Brain Res., 202:307.

Neuweiler, G., Bruns, V., and Schuller, G., 1980, Ears adapted for the detection of motion, or how echolocating bats have exploited the capacities of the mammalian auditory system, J. Acoust. Soc. Am., 68:741.

Novick, A., and Griffin, D.R., 1961, Laryngeal mechanisms in bats for the production of the orientation sounds, J. Exp. Zool., 148:125.

Novick, A., and Vaisnys, J.R., 1964, Echolocation of flying insects by the bat, Chilonycteris parnellii, Bio. Bull., 127:478.

Ostwald, J., 1980, The functional organization of the auditory cortex in the CF-FM bat Rhinolophus ferrumequinum, in: "Animal Sonar Systems," R.G. Busnel, and J.F. Fish, eds., Plenum Press, New York.

Pandya, D.N., and Kuypers, H.G.J.M., 1969, Cortico-cortical connections in the rhesus monkey, Brain Res., 13:13.

Ploog, D., Hupfer, K., Jürgens, U., and Newman, J.D., 1975,
    Neuroethologic studies of vocalization in squirrel monkeys
    with special reference to genetic differences of calling in
    two subspecies, in: "Growth and Development of the Brain,
    "M.A.B. Brazier, ed., Raven Press, New York.

Poggio, G.F., and Mountcastle, V.B., 1980, Functional organization
    of thalamus and cortex, in: "Medical Physiology," V.B.
    Mountcastle, ed., CV Mosby Co., St. Louis.

Pollak, G.D., and Bodenhamer, R.D., 1981, Specialized
    characteristics of single units in inferior colliculus of
    mustache bat: frequency representation, tuning, and discharge
    patterns, J. Neurophysiol., 46:605.

Pollak, G.D., Bodenhamer, R.D., and Zook, J.M., 1983, Cochleotopic
    organization of the mustache bat's inferior colliculus, in:
    "Advances in Vertebrate Neuroethology," J.P. Ewert, R.R.
    Capranica, and D.J. Ingle, eds., Plenum, New York.

Pollak, G.D., Henson, O.W., and Novick, A., 1972, Cochlear
    microphonic audiograms in the pure tone bat Chilonycteris
    parnellii parnellii, Science, 176:66.

Pye, J.D., 1980, Echolocation signals and echoes in air, in: "Anim
    Sonar Systems," R.G. Busnel, and J.F. Fish, eds., Plenum
    Press, New York.

Rübsamen, R., and Betz, M., 1986, Control of echolocation pulses i
    the nucleus ambiguus of the rufous horseshoe bat (Rhinolophu
    rouxi) I. Single unit recordings in the motor nucleus of the
    larynx in actively vocalizing bats, J. Comp. Physiol.,
    159:675.

Rübsamen, R., and Schuller, G., 1981, Laryngeal nerve activity
    during pulse emission in the CF-FM bat, Rhinolophus
    ferrumequinum. II. The recurrent laryngeal nerve, J. Comp.
    Physiol., 143:323.

Rübsamen, R., and Schweizer, H., 1986, Control of echolocation
    pulses in the nucleus ambiguus of the rufous horseshoe bat
    (Rhinolophus rouxi) II. Afferent and efferent connections o
    the motor nucleus of the laryngeal nerves, J. Comp. Physiol
    159:689.

Schnitzler, H-U., 1968, Die Ultraschall-Ortungslaute der Hufeisen
    Fledermause (ChiropteraRhinolophidae) in verschiedenen
    Orienter-ungssituationen, Z. vergl. Physiol., 57:376.

Schnitzler, H-U., 1970, Echoortung bei der Fledermaus Chilonycter
    rubiginosa, Z. vergl. Physiol., 68:25.

Schnitzler, H-U., 1973, Control of Doppler shift compensation in the greater horseshoe bat, Rhinolophus ferrumequinum, J. Comp. Physiol., 82:79.

Schnitzler, H-U., Hackbarth, H., Heilmann, U., and Herbert, H., 1985, Echolocation behavior of rufous horseshoe bats hunting for insects in the flycatcher style, J. Comp. Physiol., 157:39.

Schnitzler, H-U., and Flieger, E., 1983, Detection of oscillating target movements by echolocation in the Greater Horseshoe Bat, J. Comp. Physiol., 153:385.

Schnitzler, H-U., Menne, D., Kober, R., and Heblich, K., 1983, The acoustical image of fluttering insects in echolocating bats, in: "Neuroethology and Behavioral Physiology," F. Huber, and H. Markl, eds., Springer-Verlag, Berlin.

Schuller, G., 1977, Echo delay and overlap with emitted orientation sounds and Doppler-shift compensation in the bat, Rhinolophus ferrumequinum, J. Comp. Physiol., 114:103.

Schuller, G., 1979, Coding of small sinusoidal frequency and amplitude modulations in the inferior colliculus of the CF-FM bat, Rhinolophus ferrumequinum, Exp. Brain Res., 34:117.

Schuller, G., 1984, Natural ultrasonic echoes from wing beating insects are encoded by collicular neurons in the CF-FM bat, Rhinolophus ferrumequinum, J. Comp. Physiol., 155:121.

Schuller, G., Beuter, K., and Rübsamen, R., 1975, Dynamic properties of the compensation system of Doppler shifts in the bat Rhinolophus ferrumequinum, J. Comp. Physiol., 97:113.

Schuller, G., Beuter, K., and Schnitzler, H-U., 1974, Response to frequency shifted artificial echoes in the bat Rhinolophus ferrumequinum, J. Comp. Physiol., 89:275.

Schuller, G., and Pollak, G.D., 1979, Disproportionate frequency representation in the inferior colliculus of Doppler-compensating greater horseshoe bats: evidence for an acoustic fovea, J. Comp. Physiol., 132:47.

Schuller, G., and Suga, N., 1976a, Storage of Doppler-shift information in the echolocation system of the CF-FM bat, Rhinolophus ferrumequinum, J. Comp. Physiol., 105:9.

Schuller, G., and Suga, N., 1976b, Laryngeal mechanisms for the emission of CF-FM sounds in the Doppler-shift compensating bat, Rhinolophus ferrumequinum, J. Comp. Physiol., 107:253.

Schweizer, H., 1981, The connections of the inferior colliculus and
    the organization of the brain stem auditory system in the
    greater horseshoe bat (<u>Rhinolophus ferrumequinum</u>), <u>J</u>. <u>Comp</u>.
    <u>Neurol</u>., 201:25.

Schweizer, H., and Radtke, S., 1980, The auditory pathway of the
    greater horseshoe bat, <u>Rhinolophus ferrumequinum</u>, <u>in</u>: "Animal
    Sonar Systems," R.G. Busnel, and J.F. Fish, eds., Plenum
    Press, New York.

Schweizer, H., Rübsamen, R., and Ruehle, C., 1981, Localization of
    brain stem motor neurons innervating the laryngeal muscles in
    the rufous horseshoe bat, <u>Rhinolophus</u> <u>rouxi</u>, <u>Brain</u> <u>Res</u>.,
    230:41.

Suga, N., 1984, Neural mechanisms of complex-sound processing for
    echolocation, <u>Trends</u> <u>Neurosci</u>., 7:20.

Suga, N., and Jen, P.H-S., 1976, Disproportionate tonotopic
    representation for processing CF-FM sonar signals in the
    mustached bat auditory cortex, <u>Science</u>, 194:542.

Suga, N., and Jen, P.H-S., 1977, Further studies on the peripheral
    auditory system of CF-FM bats specialized for fine frequency
    analysis of Doppler-shifted echoes, <u>J</u>. <u>Exp</u>. <u>Biol</u>., 69:207.

Suga, N., O'Neill, W.E., Kujirai, K., and Manabe, T., 1983,
    Specificity of "combination sensitive" neurons for processing
    complex biosonar signals in the auditory cortex of the
    mustached bat, <u>J</u>. <u>Neurophysiol</u>., 49:1573.

Suga, N., O'Neill, W.E., and Manabe, T., 1978, Cortical neurons
    sensitive to combinations of information-bearing elements of
    biosonar signals in the mustached bat. <u>Science</u>, 200:778.

Suga, N., Schlegel, P., Shimozawa, T., and Simmons, J.A., 1973,
    Orientation sounds evoked from echolocating bats by electrical
    stimulation of the brain, <u>J</u>. <u>Acoust</u>. <u>Soc</u>. <u>Am</u>., 54:793.

Suga, N., Simmons, J.A., and Jen,P.H-S., 1975, Peripheral
    specialization for fine analysis of Doppler-shifted echoes in
    the auditory system of the CF-FM bat, <u>Pteronotus</u> <u>parnellii</u>, <u>J</u>.
    <u>Exp</u>. <u>Biol</u>., 63:161.

Suga, N., Simmons, J.A., and Shimozawa, T., 1974, Neurophysiological
    studies on echolocation systems in awake bats producing CF-FM
    orientation sounds, <u>J</u>. <u>Exp</u>. <u>Biol</u>., 61:379.

Suthers, R.A., and Fattu, J.M., 1973, Mechanisms of sound production
    by echolocating bats, <u>Amer</u>. <u>Zool</u>., 13:1215.

Sutton, D., Samson, H.H., and Larson, C.R., 1978, Brain mechanisms
    in learned phonation of Macaca mulatta, in: "Recent Advances
    in Primatology," D.J. Chivers, and J. Herbert, eds., Academic
    Press, New York.

Sutton, D., Trachy, R.E., and Lindeman, R.C., 1981, Primate
    phonation: unilateral and bilateral cingulate lesion effects,
    Behav. Brain Res., 3:99.

Trappe, M., and Schnitzler, H-U., 1982, Doppler-shift compensation
    in insect-catching horseshoe bats, Naturwissenshaften, 69:193.

Wetzel, D.M., Kelley, D.B., and Campbell, B.A., 1980, Central
    control of ultrasonic vocalizations in neonatal rats.
    I.brainstem motor nuclei, J. Comp. Physiol. Psychol., 94:596.

Yajima, Y., Hayashi, Y., and Yoshii, N., 1980, The midbrain central
    gray substance as a highly sensitive neural structure for the
    production of ultrasonic vocalization in the rat, Brain Res.,
    198:446.

EVOLUTION OF AUDIOVOCAL COMMUNICATION AS REFLECTED BY THE THERAPSID-MAMMALIAN TRANSITION AND THE LIMBIC THALAMOCINGULATE DIVISION

Paul D. MacLean

Laboratory of Clinical Science, NIMH
P.O. Box 289
Poolesville, MD   20837

In the evolutionary transition from reptiles to mammals three key developments were (1) nursing, conjoined with maternal care, (2) audiovocal communication for maintaining maternal-offspring contact, and (3) play behavior (MacLean, 1985). There is accumulating evidence that the full expression of this family related behavioral triad depended on the evolution of the thalamocingulate division of the limbic system (MacLean, 1986a). This name derives from the fact that the transitional cingulate cortex of the limbic lobe receives its main afferent connections from the thalamus. Significantly, there is no apparent counterpart of this subdivision in the reptilian brain (Clark and Meyer, 1950).

The present article deals with the neurobehavioral evolution of that component of the family related triad concerned with audiovocal communication for maintaining maternal-offspring contact. It focuses specifically on the origin and cerebral representation of the separation cry which perhaps ranks as the first and most basic mammalian vocalization.

The Therapsid-Mammalian Transition

It is commonly assumed that all land vertebrates vocalize, but this is not true of most lizards, and it may not have been true of the antecedents of mammals--the so-called mammal-like reptiles. The cactus tree in Fig. 1 depicts the lineage of mammals leading back to Permian times when the synapsids arose from the anapsid stem reptiles. The advanced mammal-like reptiles are taxonomically characterized as therapsids because the temporal fossa has a resemblance to that of true mammals. Two

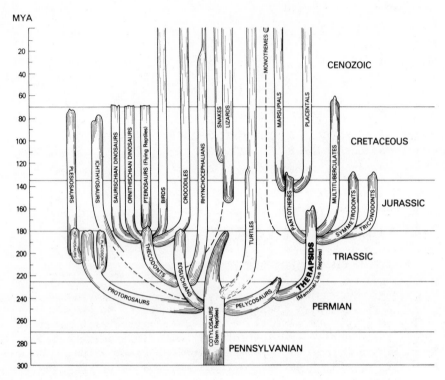

Fig. 1. Cactus tree, depicting the evolutionary radiation of
         reptiles. The rightmost branch gives emphasis to the
         therapsid line leading to mammals. MYA, million years
         ago (from MacLean, 1985).

hundred and fifty million years ago when there was but one giant
continent, now referred to by Wegener's term Pangaea (1915), the
therapsids roamed every part of it, including Antarctica, not far
from the Karroo beds of South Africa, where according to Robert
Broom (1932), there still lie the remains of 800 billion mammal-
like reptiles. Most of the therapsids were either carnivores or
herbivores (Romer, 1966). The carnivores are the presumed antecedents of mammals (see Hotton et al., 1986, for recent review).
Skeletal reconstructions suggest that they were dog-like or
badger-like in appearance. Significantly, in regard to the present topic, it is the region of the ear and jaw joint that most
clearly differentiates the therapsids from mammals. Whereas
mammals have a single articulation between the dentary and
squamous bones, therapsids had an extra articulation involving
the small quadrate and articular bones that allows the swallowing of large masses of unchewed food. The migration of these

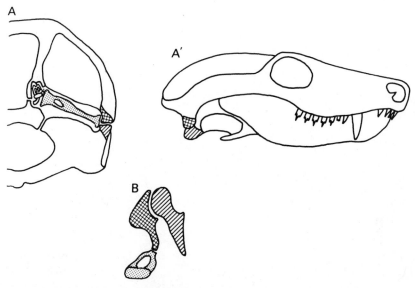

Fig. 2.   Representation of two small bones of the therapsid jaw
          joint that become transformed into the malleus and incus
          of the mammalian middle ear. A and A′, cross-section
          and lateral view of a therapsid skull showing position
          of the articular (diagonal shading) and quadrate
          (crosshatch) bones in jaw joint. B, shading identifies
          corresponding bones in mammalian middle ear (adapted
          from Romer, 1966).

two small bones to become the malleus and incus of the mammalian
ear (Fig. 2) represents, in Colbert's words, "one of the most
remarkable transformations...in the history of vertebrate evolution" (1969, p. 251).

     Because its skeleton was so lizard-like, one of the primi-
tive mammal-like reptiles is called Varanosaurus, after the
monitor lizard, of which the Komodo dragon is the most striking
example. The auditory apparatus of the synapsids generally
was also lizard-like (Barghusen, 1986), consisting of a tympanic
membrane and a stapes abutting upon the internal ear. In all
the synapsids the stapes has end-on contact with the ventral
portion of the quadrate (Fig. 3). The presence of this contact
indicates that the quadrate transmitted sound vibrations.

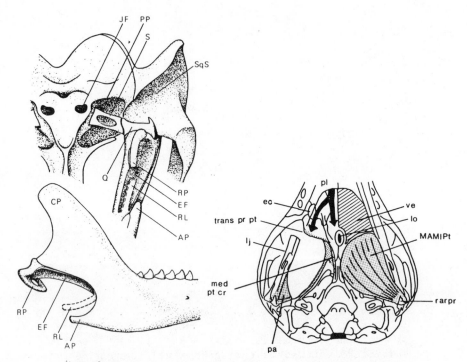

Fig. 3.   (left) Ventral view of skull of a therapsid cynodont
           (<u>Exaeretodon</u>), with lateral view of mandible underneath.
           Upper figure is used to illustrate that in all synapsids,
           the stapes (S) has an end-on contact with the ventral
           portion of the quadrate (Q). This articulation indi-
           cates that the quadrate transmitted sound vibrations.
           Other abbreviations: AP, angular process; CP, coronoid
           process of dentary; EF, external fossa of body of angu-
           lar (=tympanic); JF, jugular foramen; PP, paroccipital
           process of petrosal; RL, reflected lamina of angular;
           RP, retroarticular process of articular (=neck and
           manubrium of malleus); SqS, squamosal sulcus (from
           Allin, 1986).

Fig. 4.   (right) Ventral view of skull and lower jaw of the
           therapsid <u>Thrinaxodon</u>. The stippled area on the right
           side indicates the areas of bony attachment of the
           posterior ptyerygoid muscle (MAMIPt), respective parts
           of which are inferred to have been the origin of both
           the mammalian <u>tensor</u> <u>tympani</u> and <u>tensor</u> <u>veli</u> <u>palatini</u>.
           Arrows indicate medial and lateral air passages. Other
           abbreviations: lj, lower jaw; lo, laryngeal opening;
           med pt cr, medial ptyerygoid crest; pa, prearticular;
           r ar pr, retroarticular process of the articular; ve,
           velum (from Barghusen, 1986).

Since the ear structure of the mammal-like reptiles was comparable to that of lizards, it suggests that they were hard of hearing (Hotton, 1959; Allin, 1975) and possibly like most lizards did not vocalize. Westoll (1945, 1965), however, has suggested that the recessus mandibularis of cynodonts functioned not only as a detector of air-borne sound, but also as a vocal resonating amplifier.

A few other evolutionary details require consideration. Barghusen (1986) has provided further evidence supporting the suggestion that the reptilian pterygoideus musculature involved in movements of the jaw is the source of both the mammalian tensor tympani and tensor veli palatini muscles (Fig. 4). Here again it is to be noted that, posteriorly, the pterygoid bone of cynodonts has a configuration like that of extant lizards. Barghusen points out that the insertion of the tensor tympani on the malleus of mammals compares to the insertion of internal pterygoid on the articular bone in a cynodont therapsid. Similarly the tensor veli palatini in mammals compares to the most lateral part of the origin of the posterior pterygoid in cynodonts. Finally, Barghusen suggests that the lateral nasopharyngeal passage in cynodonts leads to the formation of the auditory tube in mammals (cf. Fig. 4). Hence, he argues that neither the tensor muscles nor the auditory tube represent de novo structures in mammals.

As Allin (1986) has commented, "Existing mammals are unique in ear structure and generally perceive sound frequencies far above the range of all other vertebrates" (p. 238). In the earliest true mammals, the middle ear compares to that of recent mammals. In other words, the articular and quadrate bones had completed their migration and become transformed into malleus and incus of the broadly tuned mammalian ear. This means that the ear had been largely liberated from noise produced by chewing movements of the jaw joint.

The presence of milk teeth in early mammals is presumptive evidence that they suckled their young. If, as now believed, the tiny, early mammals were nocturnal and avoided predators by living within the dark floor of the forest, audiovocal communication would have been a valuable adjunct to olfaction and vision in maintaining maternal-offspring contact. If that capacity existed, the separation cry characteristic of extant mammals may represent the most primitive and basic mammalian vocalization.

These considerations call attention to a great difference between the parent-offspring relationship of mammals and that of most lizards. The female lizard of most species lays her eggs and then leaves them to hatch on their own. If the little hatchlings were to announce their presence by a separation cry, their parents might search them out and eat them. The young of the Komodo dragon, for example, must escape to the trees for the first year of life lest they be cannibalized (Auffenberg, 1978). Infant mammals, on the contrary, cannot survive for long without the sustenance of a nursing mother.

Since the separation cry helps to establish bonding between parent and offspring, and since it is used later in life as a means of maintaining contact among members of a group, it is of fundamental interest to obtain an understanding of its evolutionary development and cerebral representation.

Relevent Aspects of Forebrain Evolution

Based on the few available cranial endocasts, the cerebral hemispheres of fairly advanced therapsids were relatively long and narrow and accordingly more reptilian than mammalian in configuration. Elsewhere I have discussed some of the possible cortical changes that may have accounted for the broadening of the brain seen in a primitive mammal (MacLean, 1986b), as illustrated by comparison of a cranial endocast prepared by Simpson (1927) with one of a cynodont described by Watson (1913).

In its continued evolution, the mammalian forebrain has developed as a triune amalgamation of three neural assemblies (Fig. 5) that anatomically and chemically reflect an ancestral relationship to reptiles, early mammals, and late mammals (MacLean, 1970, 1973). The counterpart of the protoreptilian forebrain comprises parts of the so-called basal ganglia, including the olfactostriatum and corpus striatum. The part of the forebrain identified with early mammals corresponds to the so-called limbic system (MacLean, 1952) represented predominately by the cortex of the great limbic lobe and structures of the brainstem with which it has primary connections. In reptiles and birds the limbic cortex is rudimentary and only partially represented. The neomammalian brain comprises the neocortex and structures of the brainstem with which it is primarily connected. (Some anatomists regard the subcortical ganglionic masses in the dorsal ventricular ridge of reptiles and birds as neocortex.)

Contrary to the traditional view that the protoreptilian complex is simply part of the motor apparatus, we have found that in animals as diverse as lizards and monkeys this complex is essential for the evocation of displays used in animal communication (MacLean, 1978; Greenberg et al., 1979). Other evidence indicates that it is vital for the orchestration of the daily master routine and subroutines (see MacLean, 1985).

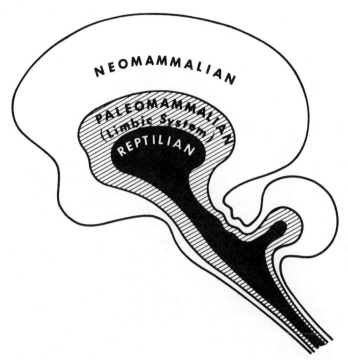

Fig. 5.   Schematic of triune evolution of the mammalian brain.
The three basic neural assemblies that anatomically and
biochemically reflect an ancestral relationship to
reptiles, early mammals, and late mammals are labeled
at the level of the forebrain (from MacLean, 1967).

As schematized in Fig. 6, the limbic system comprises three
main cortico-subcortical subdivisions (MacLean, 1973). The two
divisions associated, respectively, with telencephalic nuclei
of the amygdala and septum are closely related to the olfactory
apparatus. The amygdala division has been shown to be involved
in self-preservation as it pertains to feeding and the struggle
to obtain food, whereas the septal division mediates sexual
functions requisite for the survival of the species.

As mentioned in the introduction, the third division referred
to as the thalamocingulate division appears to have a representation of three forms of behavior not found in lizards--namely,
nursing conjoined with maternal care; audiovocal communication for
maintaining maternal-offspring contact; and play. Significantly

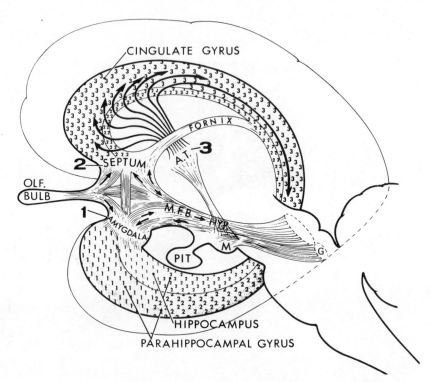

Fig. 6.   Diagram of three main cortico-subcortical divisions
          of the limbic system identified by the numerals 1, 2,
          and 3. The present focus is on the thalamocingulate
          division and its functions pertaining to family related
          behavior, including the separation cry. Abbreviations:
          AT, anterior thalamic nuclei; G, dorsal and ventral
          tegmental nuclei of Gudden; HYP, hypothalamus; MFB,
          medial forebrain bundle; PIT, pituitary; OLF, olfac-
          tory (after MacLean, 1973).

in this regard, as was also noted, there appears to be no counterpart of this division in the reptilian brain.

Cerebral Representation of Separation Cry

     Given this background, we focus now on the part of our topic
concerned with the cerebral representation of the separation cry.
Infant mammals of all species examined thus far have been found
to emit separation cries. It was first recognized in 1954
(Anderson, 1954) that the separation calls of some small rodents
are ultrasonic, serving perhaps to avert detection by predators
such as owls (Okon, 1972; Smith and Sales, 1980). As illustrated
in Fig. 7 by the spectrograms of a squirrel monkey, macaque,

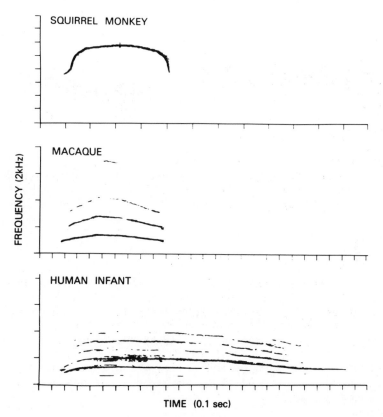

Fig. 7. Sound spectrograms of separation cries of a squirrel
monkey, a macaque, and a human infant. In primates,
such cries have the basic pattern of a slowly changing
tone (adapted from Newman 1985a; from MacLean, 1985).

and human infant, the separation cries of primates have the characteristic of a slowly changing tone (Newman, 1985a). According
to Newman (1985a), this characteristic is indicative of a
"conservative evolutionary history."

    In neurobehavioral studies on species-typical behavior I
have used two varieties of squirrel monkeys that I originally
identified as "gothic" and "roman" because of the shape of the
circumocular patch (MacLean, 1964). Hershkovitz (1984) has
concluded that these varieties represent two main species that
he designates as Saimiri sciureus and Saimiri boliviensis. These
monkeys show distinctive differences in their displays (MacLean,
1964). As illustrated by Fig. 8, the late Peter Winter (1969)
found that these same varieties could be just as readily distinguished by differences in their separation cries (or isolation
peeps as termed by Winter et al., 1966). There is evidence that
these differences are genetically determined (Newman, 1985b).

14 k Hz
12
10
8
6

500 msec

Fig. 8.   Sound spectrograms of separation cries of a gothic- and
roman-type monkeys. Their spectrograms are respectively
distinguished by the downward and upward terminations
(recordings by Newman from MacLean, 1985).

Since adult squirrel monkeys emit separation cries under
experimental conditions, Newman and I have used these animals
in our studies on the cerebral representation of such calls.
We test adult monkeys for their ability to produce separation
cries before and after ablation of different parts of the brain.
Criterion performance is the production of 20 or more spontaneous
calls during a 15-minute period of isolation in a sound-reducing
chamber. Under these conditions such vocalizations are referred
to as isolation calls.

In the initial study we found that electrocoagulation of
structures at the thalamo-midbrain junction resulted in an alteration of the structure of the call (Newman and MacLean, 1982).
Lesions of the ventral central gray and contiguous parts of the
central tegmental tract were followed by a marked reduction in
the production of the call, but no alteration in its structure.
The question then arose as to what parts of the forebrain influence the production of the call. Since the original findings
of Wilbur Smith in 1945, it has been recognized that the rostral
cingulate cortex is the most effective cortical locus for eliciting vocalization in the rhesus monkey (Kaada, 1951; Robinson,
1967). Stimulation involving this region also elicits vocalization in the squirrel monkey (Dua and MacLean, 1964; Jürgens and
Ploog, 1970). It deserves emphasis that in the monkey stimulation of any part of the neocortex fails to elicit vocalization
(see Ploog, 1981, p. 37).

Consequently, Newman and I focused next on the midline
frontolimbic cortex. By the process of elimination, we have
identified a continuous band of limbic cortex implicated in the
spontaneous production of the isolation call (Newman and MacLean,

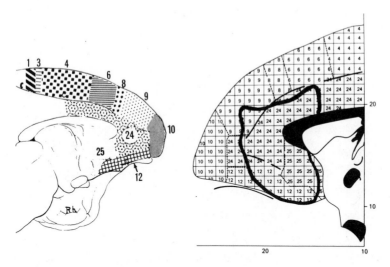

Fig. 9. Representations of midline frontal cortex of squirrel
monkey, with numbers for Rosabal's (1967) cytoarchitectural areas (A) inserted into mm squares (B) conforming to
planes of brain atlas (Gergen and MacLean, 1962). B,
encircled region shows extent of ablation (largely
limited to limbic areas 24, 25, and 12) requisite for
elimination of the spontaneous isolation call (separation cry). (A, adapted from Rosabal, 1967; B, adapted
from MacLean and Newman, 1988.)

1985; MacLean and Newman, 1988). Pregenual lobotomy or lobectomy, but not prefrontal lobectomy, resulted in failure to
produce spontaneous isolation calls. The results of the pregenual lesions did not answer the question as to whether or not
severance of connections with the midline or lateral cortex
rostral to the lesions, or the midline cortex caudal to the
lesions, accounts for the deficit. Hence, it was significant
that in one subject, a large bilateral ablation of the midline
cortex was sufficient to eliminate the call. In this animal,
an ablation of a large part of areas 8 and 9 together with
limbic areas 24, 25, and caudal part area 12, resulted in a
virtual elimination of the isolation call during the 8 months
of testing before sacrifice. In another case in which the
ablation was further limited to the supragenual, pregenual,
subcallosal, and preseptal limbic cortex (Fig. 9B), the subject
failed in calling during the 16 successive weeks in which it
was tested. Significantly, aspiration of all the midline neocortex peripheral to this zone was soon followed by recovery of
calling at the preoperative level. It must also be emphasized
that ablations of parts of the limbic zone in question had no

enduring effect on the call. Consequently, the findings indicate
that the spontaneous call depends on the concerted action of a
continuous band of frontolimbic cortex comprising parts of
areas 24, 25, and 12.

Questions Hinging on Answers Regarding Thalamic Connections

        It has long been recognized that, with the exception of the
midline polar area, ablations of the midline frontal cortex fail
to result in clearly defined retrograde degeneration in the thalamus. In 1964, for example, Akert commented: "The existence in
rhesus monkey of athalamic frontal areas is already suggested by
the work of Walker (1938, Fig. 39)....[F]rontal granular cortex
consists of two principal regions: one (lateral-ventral) which
receives essential projections from the medial dorsal nucleus,
and another (dorsal-medial) which receives no essential projections from the thalamus and at most may be supplied by sustaining
ones" (pp. 380-81). Because of this I am employing cytochemical
tracing techniques to obtain clarification of this matter. In
the first phase of the work, it has been the purpose to demonstrate the presence or absence of midline limbic and neocortical
areas with the thalamus, using wheat germ agglutinin conjugated
to horseradish peroxidase (WGA-HRP). The results obtained with
this substance support, in general, what others have found upon
application of HRP alone to the anterior cingulate cortex in the
squirrel monkey (Jürgens, 1983) and the macaque (Baleydier and
Mauguiere, 1980). On the basis of my own additional findings
on the subcallosal cortex, it would appear as a generalization
that the area of limbic cortex implicated in the separation cry
receives connections from the following thalamic nuclei: reuniens,
anterior medial and ventral, densocellularis, parataenial,
superolateral central, dorsal and caudal parts of medial dorsal,
medial pulvinar, limitans, parafascicularis, and the magnocellular
part of ventralis anterior (VAmc) and medial part of ventralis
lateralis (VLm).

        It will be recalled that the last-mentioned nuclei (VAmc
and VLm) receive connections from the substantia nigra, while
the principal part of VA and oral portion of VL are innervated
by the medial segment of the globus pallidus (see Carpenter, 1976,
for review). When neurosurgical procedures were being used for
the treatment of Parkinson's disease, it was found that stimulation of the inner pallidum or of VL elicited laughing (Hassler,
1961), whereas coagulations of the pallidum on one side and VL
on the other resulted in pathological crying (Krayenbühl et al.,
1961). Based on the new anatomical findings and an assortment
of clinical data in regard to limbic epilepsy, I have suggested
that there exists a linkage of thalamocingulate, striopallidoni-
gral, and cerebellar mechanisms implicated in both the feeling
and expression of crying and laughter (MacLean, 1987).

The finding of parafascicular connections with the medial
frontolimbic cortex is of interest to consider in regard to the
distressful (or what otherwise might be called "painful") nature
of the separation cry, both as it applies to infants and adults.
In this respect, it may be significant that according to the
findings and illustrations in one report (Wise and Herkenham,
1982) there is a high concentration of opiate receptors in the
cingulate cortex of the rhesus monkey. As Panksepp (1981) and
others have shown in non-primate mammals, Newman and co-workers
(1982) have found that small doses of morphine sulphate suppress
the separation cry of squirrel monkeys, whereas the antagonist
Naloxone, restores the cry. In 1957 Foltz and White reported
that ablations of the anterior cingulate cortex alleviated the
symptoms of morphine withdrawal. Such considerations suggest
that more than the fleeting effects of euphoria, those suffering
from opiate addiction may seek release from ineffable feelings
of loneliness, alienation, and isolation (MacLean, 1986a).

Finally, in connection with the present discussion, the earlier consideration of the therapsid-mammalian transition invites
reflection regarding what is referred to as directional evolution.
As Crompton and Jenkins (1973) have commented, it is remarkable
that "the incorporation of the quadrate and articular into the
middle ear must have occurred independently in therian and non-
therian lines" (p. 139). In like vein, one could cite several
other examples of such directional evolution among different
lines spanning the therapsid-mammalian transition (see MacLean,
1986b, for further discussion). In regard to the present topic
and the evolution of Recent mammals, there are neuroanatomic
indications of directional evolution pertaining to the frontal
cortex and its thalamic connections, particularly as reflected
in primates. Although the medial dorsal nucleus might in some
respects be regarded as the most typical mammalian thalamic
nucleus, I will focus here on the frontal connections of the VA
complex (see Carmel, 1970). With injections of WGA-HRP further
and further towards the frontal pole and then backwards in the
neocortex to the rostral supplementary area (MacLean, unpublished;
see also Jürgens, 1984, re supplementary area), the labeling in
the VA complex appears to extend more and more laterally, as
though, in a figurative sense, one were unrolling a scroll or
opening a fan. Such connections help to clarify the verified
findings of Starzl and Magoun (1951) more than 35 years ago that
VA appeared to be central to a short-latency, diffuse thalamic
projecting system affecting predominantly the frontal cortex,
but also accounting for widespread cortical responses elsewhere.
Hence the present studies apply not only to mechanisms of crying
and laughter, but also to global functions of the frontal lobe,
including functions depending on an integration of past memory,
memory of on-going experience, and "memory of the future."
Judged by human behavior, it was as though there were a directional

evolution towards the development of a concern not only for the feelings and future welfare of human beings, but also for all living things.

References

Akert, K., 1964, Comparative anatomy of frontal cortex and thalamofrontal connections, in: "The Frontal Granular Cortex and Behaviour," J.M. Warren and K. Akert eds., McGraw-Hill.

Allin, E.F., 1975, Evolution of the mammalian middle ear, J. Morph. 147:403.

Allin, E.F., 1986, The auditory apparatus of advanced mammal-like reptiles and early mammals, in: "The Ecology and Biology of Mammal-like Reptiles," N. Hotton III, P.D. MacLean, J.J. Roth, and E.C. Roth eds., Smithsonian Institution Press, Washington/London.

Anderson, J.W., 1954, The production of ultrasonic sounds by laboratory rats and other mammals, Science 119:808.

Auffenberg, W., 1978, Social and feeding behavior in Varanus komodoensis, in: "The Behavior and Neurology of Lizards," N. Greenberg and P.D. MacLean eds., U.S. Government Printing Office, Washington, DHEW Publication, No. (ADM) 77-491.

Baleydier, C. and Mauguiere, F., 1980, The duality of the cingulate gyrus in monkey. Neuroanatomical study and functional hypothesis, Brain 103:525.

Barghusen, H.R., 1986, On the evolutionary origin of the therian tensor veli palatini and tensor tympani muscles, in: "The Ecology and Biology of Mammal-like Reptiles," N. Hotton III, P.D. MacLean, J.J. Roth, and E.C. Roth eds., Smithsonian Institution Press, Washington/London.

Broom, R., 1932, "The Mammal-like Reptiles of South Africa and the Origin of Mammals," H.F. and G. Witherby, London.

Carmel, P.W., 1970, Efferent projections of the ventral anterior nucleus of the thalamus in the monkey, Am. J. Anat. 128:159.

Carpenter, M.B., 1976, Anatomical organization of the corpus striatum and related nuclei, in: "The Basal Ganglia," Res. Publ. Ass. Res. Nerv. Ment. Dis., 55:1.

Clark, W.E.LeG. and Meyer, M., 1950, Anatomical relationships between the cerebral cortex and the hypothalamus, Brit. Med. Bull. 6:341.

Colbert, E.H., 1969, "Evolution of the Vertebrates," John Wiley & Sons, Inc., New York.

Crompton, A.W. and Jenkins, F.A. Jr., 1973, Mammals from reptiles: A review of mammalian origins, Ann. Rev. Earth Plan. Sci. 1:131.

Dua, S. and MacLean, P.D., 1964, Localization for penile erection in medial frontal lobe, Amer. J. Physiol. 207:1425.

Foltz, E.L. and White, L.E., Jr., 1957, Experimental cingulumotomy and modification of morphine withdrawal, J. Neurosurg. 14:655.

Greenberg, N., MacLean, P.D., and Ferguson, L., 1979, Role of
    the paleostriatum in species-typical display behavior of the
    lizard (Anolis carolinensis), Brain Res. 172:229.
Gergen, J.A. and MacLean, P.D., 1962, "A Stereotaxic Atlas of the
    Squirrel Monkey's Brain (Saimiri sciureus)", U.S. Government
    Printing Office, Washington, PHS Publication No. 933.
Hassler, R., 1961, Motorische und sensible Effekte umschriebener
    Reizungen und Ausschaltungen im menschlichen Zwischenhirn,
    Deutsche Zeitschrift für Nervenheilkunde 183:148.
Hershkovitz, P., 1984, Taxonomy of squirrel monkeys genus
    Saimiri (Cebidae, Platyrrhini): A preliminary report with
    description of a hitherto unnamed form, Amer. J. of Primatology
    7:155.
Hotton, N., III, 1959, The pelycosaur tympanum and early evolu-
    tion of the middle ear, Evolution 13:99.
Hotton, N., III, MacLean, P.D., Roth, J.J., and Roth, E.C., 1986,
    "The Ecology and Biology of Mammal-Like Reptiles," Smithsonian
    University Press, Washington/London.
Jürgens, U., 1983, Afferent fibers to the cingular vocalization
    region in the squirrel monkey, Experimental Neurology 80:395.
Jürgens, U., 1984, The efferent and afferent connections of the
    supplementary motor area, Brain Res. 300:63.
Jürgens, U. and Ploog, D., 1970, Cerebral representation of vo-
    calization in the squirrel monkey, Exp. Brain Res. 10:532.
Kaada, B.R., 1951, Somato-motor, autonomic and electrocortico-
    graphic responses to electrical stimulation of 'rhinencephalic'
    and other structures in primates, cat, and dog. A study of
    responses from the limbic, subcallosal, orbito-insular, piri-
    form and temporal cortex, hippocampus-fornix and amygdala,
    Acta Physiol. Scand. 23:Suppl. 83, 1.
Krayenbühl, H., Wyss, O.A.M., and Yasargil, M.G., 1961, Bilateral
    thalamotomy and pallidotomy as treatment for bilateral Par-
    kinsonism, J. Neurosurg. 18:429.
MacLean, P.D., 1952, Some psychiatric implications of physiolog-
    ical studies on frontotemporal portion of limbic system
    (visceral brain), Electroencephalogr. Clin. Neurophysiol. 4:407.
MacLean, P.D., 1964, Mirror display in the squirrel monkey,
    Saimiri sciureus, Science 146:950.
MacLean, P.D., 1967, The brain in relation to empathy and
    medical education, J. Nerv. Ment. Dis. 144:374.
MacLean, P.D., 1970, The triune brain, emotion, and scientific
    bias, in: "The Neurosciences Second Study Program," F.O.
    Schmitt, ed., The Rockefeller University Press, New York.
MacLean, P.D., 1973, A triune concept of the brain and behavior.
    Lecture I. Man's reptilian and limbic inheritance; Lecture II.
    Man's limbic brain and the psychoses; Lecture III. New trends
    in man's evolution, in: "The Hincks Memorial Lectures,"
    T. Boag and D. Campbell eds., University of Toronto Press,
    Toronto.

MacLean, P.D., 1978, Effects of lesions of the globus pallidus on species-typical display behavior of squirrel monkeys, Brain Res. 149:175.

MacLean, P.D., 1985, Brain evolution relating to family, play, and the separation call, Arch. Gen. Psychiatry 42:405.

MacLean, P.D., 1986a, Culminating developments in the evolution of the limbic system: the thalamocingulate division, in: "The Limbic System: Functional Organization and Clinical Disorders," B.K. Doane and K.F. Livingston, eds., Raven Press, New York.

MacLean, P.D., 1986b, Neurobehavioral significance of the mammal-like reptiles (therapsids), in: "The Ecology and Biology of the Mammal-like Reptiles," Hotton, N., MacLean, P.D., Roth, J.J., and Roth, E.C. eds., Smithsonian Institution Press, Washington/London.

MacLean, P.D., 1987, The midline frontolimbic cortex and the evolution of crying and laughter, in: "The Frontal Lobes Revisited," E. Perecman, ed., The IRBN Press, New York.

MacLean, P.D. and Newman, J.D., 1988, Role of midline fronto-limbic cortex in production of the isolation call of squirrel monkeys, Brain Res. 450:111.

Newman, J.D., 1985a, The infant cry of primates. An evolutionary persepctive, in: "Infant Crying: Theoretical and Research Perspectives," B.M. Lester and C.F.Z. Boukydis, eds., Plenum Press, New York.

Newman, J.D., 1985b, Squirrel monkey communication, in: "Handbook of Squirrel Monkey Research," L.A. Rosenblum and C.L. Coe, eds., Plenum Press, New York.

Newman, J.D. and MacLean, P.D., 1982, Effects of tegmental lesions on the isolation call of squirrel monkeys, Brain Res. 232:317.

Newman, J.D. and MacLean, P.D., 1985, Importance of medial frontolimbic cortex in production of the isolation call of squirrel monkeys, Neurosci. Abstr. 16:495.

Newman, J.D., Murphy, M.R., and Harbaugh, C.R., 1982, Naloxone-reversible suppression of isolation call production after morphine injections in squirrel monkeys, Neurosci. Abstr. 8:940.

Okon, E.E, 1972, Factors affecting ultrasonic production in infant rodents, J. Zool. (Lond.) 168:139.

Panksepp, J., Herman, B., Conner, R., Bishop, P., and Scott, J.P., 1978, The biology of social attachments: Opiates alleviate separation distress, Biol. Psychiat. 13:607.

Ploog, D.W., 1981, Neurobiology of primate audio-vocal behavior, Brain Res. Rev. 3:35.

Robinson, B.W., 1967, Vocalization evoked from forebrain in Macaca mulatta, Physiol. Behav. 2:345.

Romer, A.S., 1966, "Vertebrate Paleontology," University of Chicago, Chicago.

Rosabal, F., 1967, Cytoarchitecture of the frontal lobe of
the squirrel monkey, J. Comp. Neurol., 130:87.

Simpson, G.G., 1927, Mesozoic mammalia, IX. The brain of
Jurassic mammals, Am. J. Sci. 214:259.

Smith, J.C. and Sales, G.D., 1980, Ultrasonic behavior and
mother-infant interactions in rodents, in: "Maternal Influences and Early Behavior," Bell, R.W. and Smotherman, W.P.,
eds., S.P. Medical and Scientific Books, New York/London.

Smith, W.K., 1945, The functional significance of the rostral
cingular cortex as revealed by its responses to electrical
excitation, J. Neurophysiol. 8:241.

Starzl, T.E. and Magoun, H.W., 1951, Organization of the diffuse
thalamic projection system, J. Neurophysiol. 14:133.

Walker, A.E., 1938, "The Primate Thalamus," University of Chicago
Press, Chicago.

Watson, D.M.S., 1913, Further notes on the skull, brain, and
organs of special sense of Diademodon, Ann. Mag. Nat. Hist.
12(8):217.

Wegener, A.L., 1915, Die Entstehung der Kontinente und Ozeane,
F. Vieweg, Braunschweig.

Westoll, T.S., 1945, The hyomandibular of Eusthenopteron and
the tetrapod middle ear, Proc. Roy. Soc. (Lond.)B 131:393.

Westoll, T.S., 1945, The mammalian middle ear, Nature (Lond.)
155:114.

Winter, P., 1969, Dialects in squirrel monkeys: Vocalization
of the roman arch type, Folia primatol. 10:216.

Winter, P., Ploog, D., and Latta, J., 1966, Vocal repertoire of
the squirrel monkey (Saimiri sciureus) its analysis and
significance, Exp. Brain Res. 1:359.

Wise, S.P. and Herkenham, M., 1982, Opiate receptor distribution
in the cerebral cortex of the rhesus monkey, Science 218:387.

STRUCTURE AND CONNECTIONS OF THE CINGULATE VOCALIZATION REGION IN

THE RHESUS MONKEY

Brent A. Vogt and Helen Barbas

Departments of Anatomy and Physiology
Boston University School of Medicine
Department of Health Sciences
Boston University
Boston, MA, and Veterans Hospital, Bedford, MA

INTRODUCTION

Many primate utterances are simple vocalizations that may be associated with brainstem activity and contain limited information about the internal state of the animal. Sequences of tone and amplitude modulated vocalizations which have associative content form the basis for more complex communication within a species. These complex vocalizations are organized at suprabulbar levels, including the cerebral cortex.

In nonhuman primates and cats the anterior cingulate and supplementary motor cortices have been implicated in vocalization. It is not clear at present what the specific role of these cortices is in vocalization. In the human there is the additional contribution of Wernicke's and Broca's areas for the comprehension and production of speech. As will be discussed later, a number of studies support the view that species-specific vocalizations are dependent on auditory association cortices. However, projections of auditory association areas to the cingulate vocalization region have not been analyzed and auditory projections to cingulate cortex may not be necessary to initiate vocalization but rather for modulation of vocal output. Internal states seem to be responsible for emitted sounds in nonhuman primates and thus may be more effective in evoking vocalization. As a major component of the limbic system, cingulate cortex seems to be involved in monitoring internal states. Thus, specific connections among limbic structures associated with the cingulate vocalization region may have a role in triggering vocalizations associated with emotional states.

The goal of the present chapter is to analyze the corticocortical connections of anterior cingulate cortex which may account for its role in vocalization and communication in primates. This effort will concentrate on the following issues. First, since the vocalization field in cingulate cortex crosses cytoarchitectonic borders, what are the common connections of these areas? Second, in view of the fact that vocalizations in primates are often made in response to noxious stimuli, and in light of evidence that vocalization is modulated by opiate compounds, where does cingulate cortex interface with pathways associated with the pain systems? Third, what are the sources of direct and indirect auditory inputs to the cingulate vocalization region? Fourth, what are the connections of cingulate cortex with the motor system necessary to carry out the act of vocalization? Finally, a qualitative model will be presented which integrates the various cingulate connections that might subserve triggering and modulation of vocalization.

THE CINGULATE VOCALIZATION REGION

Smith (1945) reported that the most prominent response obtained from electrical stimulation of monkey anterior cingulate cortex was vocalization. Although he outlined a broad region of responsive cortex, subsequent electrical stimulation studies by Kaada (1951), Jürgens and Ploog (1970), Jürgens (1976) and Müller-Preuss at al. (1980) suggest a more limited region in rostral cingulate cortex (Fig. 1). Ablation studies support this localization since phonation is severely disrupted when lesions are centered in cortex rostral to the genu of the corpus callosum (Sutton et al., 1974; Aitken, 1981; Fig. 2A). Animals with such lesions have limited spontaneous as well as discriminatively-conditioned vocalizations (Aitken, 1981). Moreover, ablation of anterior cingulate cortex in young monkeys abolishes the characteristic cry emitted when an infant monkey is separated from its mother (MacLean, 1985). In contrast, lesions of lateral neocortical areas appear to have no influence on the production of vocalizations (Fig. 2B).

Precise localization of vocalization areas on the medial surface of the human brain is difficult. Notwithstanding, the following observations appear justified in comparing the role of anterior cingulate cortex in the human to that of other primates in vocalization. First, no vocalization or language disturbances have been reported for cases in which limited lesions were made in area 24 dorsal to the corpus callosum. These include observations made after neurosurgical intervention for relief of intractable pain, drug addiction, or psychiatric disorders (Le Beau, 1952; Tow and Whitty, 1953; Ballantine et al., 1967; Foltz and White, 1968; Kanaka

A. CYTOARCHITECTURE

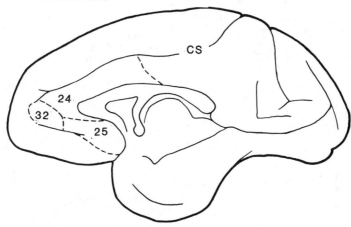

B. ELECTRICAL STIMULATION

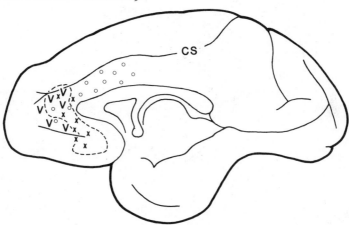

Fig. 1. A. Cytoarchitectural areas in anterior cingulate cortex of the rhesus monkey; B. Composite of points where electrical stimulation has been previously reported to evoke vocalization; CS refers to the cingulate sulcus. Symbols in B refer to the following studies: o, Smith (1945); v, Kaada (1951); dashed line, Jürgens and Ploog (1970); x, Müller-Preuss et al. (1980).

A. MEDIAL SURFACE

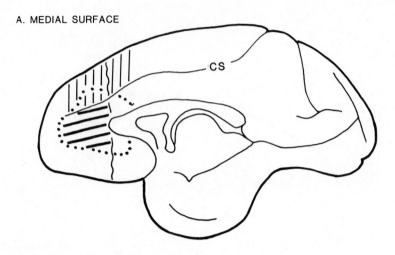

B. LATERAL SURFACE

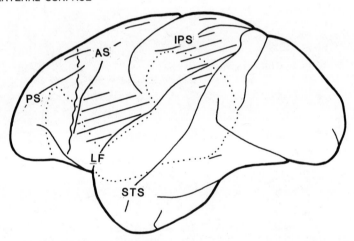

Fig. 2. A. Summary of the extent of ablations that interfered with
        vocalization as reported in previous studies. These
        included lesions which affected performance of
        discriminative calls (Sutton et al., 1974; large dots),
        those which severely disrupted conditioned and spontaneous
        vocal behavior (Aitken, 1981; heavy oblique lines), lesions
        in the supplementary motor area which increased the latency
        of a vocal response (Sutton et al., 1985; vertical lines),
        and a prefrontal lobectomy extending to wavy vertical line
        (Franzen and Myers, 1973), extrapolated from the lateral to
        the medial surface. B. Ablations of lateral cortical areas
        which did not affect vocalization as reported by Sutton et
        al. (1974; area within dotted line) and Aitken (1981; thin
        oblique lines). AS, arcuate sulcus; IPS, intraparietal
        sulcus; LF, lateral fissure; PS, principal sulcus; STS,
        superior temporal sulcus.

and Balasubramaniam, 1978). In addition, Talairach et al. (1973)
failed to evoke vocalization with electrical stimulation of caudal
area 24. Second, bilateral infarction of anterior cingulate cortex
including cortex anterior to the rostrum of the corpus callosum
results in akinetic mutism (Nielsen and Jacobs, 1951; Barris and
Schuman, 1953) but within 10 weeks speech is restored (Jürgens and
von Cramon, 1982). In the latter instance, speech was characterized
by monotonous intonation and these authors suggested that anterior
cingulate cortex is involved in "volitional control of emotional
vocal utterances". Furthermore, infarcts of medial cortex likely
involving both cingulate and supplementary motor cortices produce a
form of transcortical motor aphasia in which spontaneous
conversational speech is disrupted, but repetition, naming, and
comprehension are preserved (Rubens, 1975; Goldberg et al., 1981).
This differs from monkey cases in which both spontaneous and
conditioned vocalizations are disrupted by rostral cingulate
lesions.

Observations based on electrical stimulation and ablation of
medial cortex in the rhesus monkey (summarized in Figs. 1B and 2A)
suggest that the cortex which is critical for vocalization lies
around the rostrum of the corpus callosum. Although the cingulate
sulcus borders this region dorsally, there are no landmarks that
define its rostral and ventral extents. A number of
cytoarchitectonic classifications have been made of the primate
anterior cingulate region (Brodmann, 1909; von Economo, 1929; Rose,
1927; von Bonin and Bailey, 1947; Vogt et al., 1987). Comparison of
these maps with the area which is involved in vocalization indicates
that the latter region is structurally heterogeneous. Figure 1A
depicts the topography of cytoarchitectonic areas in anterior
cingulate cortex. It is evident that vocalization can be evoked
from cortex which lies at the confluence of three regions: areas 24,
32, and 25. In light of these observations the following question
arises: if vocalization is a function of more than one
cytoarchitectonic area, what is the basis for the common function?
It is likely that there are connections that are shared by each area
which operate to form a functional unit which can be referred to as
the cingulate vocalization region.

COMMON CONNECTIONS OF CINGULATE AREAS INVOLVED IN VOCALIZATION

The search for afferent connections that functionally unify
areas in the cingulate vocalization region may be guided by the
following considerations. Projections from extrinsic sources may be
selective for the cingulate vocalization region or a number of
larger projection fields could overlap to functionally unify the
region. A common output from the cingulate vocalization region
could be generated from an overlap by two or more widespread
connections. Connections which are particularly dense in the

cingulate vocalization region are of more interest than are light and topographically limited connections. Finally, it should be noted that injections are usually limited in extent in experimental cases and so the observations from selected cases cannot be viewed as necessarily representing an entire connection. Three classes of connections stand out as being particularly important to integrating activity of the cingulate vocalization region: those that interconnect the cingulate vocalization subdivisions; those originating in the amygdala; and those arising from superior temporal cortices. In addition, a final common output of the anterior cingulate areas to the periaqueductal gray may serve to unify the functions of these areas.

Intracingulate Connections

In the rhesus monkey areas 32, 24, and 25 are interconnected as demonstrated in both radiolabeled amino acid and enzyme transport studies (Pandya et al., 1981; Vogt and Pandya, 1987). These connections arise primarily from layer III and layer V pyramidal neurons. The distribution of retrogradely labeled neurons following an area 32 horseradish peroxidase (HRP) injection is presented in Figure 4 in another context; however, it can be seen that both rostral area 24 and area 25 had many labeled neurons. Similar connections have been reported for a part of this region in the squirrel monkey by Jürgens (1983). The intracingulate connections of these pyramidal neurons could serve as the basis for coordinating the output of the three subdivisions of the vocalization region.

Connections with the Amygdala

Electrical stimulation of the amygdala can produce vocalizations (Jürgens and Ploog, 1970). Although these responses could be associated with the reinforcing properties of the stimulus (Jürgens, 1976), evidence is presented in this volume by Lloyd and Kling that the amygdala is involved in coding the "affective content" of conspecific vocalizations. Since cingulate cortex also has been implicated directly in coding of the emotional significance of stimuli (Gabriel et al., 1980), it is likely that the joint action of the cingulate vocalization region and the amygdala is important for the affective component of some vocalizations. The amygdala stands out from other brain regions from a hodological viewpoint because its medial cortical projections seem to be directed primarily to the cingulate vocalization region.

The accessory basal and lateral basal amygdaloid nuclei have strong projections to inner layer I and layer II of cingulate cortex (Porrino et al., 1981; Jürgens, 1983; Amaral and Price, 1984). In addition area 24, at least, projects to the lateral basal nucleus (Pandya et al., 1973). It is important to note that the projection from the amygdala is one of the clear instances in which the vocalization region is fully included by a major afferent projection (Vogt and Pandya, 1987). Therefore, although the amygdala may not be directly involved in producing vocalization, it may transmit signals to rostral cingulate cortex associated with certain emotional states and thus lower the threshold for eliciting vocalization from anterior cingulate cortex.

Superior Temporal Connections

Projections of temporal cortex will be described in more detail shortly; however, two points are of particular note at this juncture. First, projections from the superior temporal cortex to the medial surface are preferentially directed to the cingulate vocalization region (Fig. 3A). Second, projections from hippocampal (Rosene and Van Hoesen, 1977) and parahippocampal areas TL and TF (Vogt and Pandya, 1987) to the vocalization region appear quite sparse. This suggests that the hippocampus may not be involved in vocalization.

Periaqueductal Gray

Of pivotal importance to evoking vocalization is the final common pathway by which activity in areas of the cingulate vocalization region is relayed to the laryngeal motor neurons. Kelly et al. (1946) showed that facio-vocal control was spared following ablations of the mesencephalic/diencephalic junction but not after those in the periaqueductal gray and the adjacent tegmentum. A study by Jürgens and Pratt (1979) clarified these findings in a critical way by demonstrating that periaqueductal gray lesions abolished vocalization produced by electrical stimulation of anterior cingulate cortex. In all mammals studied, it appears that layer V pyramidal neurons in anterior cingulate cortex project to the periaqueductal gray (Morrell et al., 1981; Mantyh, 1982; Wyss and Sripanidkulchai, 1984). Thus it is likely that the neurons that conduct impulses from the cingulate vocalization region concerning the internal state of the animal and/or responses of specific stimuli, directly activate brainstem vocalization pathways.

In conclusion, the part of anterior cingulate cortex which is involved in vocalization is cytoarchitectonically heterogeneous and includes parts of areas 25, 24, and 32. This cingulate vocalization region may be consolidated as a functional unit by intrinsic connections as well as afferents from the amygdala and superior temporal cortex. Furthermore, the common pathway by which vocalization is evoked via the cingulate vocalization region is centered on layer V pyramidal neurons which project to the periaqueductal gray.

NOXIOUS STIMULI: A POSSIBLE TRIGGER FOR VOCALIZATION

As a general rule a limited number of essential functions are attributed to a single cortical area or connection. The cingulate vocalization region stands apart from this perspective because it is not composed of a single cytoarchitectonic area, no single input to this region can be ascribed a function primarily in vocalization, and numerous other functions have been attributed to this region in addition to vocalization. Other functions of the anterior cingulate cortex include a role in autonomic and other somatic motor activity (Kaada, 1951), affective responses to painful stimuli (Ballantine et al., 1967; Foltz and White, 1968), attention (Watson et al., 1973), significance coding of sensory stimuli (Gabriel et al., 1980), maternal and play behaviors (Murphy et al., 1981) and monitoring internal states (Bachman et al., 1977). In this context it appears that vocalization at the cortical level may be triggered by a number of inputs to the cingulate vocalization region. These inputs may be most effective during alteration in the internal state of the animal. Painful stimuli alter internal states and may be thus quite effective in evoking vocalization. Secondary responses to stimulation of nociceptors could include those associated with a withdrawal reflex organized in the spinal cord, and autonomic responses due to activation of sympathetic afferents which may reach the vocalization region via polysynaptic pathways. All of these activities could occur within seconds of nociceptor activation to produce vocalization.

Although the cellular mechanisms for each of the above noted events have not been defined yet, there is evidence that anterior cingulate cortex is involved in affective responses to noxious stimuli (Ballantine et al., 1967; Foltz and White, 1962). Vocalization may be a part of this response. Although the cingulotomy procedure which involves ablations of dorsal area 24 and/or the underlying white matter does not interfere with vocalization or speech, it does alter responses to painful stimuli. As stated by Foltz and White (1962) one patient reported after such an operation, that the pain was still present but did not concern her. It is likely that this patient's threshold for vocalization in response to painful stimuli was altered.

One of the primary behavioral roles of cingulate cortex is in coding of significant stimuli as a part of learning (Gabriel et al., 1980), an aspect of which is learning to avoid noxious stimuli. Ablations of cingulate cortex in experimental animals interfere with the ability to learn to avoid shock, i.e. active avoidance learning (Peretz, 1960; Thomas and Slotnick, 1963; Lubar, 1964). Lesions of the parafascicular nucleus in cats also disrupt this learning (Kaelber et al., 1975). The parafascicular nucleus projects to the cingulate cortex of both cats (Robertson and Kaitz, 1981) and monkeys (Vogt et al., 1979, 1987). Thus far one source of putative nociceptor input can be proposed for the cingulate vocalization region and that is from the parafascicular and centrolateral divisions of the intralaminar thalamus. Neurons in these nuclei respond in a graded fashion to noxious stimuli and there is little or no somatotopic organization in their receptive fields (Casey, 1966; Dong et al., 1978; Peschanski et al., 1981). Thalamic nuclei such as those of the midline region, including the centrodensocellular, rhomboid and paraventricular nuclei, which are associated with limbic cortices including cingulate cortex, also may have a role in nociception, but there are no physiological studies addressing this issue.

Vocalizations emitted during distress, associated with separation of infant monkeys from their mothers, and those produced by electrical stimulation of the thalamus in guinea pigs are enhanced with naloxone, an opiate receptor antagonist (Herman and Panksepp, 1978, 1980). It is striking that layer V of anterior cingulate cortex in monkey has particularly high opiate receptor binding (Wamsley et al., 1982). The most direct way to modulate vocalization at the cortical level is likely through opiate receptors located on layer V pyramidal neurons that project to the periaqueductal gray. However, the localization of opiate receptors has not yet been accomplished with this level of resolution. Some interneurons in rodent cingulate cortex are immunoreactive for enkephalin and appear to form synapses with layer V pyramids (Sar et al., 1978). Additionally, axosomatic synapses are formed between multipolar and pyramidal neurons which are symmetric and so are likely inhibitory in function (Peters and Proskauer, 1979). Thus it is proposed that interneurons containing opioid compounds may be capable of directly inhibiting pyramidal cells which project to the periaqueductal gray.

Responses to noxious stimuli may not be dependent solely on cingulate cortex, and it is proposed here that the amygdala operates in conjunction with cingulate cortex to produce these responses. This suggestion is made because the amygdala has receptors and connections that are similar to those of cingulate cortex. For example, like cingulate cortex, opiate receptors are concentrated in the amygdala, particularly in the lateral basal nucleus which projects to cingulate cortex (Wamsley et al., 1982). Thalamic projections to the amygdala, like those to cingulate cortex, arise from the paraventricular, central superior, centrodensocellular, reuniens and paracentral nuclei (Aggleton et al., 1980). It is also interesting to note that these thalamic nuclei which project to both the amygdala and cingulate cortex also have high binding of opiate compounds (Wamsley et al., 1982). Thus it would appear that both the amygdala and the cingulate vocalization region are involved in affective responses to painful stimuli and associated vocalizations. The hypothesis of a joint role of these structures may explain why opiate antagonists are so potent in enhancing distress vocalizations.

In conclusion, it is possible that a number of inputs associated with sensory responses such as painful ones including resultant activity in the thalamus and amygdala could summate to evoke vocalization. In addition, a direct role of the opiate system in vocalization can be postulated whereby enkephalinergic interneurons may inhibit the activity in layer V neurons thus inactivating control of vocalization by the cingulate vocalization region. Finally, the cingulate vocalization region and lateral basal nucleus of the amygdala may operate jointly in producing vocalization and each would be an important site for the actions of opiate antagonists.

AUDITORY AFFERENTS: MODULATION OF THE VOCALIZATION REGION'S OUTPUT

Although it is possible that auditory stimuli directly trigger vocalization in some species, it is more likely that projections from auditory cortices provide feedback for modulation of tonal qualities. The possible role of auditory cortex in modulating vocalization responses is supported by observations that neurons in the superior temporal gyrus respond to species-specific vocalizations (Newman and Wollberg, 1973) and bilateral ablations of auditory cortex interfere with discrimination of these vocalizations (Hupfer et al., 1977; Heffner and Heffner, 1984, 1986). There have been no systematic studies of auditory projections to the cingulate vocalization region. Auditory input could reach this part of the brain directly from auditory association cortices or indirectly through the prefrontal cortex.

Direct Auditory Connections

In the rhesus monkey a tritiated amino acid injection into the dorsal temporal proisocortex and TS1 of Galaburda and Pandya (1983) resulted in labeling over much of the cingulate vocalization region (Fig. 3A). This included rostral area 24, caudal and ventral parts of area 32 and rostral area 25 in addition to parts of area 14. An injection of HRP into area 32 and adjacent area 14 is presented in Figure 4. This area received 17% of its cortical input from auditory association cortices based on the distribution of all HRP labeled neurons in the cortex. More than 60% of these labeled neurons in auditory cortices came from TS1, while most of the remainder were in areas Pro, TS2 and TS3. It has also been observed that there are projections from the cingulate vocalization region back to auditory cortex in the squirrel monkey (Müller-Preuss et al., 1980).

Indirect Auditory Connections

There is evidence of impairment of auditory discrimination following dorsolateral prefrontal ablations (Weiskrantz and Mishkin, 1958; Gross and Weiskrantz, 1962). The possible role of auditory

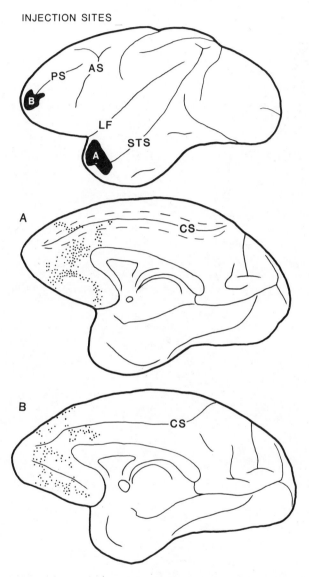

Fig. 3. Tritiated amino acid injections into rostral superior
temporal cortex including areas Pro and TS1 (A, black
area) and into frontal polar area 10 (B, black area). In
each instance there were labeled terminals in the
cingulate vocalization region as shown on the medial side
of the hemisphere in A and B (dots).

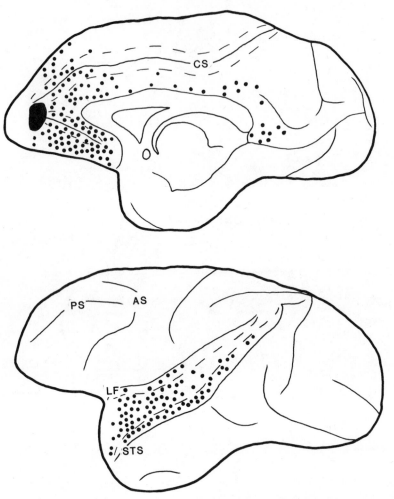

Fig. 4.   Distribution of labeled neurons following an HRP injection
          into area 32.   A preponderance of labeled neurons was in
          auditory association areas and rostral cingulate areas 24
          and 25.

responsive neurons in prefrontal cortex in vocalization is supported
by the observations of Newman and Lindsley (1976) who showed that
cells around the principal sulcus responded to species-specific
vocalizations in addition to other auditory stimuli.   There are
several sites within the prefrontal cortex that receive input from
auditory association regions.   These include periarcuate (area 8),
peri-principalis (areas 46 and 10) and ventrolateral area 12 (Barbas

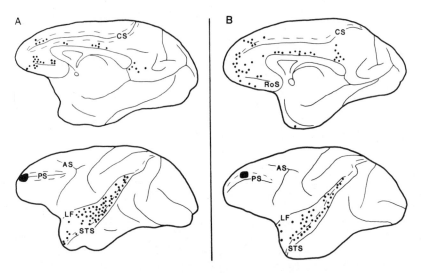

Fig. 5. Distribution of labeled neurons following HRP injections into rostral area 10 (A.) and dorsal area 46 (B.). Each case had extensive HRP labeling of neurons in auditory association cortices along the superior temporal gyrus as well as in parts of the cingulate vocalization region.

and Mesulam, 1981, 1985; Barbas, in preparation; Chavis and Pandya, 1976; Jones and Powell, 1970).

An analysis of the proportion of retrogradely labeled neurons in auditory association areas after an HRP injection within the prefrontal cortex revealed that of all known auditory recipient prefrontal regions at least two appear to be major targets of auditory projections. In other words these latter regions received 15% or more of all their cortical connections from auditory areas. Thus, a dorsolateral region at the tip of the principal sulcus (area 10) received 25% of its total cortical connections from auditory association regions (Fig. 5A). In addition, a mid-dorsal, peri-principalis region (dorsal area 46) received more than 15% of its total cortical projections from auditory association regions (Fig. 5B). In these cases, most projections originated in auditory association areas TS1, TS3, TS2, PaAlt and Tpt described by Galaburda and Pandya (1983). However, the majority of auditory projections to dorsal areas 46 and 10 originated in areas TS1-TS3 (70%), and fewer came from more caudal and architectonically more differentiated auditory association areas PaAlt and Tpt.

Both of the dorsolateral prefrontal areas that appear to be major targets of cortical auditory association projections, in turn, are closely related anatomically with the cingulate vocalization region. Thus dorsal area 46 projects to medial area 32. The frontal polar area 10 projects to components of all cingulate areas associated with vocalization, including areas 32, 25 and rostral area 24 (Fig. 3B). Auditory projections, therefore reach the cingulate vocalization region both directly and indirectly. Direct projections from auditory association cortices reach areas 32 and 25, while indirect auditory input may reach the cingulate vocalization region via auditory recipient prefrontal areas 46 and 10.

CONNECTIONS BETWEEN THE VOCALIZATION REGION AND DORSAL AREA 24

Although electrical stimulation of dorsal and caudal parts of area 24, i.e. above the corpus callosum, does not evoke vocalization, it is possible that this area modulates the activity of the cingulate vocalization region. For example, Foltz and White (1968) found that cingulotomies for relief of pain improved verbal communication in two aphasic patients. Cats with ablations in a similar place showed significantly more vocalization (Lubar and Perachio, 1965). Suppression of attack evoked by electrical stimulation of the hypothalamus has been possible also with electrical stimulation of dorsal area 24 in cats (Siegel and Chabora, 1971). Finally large lesions of dorsal area 24 in monkeys (Showers, 1959) resulted in hyperkinetic animals and almost constant vocalization. These latter calls seemed to have no apparent association with other animals in the colony or its surroundings. Thus, it appears possible that dorsal area 24 plays a role in inhibiting vocalizations generated within the more ventrally situated cingulate region.

Although direct connections between the vocalization region and dorsal area 24 are not extensive, such connections have been reported. Pandya et al. (1981) showed that area 24 projects to area 25. In addition, in Figure 4, it can be seen that there are retrogradely labeled neurons in dorsal area 24 following an HRP injection in area 32. This connection will assume more importance when discussing the supplementary motor area and its role in vocalization, because it is this dorsal part of area 24 which is most heavily interconnected with the supplementary motor area. Interactions at the cortical level between the supplementary motor area and the vocalization region are likely mediated by dorsal area 24.

CONNECTIONS OF THE VOCALIZATION REGION WITH SUPPLEMENTARY MOTOR CORTEX

The supplementary motor area is thought to be involved in intentional or preparative motor processes (Goldberg, 1985).

Although it has been implicated clinically in speech in a number of reports, its role at a mechanistic level in the human is unclear as is its role in vocalization in nonhuman primates. Most clinical reports of patients with supplementary motor area infarction due to occlusion of the anterior cerebral artery have concomitant involvement of the cingulate vocalization region. In these cases there is marked reduction or absence of spontaneous speech and difficulty in initiating speech (Racy et al., 1979; Alexander and Schmitt, 1980; Brust et al., 1982). In only one case was there limited involvement of area 24 in addition to the supplementary motor area (Masdeu et al., 1978). In this latter case reduced spontaneous speech and word recall were reported one month following the infarct. Laplane et al. (1977) reported another series of patients who had undergone surgical ablations of the medial cortical surface involving the supplementary motor area, dorsal parts of area 24 and medial parts of areas 6 and 9. These individuals initially had an arrest of speech followed by a reduction in spontaneous speech. Within 8 to 15 months these clinical signs had subsided.

Two other observations implicate the supplementary motor area in the initiation of speech. First, electrical stimulation of this area interrupted speaking or evoked vocalization of short syllables (Penfield and Jasper, 1954). Second, spontaneous speech increases blood flow in supplementary motor cortex (Larsen et al., 1978). In light of the above clinical observations it is reasonable to state that the supplementary motor area is involved in speech by initiating the production of its basic components such as syllables and vowels. It appears that the affective component of speech is not a function of this area in humans.

The role of the supplementary motor area in vocalization in nonhuman primates is not yet resolved. Smith (1945) could evoke vocalization in monkey by electrical stimulation of this area only immediately after evoking it from rostral cingulate cortex. Sutton et al. (1985) ablated the supplementary motor area and areas 9 and 6 (Fig. 2A) and found that there was an increase in the latency of vocal responses but not in the "efficiency" of vocal and nonvocal responses. Finally, Kennard's (1955) presumptive cingulate cortex lesions in cats were likely in supplementary motor cortex and the cats "purred more and seemed to do so inappropriately and at all times."   Thus, there may be a functional link between the supplementary motor and cingulate vocalization regions but its precise role is not yet clear.

There is no evidence of direct connections between the supplementary motor and cingulate vocalization regions. Limited connections do exist, however, between the supplementary motor area and area 24 dorsal to the corpus callosum. Damasio and Van Hoesen (1980) have reported reciprocal connections between anterior cingulate and supplementary motor cortices in rhesus monkey. In

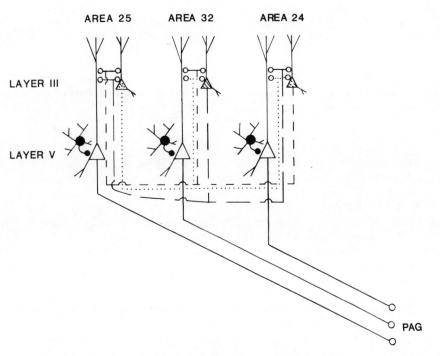

Fig. 6. Architecture and intrinsic connections of the cingulate
vocalization region. Large layer V pyramidal neurons which
project to the periaqueductal gray (PAG) are the primary
components of this model. Intracingulate connections of
layer III and layer V neurons and inhibitory interneurons
modulate the activity of the largest projection cells.

addition, Pandya et al. (1981) presented a case in which a large injection of tritiated amino acids was made into area 24 and had anterograde transport into the supplementary motor area. The critical part of area 24 that is involved in these connections is a dorsal and caudal part of area 24 (Van Hoesen, personal communication).

In conclusion, if the supplementary motor area influences the cingulate vocalization region at the cortical level, it would have to be primarily through a series of corticocortical connections mediated by dorsal area 24. This indirect linking might be the reason for the limited role that the supplementary motor cortex plays in nonhuman primate vocalization.

STRUCTURAL MODEL OF THE VOCALIZATION EVENT

Statements in this chapter about the role of anterior cingulate cortex in vocalization and its specific connections can be presented as a model with three essential components. First, the intrinsic structure of the cingulate vocalization region and its projections to the periaqueductal gray. Second, connections associated with nociceptive pathways and the amygdala for triggering activity in the cingulate vocalization region. Third, connections with auditory association cortices for modulation of activity in the vocalization region.

In the circuit model in Figure 6 a large layer V pyramidal neuron which projects to the periaqueductal gray is presented for each area in the cingulate vocalization region. Activity in the vocalization region is integrated by excitatory activity in layer III and layer V pyramidal neurons which project among the three areas. In addition, enkephalinergic interneurons (filled cells) are incorporated in each area to provide for direct inactivation of vocalization by inhibiting the layer V pyramidal neurons.

Putative nociceptor input is transmitted via the parafascicular and centrolateral nuclei of the thalamus to pyramidal cells with dendrites mainly in deep layer III as shown in Figure 7. Limbic system projections relating to significance coding of vocal events may arise in the amygdala and terminate in layers superficial to the thalamic input. The summation of activity in the layer V projection neurons could lead to their discharge and activation of vocalization via the periaqueductal grey. Finally, numerous corticocortical connections are in place for modulating the basic vocalization response. Of greatest importance are those of direct origin in auditory association cortices and indirect origin in prefrontal cortices.

(We thank Ms. Michelle Richmond for typing the manuscript. This work was supported by NIH grants NS18745 and 24760.)

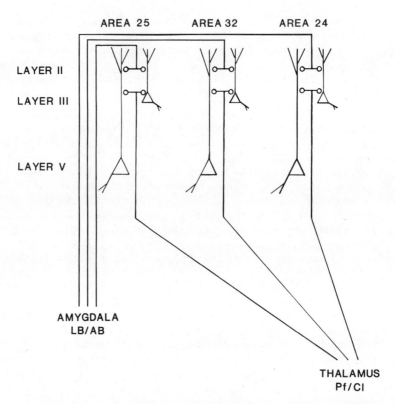

Fig. 7.   Connections critical for triggering vocalization are those
          associated with nociceptor activation, the output of which
          is transmitted to cingulate cortex via the parafascicular
          (Pf) and centrolateral (Cl) nuclei of the thalamus.
          Projections from the amygdala to the vocalization areas
          terminate superficial to the thalamic inputs.   Projections
          from the amygdala may be involved in affective responses to
          painful stimuli and determine the emotional significance of
          associated vocalizations.

REFERENCES

Aggleton, J. P., Burton, M. J., and Passingham, R. E., 1980, Cortical and subcortical afferents to the amygdala of the rhesus monkey (Macaca mulatta), Brain Res., 190:347.

Aitken, P. G., 1981, Cortical control of conditioned and spontaneous vocal behavior in rhesus monkeys, Brain and Lang., 13:171.

Alexander, M. P., and Schmitt, M. A., 1980, The aphasia syndrome of stroke in the left anterior cerebral artery territory, Arch. Neurol., 37:97.

Amaral, D. G., and Price, J. L., 1984, Amygdalo-cortical projections in the monkey (Macaca fascicularis), J. Comp. Neurol., 230:465.

Bachman, D. S., Hallowitz, R. A., and MacLean, P. D., 1977, Effects of vagal volleys and serotonin on units of cingulate cortex in monkeys, Brain Res., 130:253.

Ballantine, H. T., Cassidy, W. L., Flanagan, N. B., and Marino, R.,Jr., 1967, Stereotaxic anterior cingulotomy for neuropsychiatric illness and intractable pain, J. Neurosurg., 26:488.

Barbas, H., and Mesulam, M-M., 1981, Organization of afferent input to subdivisions of area 8 in the rhesus monkey, J. Comp. Neurol., 200:407.

Barbas, H., and Mesulam, M-M., 1985, Cortical afferent input to the principalis region of the rhesus monkey, Neurosci., 15:619.

Barris, R. W., and Schuman, H. R., 1953, Bilateral anterior cingulate gyrus lesions: syndrome of the anterior cingulate gyri, Neurology, 3:44.

Bonin, G. von, and Bailey, P., 1947, "The Neocortex of Macaca Mulatta", The University of Illinois Press, Urbana.

Brodmann, K., 1909, "Vergleichende Lokalisationslehre der Grosshirenrinde in ihren Prinzipien dargestellt auf Grund des Zellenbaues," J. A. Barth, Leipzig.

Brust, J. C. M., Plank, C., Burke, A., Guobadia, M. M. I., and Healton, E. B., 1982, Language disorder in a right-hander after occlusion of the right anterior cerebral artery, Neurology, 32:492.

Casey, K. L., 1966, Unit analysis of nociceptive mechanisms in the thalamus of the awake squirrel monkey, J. Neurophysiol., 29:727.

Chavis, D. A., and Pandya, D. N., 1976, Further observations on corticofrontal connections in the rhesus monkey, Brain Res., 117:369.

Damasio, A. R., and Van Hoesen, G. W., 1980, Structure and function of the supplementary motor area, Neurology, 30:359.

Dong, W. K., Ryu, H. and Wagman, I. H., 1978, Nociceptive responses of neurons in medial thalamus and their relationship to spinothalamic pathways, J. Neurophysiol., 41:1592.

Economo, C. von, 1929, "The Cytoarchitectonics of the Human Cerebral Cortex", University Press, Oxford.

Foltz, E. L., and White, L. E., 1962, Pain "relief" by frontal cingulumotomy, J. Neurosurg., 19:89.

Foltz, E. L., and White, L. E., 1968, The role of rostral cingulumotomy in "pain" relief, Int. J. Neurol., 6:353.

Franzen, E. A., and Myers, R. E., 1973, Age effects on social behavior deficits following prefrontal lesions in monkeys, Brain Res., 54:277.

Gabriel, M. K., Foster, K., Orona, E., Saltwick, S. E., and Stanton, M., 1980, Neuronal activity of cingulate cortex, anteroventral thalamus, and hippocampal formation in discriminative conditioning: encoding and extraction of the significance of conditioned stimuli, in: "Progress in Psychobiology and Physiological Psychology," vol. 9, J. Sprague and A. N. Epstein, Academic Press, New York.

Galaburda, A. M., and Pandya, D. N., 1983, The intrinsic architectonic and connectional organization of superior temporal region of the rhesus monkey, J. Comp. Neurol., 221:169.

Goldberg, G., 1985, Supplementary motor area structure and function: Review and hypotheses, Behavioral and Brain Sciences, 8:567.

Goldberg, G., Mayer, N. H., and Toglia, J. U., 1981, Medial frontal cortex infarction and the alien hand sign, Arch. Neurol., 38:683.

Gross, C. G., and Weiskrantz, L., 1962, Evidence for dissociation of impairment on auditory discrimination and delayed response following lateral frontal lesions in monkeys, Expl. Neurol., 5:453.

Heffner, H. E., and Heffner, R. S., 1984, Temporal lobe lesions and perception of species-specific vocalizations by macaques, Science, 226:75.

Heffner, H. E., and Heffner, R. S., 1986, Effect of unilateral and bilateral auditory cortex lesions on the discrimination of vocalizations by Japanese macaques, J. Neurophysiol., 56:683.

Herman, B. H., and Panksepp, J., 1978, Effects of morphine and naloxone on separation distress and approach attachment: evidence for opiate mediation of social affect, Pharmacol. Biochem. Behav., 9:213.

Herman, B. H., and Panksepp, J., 1980, Ascending endorphin inhibition of distress vocalization, Science, 211:1060.

Hupfer, K., Jürgens, U., and Ploog, D., 1977, The effect of superior temporal lesions on the recognition of species-specific calls in the squirrel monkey, Exp. Brain Res., 30:75.

Jones, E. G., and Powell, T. P. S., 1970, An anatomical study of converging sensory pathways within the cerebral cortex of the monkey, Brain, 93:793.

Jürgens, U., 1976, Reinforcing concomitants of electrically elicited vocalizations, Exp. Brain Res., 26:203.

Jürgens, U., 1983, Afferent fibers to the cingular vocalization region in the squirrel monkey, Exp. Neurol., 80:395.

Jürgens, U., and Ploog, D., 1970, Cerebral representation of vocalization in the squirrel monkey, Exp. Brain Res., 10:532.

Jürgens, U., and Pratt, R., 1979, Role of the periaqueductal grey in vocal expression of emotion, Brain Res., 167:367.

Jürgens, U., and Cramon, D. von, 1982, On the role of the anterior cingulate cortex in phonation: a case report, Brain and Lang., 15:234.

Kaada, B. R., 1951, Somato-motor autonomic and electrocorticographic responses to electrical stimulation of 'rhinencephalic' and other structures in primates, cat and dog, Acta Physiol. Scand., 24, suppl. 83:1.

Kaelber, W. W., Mitchell, C. L., Yarmat, A. J., Afifi, A. K., and Lorens, S. A., 1975, Centrum medianum-parafascicularis lesions and reactivity to noxious and non-noxious stimuli, Exp. Neurol., 46:282.

Kanaka, T. S., and Balasubramaniam, V., 1978, Stereotactic cingulumotomy for drug addiction, Appl. Neurophysiol., 41:86.

Kelly, A. H., Beaton, L. E., and Magoun, H. W., 1946, A midbrain mechanism for facio-vocal activity, J. Neurophysiol., 9:181.

Kennard, M. A., 1955, Effect of bilateral ablation of cingulate area on behavior of cats, J. Neurophysiol., 18:159.

Laplane, D., Talairach, J., Meininger, V., Bancaud, J., and Orgogozo, J. M., 1977, Clinical consequences of corticectomies involving the supplementary motor area in man, J. Neurol. Sci., 34:301.

Larsen, B., Skinhoj, E., and Lassen, N. A., 1978, Variations in regional cortical blood flow in the right and left hemispheres during automatic speech, Brain, 101:193.

Le Beau, J., 1952, The cingular and precingular areas in psychosurgery (agitated behavior, obsessive compulsive states, epilepsy), Acta Psychiat. Neurol., 27:305.

Lubar, J. F., 1964, Effect of medial cortical lesions on the avoidance behavior of the cat, J. Comp. Physiol. Psychol., 58:38.

Lubar, J. F., and Perachio, A. A., 1965, One-way and two-way learning and transfer of an active avoidance response in normal and cingulectomized cats, J. Comp. Physiol. Psychol., 60:46.

MacLean, P. D., 1985, Brain evolution relating to family, play, and the separation call, Arch. Gan. Psych., 42:405.

Mantyh, P. W., 1982, Forebrain projections to the periaqueductal gray in the monkey, with observations in the cat and rat, J. Comp. Neurol., 206:146.

Masdeu, J. C., Schoene, W. C., and Funkenstein, H., 1978, Aphasia following infarction of the left supplementary motor area, a clinicopathologic study, Neurology, 28:1220.

Morrell, J. I., Greenberger, L. M., and Pfaff, D. W., 1981, Hypothalamic, other diencephalic, and telencephalic neurons

that project to the dorsal midbrain, J. Comp. Neurol.,
201:589.

Müller-Preuss, P., Newman, J. D., and Jürgens, U., 1980, Anatomical
and physiological evidence for a relationship between the
'cingular' vocalization area and the auditory cortex in the
squirrel monkey, Brain Res., 202:307.

Murphy, M. R., MacLean, P. D., and Hamilton, S. C., 1981, Species
typical behavior of hamsters deprived from birth of the
neocortex, Science, 213:459.

Newman, J. D., and Lindsley, D. F., 1976, Single unit analysis of
auditory processing in squirrel monkey frontal cortex, Exp.
Brain Res., 25:169.

Newman, J. D., and Wollberg, Z., 1973, Multiple coding of species-
specific vocalizations in the auditory cortex of squirrel
monkeys, Brain Res., 54:287.

Nielsen, J. M., and Jacobs, L.L., 1951, Bilateral lesions of the
anterior cingulate gyri, Bull. Los Angeles Neurol. Soc.,
16:231.

Pandya, D. N., Van Hoesen, G. W., and Domesick, V. B., 1973, A
cingulo-amygdaloid projection in the rhesus monkey, Brain
Res., 61:369.

Pandya, D. N., Van Hoesen, G. W., and Mesulam, M. M., 1981, Efferent
connections of the cingulate gyrus in the rhesus monkey, Exp.
Brain Res., 42:319.

Penfield, W., and Jasper, H., 1954, "Epilepsy and the functional
anatomy of the human brain", Little, Brown, and Company,
Boston.

Peretz, E., 1960, The effects of lesions of the anterior cingulate
cortex on the behavior of the rat, J. Comp. Physiol.
Psychol., 53:540.

Peschanski, M., Guilbaud, G., and Gautron, M., 1981, Posterior
intralaminar region in rat: neuronal responses to noxious
cutaneous stimuli, Exp. Neurol., 72:226.

Peters, A., and Proskauer, C. C., 1979, A combined Golgi-EM study of
the synaptic relationship between a smooth stellate cell and
a pyramidal neuron in the rat visual cortex, Neurosci., Abs.,
5:119.

Porrino, L. J., Crane, A. M., and Goldman-Rakic, P. S., 1981, Direct
and indirect pathways from the amygdala to the frontal lobe
in rhesus monkeys, J. Comp. Neurol., 198:121.

Racy, A., Jannotta, F. S., and Lehner, L. H., 1979, Aphasia
resulting from occlusion of the left anterior cerebral
artery; report of a case with an old infarct in the left
rolandic region, Arch. Neurol., 36:221.

Robertson, R. T., and Kaitz, S. S., 1981, Thalamic connections with
limbic cortex. I. Thalamocortical projections, J. Comp.
Neurol., 195:501.

Rose, M., 1927, Gyrus limbicus anterior und Regio retrosplenialis
(Cortex holoprotoptychos quinquestratificatus) Vergleishende
Architectonik bei Tier und Mensch J. Psych. Neurol., 35:65.

Rosene, D. L., and Van Hoesen, G. W., 1977, Hippocampal efferents reach widespread areas of cerebral cortex and amygdala in the rhesus monkey, Science, 198:315.

Rubens, A. B., 1975, Aphasia with infarction in the territory of the anterior cerebral artery, Cortex, 11:239.

Sar, M., Stumpf, W. E., Miller, R. J., Chang, K.-J., and Cuatrecasas, P., 1978, Immunohistochemical localization of enkephalin in rat brain and spinal cord, J. Comp. Neurol., 182:17.

Showers, M. J. C., 1959, The cingulate gyrus: additional motor area and cortical autonomic regulator, J. Comp. Neurol.,112:231.

Siegel, A., and Chabora, J., 1971, Effects of electrical stimulation of the cingulate gyrus upon attack behavior elicited from the hypothalamus in the cat, Brain Res., 32:169.

Smith, W. K., 1945, The functional significance of the rostral cingular cortex as revealed by its responses to electrical excitation, J. Neurophysiol., 8:241.

Sutton, D., Larson, C., and Lindeman, R. C., 1974, Neocortical and limbic lesion effects on primate phonation, Brain Res., 71:61.

Sutton, D., Trachy, R. E., and Lindeman, R. C., 1985, Discriminative phonation in macaques: effects of anterior mesial cortex damage, Exp. Brain Res., 59:410.

Talairach, J., Bancaud, J., Geier, S., Bordas-Ferrer, M., Bonis, A., Szikla, G., and Rusu, M., 1973, The cingulate gyrus and human behaviour, EEG. Clin. Neurophysiol., 34:45.

Thomas, G. J., and Slotnick, B. M., 1963, Impairment of avoidance responding by lesions in cingulate cortex in rats depends on food drive, J. Comp. Physiol. Psychol., 56:959.

Tow, P. M., and Whitty, C. W. M., 1953, Personality changes after operations on the cingulate gyrus in man, J. Neurol. Neurosurg. Psychiat., 16:186.

Vogt, B. A., and Pandya, D. N., 1987, Cingulate cortex of rhesus monkey. II. Cortical afferents, J. Comp. Neurol., in press.

Vogt, B. A., Pandya, D. N., and Rosene, D. L., 1987, Cingulate cortex of rhesus monkey. I. Cytoarchitecture and thalamic afferents, J. Comp. Neurol., in press.

Vogt, B. A., Rosene, D. L., and Pandya, D. N., 1979, Thalamic and cortical afferents differentiate anterior from posterior cingulate cortex in the monkey, Science, 204:205.

Wamsley, J. K., Zarbin, M. A., Young, W. S., III, and Kuhar, M. J., 1982, Distribution of opiate receptors in the monkey brain: an autoradiographic study, Neuroscience, 7:595.

Watson, R. T., Heilman, K. M., Cauthen, J. C., and King, F. A., 1973, Neglect after cingulectomy, Neurology, 23:1003.

Weiskrantz, L., and Mishkin, M., 1958, Effects of temporal and frontal cortical lesions on auditory discrimination in monkeys, Brain, 81:406.

Wyss, J. M., and Sripanidkulchai, K., 1984, The topography of the mesencephalic and pontine projections from the cingulate cortex of the rat, Brain. Res., 293:1.

CINGULATE GYRUS AND SUPPLEMENTARY MOTOR CORRELATES

OF VOCALIZATION IN MAN

Jason W. Brown

New York University Medical Center
530 First Avenue
New York, N.Y. 10016

INTRODUCTION

Historically, study of the pathology and physiology of the speech areas on the frontal convexity, and the analysis of patterns of motor aphasia resulting from damage to these areas, have formed the basis for our understanding of processes underlying speech production. However, from the earliest days of research on central speech disorders there have been hints that regions on the mesial surface of the frontal lobes played an equally important role. This paper reviews current knowledge of the functions of these regions, the anterior cingulate gyrus (AC) and the supplementary motor area (SMA), from the standpoint of the clinical effects of brain pathology. The different forms of speech disturbance and action disorder observed with lesions of these areas, seizure discharge or electrical stimulation, provide data relevant to a theory on the microtemporal processing of an action sequence, according to which AC and SMA mediate early stages in the entrainment of action components.

ANTERIOR CINGULATE GYRUS

Destructive Lesions

A bilateral lesion of the anterior cingulate gyrus (Brodmann area 24) leads to mutism which may be accompanied by akinesia. Nielsen and Jacobs (1951) described the first such case, a 46 year old woman with sudden onset of stupor, incontinence, mutism, inattention and weakness or akinesia of all limbs, with embolic lesions in both anterior cingulate gyri (Fig. 1). The patient was described as lying in bed "staring at the

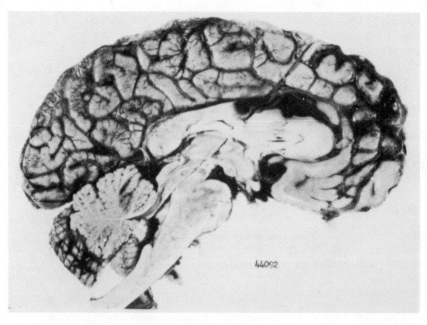

Fig. 1. Lesion of the rostral callosum and anterior cingulate gyrus in a case of akinetic mutism (Nielsen and Jacobs, 1951). There is a similar lesion in the opposite hemisphere.

ceiling, not asking for water or food, and never speaking spontaneously...(nor did she) display any emotional reaction. When her extremely painful left hip was manipulated she would grimace and attempt to remove the examiner's hand but she never cried out with pain."

Soon after, another case was described by Barris and Schuman (1953), a 40 year old man, incontinent with eyes open, "mute, akinetic (and) indifferent to painful stimuli." The autopsy findings (Fig. 2) were similar to those of Nielsen and Jacobs (1951). Additional cases with more extensive lesions were described by Faris (1969) and Freemon (1971). The review by Buge, et al. (1975) reports 3 cases and documents previous clinical descriptions of a state of vigilance with open eyes, incontinence, lack of response to pain and partial or complete mutism and akinesis. In some of these cases, the lesions were not as well localized as in the initial case studies and extended to supplementary motor area (Fig. 3).

This was also true for the case of Jürgens and von Cramon (1982), a 41 year old akinetic mute, aphonic except for occasional groans. This patient recovered through a stage of whispering. Of interest is the report by Bogen (1976) that patients with mutism following section of the corpus callosum, presumably an effect of damage in surgery to the cingulate gyrus, recover through a non-aphasic stage of hoarseness.

Akinetic mutism may also occur in cases of tumor (glioma) or degeneration of the mid-callosum.   Nielsen (1951) described a case with Marchiafava-Bignami disease and central necrosis of the corpus callosum who "never moved or spoke spontaneously, was completely apathetic but when aroused for short periods of time was not aphasic." In addition to the callosal degeneration, there was bilateral destruction of area 24.   He reviewed 9 other previous reports with anterior and central callosal degeneration and noted two stages in the course of the disease; an early stage with excitation and/or psychosis and a later stage of apathy, akinesia and mutism.   The akinetic mutism was attributed to "undermining" of the anterior cingulate gyri and loss of the emotional motivation for activity.   Akinetic mutism can occur in the M.-B. syndrome, especially in acute cases, though it appears to be more infrequent than dysarthria and hypertonicity (Castaigne et al., 1971).

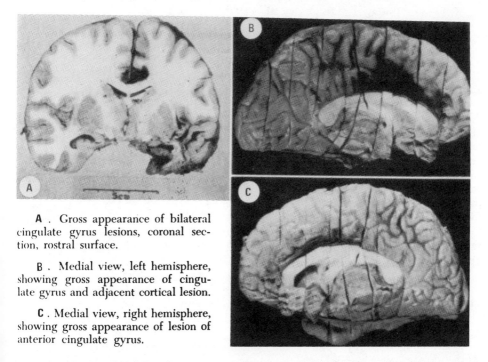

A . Gross appearance of bilateral cingulate gyrus lesions, coronal section, rostral surface.

B . Medial view, left hemisphere, showing gross appearance of cingulate gyrus and adjacent cortical lesion.

C . Medial view, right hemisphere, showing gross appearance of lesion of anterior cingulate gyrus.

Fig. 2.   Lesion of anterior cingulate gyrus in the case of Barris and Schuman (1953).

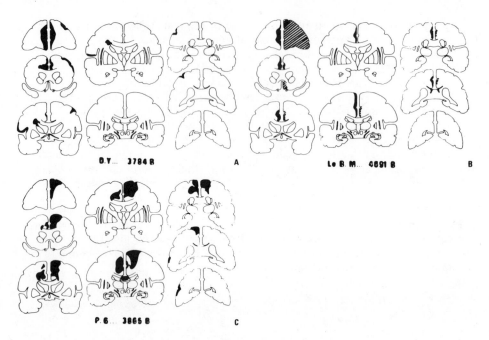

Fig. 3   Diagram of the distribution of lesions in 3 cases of akinetic mutism reported by Buge et al. (1975).

In sum, the clinical picture in the more severe cases of bilateral anterior cingulate lesion is that of sudden or progressive akinetic mutism, characterized by lack of limb and body movement, open eyes with a tendency for a fixed staring gaze, and aphonia with no attempt at vocalization. The patient does not sob or cry out to painful stimulation and only exceptionally is there moaning.   There is no evidence of comprehension, and no response to verbal commands or imitation. Limb tone is usually normal, though reflex changes may be present.   In some instances, the akinetic mutism is punctuated by bouts of excitement, differing in this way from other forms of akinetic mutism (Segarra, 1970), and resembling, perhaps, the excited phases that occur in psychiatric patients with catatonic stupor.   With recovery, speech returns through whispering or hoarseness rather than dysarthria or aphasia.

Bilateral pathology appears necessary to produce this clinical state. The only unilateral case appears to be the report by Botez and Carp (1968) of mutism without akinesia in a 12 year old with a small hematoma in the right cingulate gyrus.   In children, however, mutism is a common form of aphasia and occurs with lesions that are perhaps more widely distributed than in adults.

Akinetic mutism appears to require not only bilateral pathology in the anterior cingulate region but extensive damage.   Small stereotactic lesions as in cingulotomy give placidity with little in the way of language, motor or cognitive deficit (Corkin et al., 1979).   Placidity has been reported in animals with destruction of anterior cingulum (Ward, 1948) and in humans with naturally occurring lesions (Poeck and Kerschensteiner, 1975).   These effects may represent a partial expression of the pronounced akinetic disorder with extensive ablations.

Related Studies

In monkey, there is evidence from ablation, stimulation and recording that the anterior cingulate gyrus plays a role in vocalization. Destruction of anterior cingulate cortex impairs trained vocalization in monkey, and recordings from units in anterior cingulate gyrus indicate that activity associated with vocalization occurs early in the phonation process (Sutton et al., 1978).   Stimulation studies have demonstrated that anterior cingulate gyrus is part of a limbic and brainstem system mediating vocalization (e.g., Jürgens and Pratt, 1979).   In man, stimulation of anterior cingulate gyrus produces integrated motor behavior and affective changes (Fig. 4).   Movements induced by stimulation of cingulate cortex are largely contralateral, though bilateral and ipsilateral movements occur.   Integrated oral movements, postural distortions, reactions of fear and hallucination have also been described.   From such observations, Bancaud et al. (1976) conclude that the region mediates a primitive or archaic level of behavior.

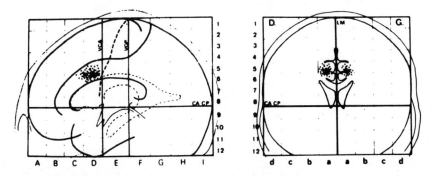

Fig. 4.   Location of 116 stimulations in 80 subjects (Bancaud et al., 1976). Responses include alerting without object orientation, simple integrated movements of the hands and legs (contralateral > ipsilateral = bilateral), synergic oral movements and affective responses.

The Role of Cingulate Gyrus in Vocalization: an Interpretation

The view of Bancaud et al. (1976), that the anterior cingulate gyrus mediates an archaic stage in behavior, is consistent with the microgenetic interpretation that this area supports a preliminary stage in the microtemporal unfolding of an action, a stage organized about the axial musculature in the space of the body midline and in relation to a level of instinctual drive in the microgeny of affect (Brown, 1977). This stage, that of a motor envelope, embraces all of the incipient vocal, limb and somatic elements of the to-be-completed motor act. The vocal component is at a prelinguistic level and presumably develops out of a still deeper rhythmic (e.g., respiratory) process which forms the motor underpinnings of phonation. Non-vocal limb or body movement is derived from postural and locomotor systems of basal ganglia and brainstem, in relation to vestibular and orienting mechanisms, and provides a background out of which the forming proximal and distal limb actions individuate. Akinetic mutism, a global inertia that affects emerging partial actions that are as yet undifferentiated, points to an early stage in the unfolding of an action that is exposed prematurely by pathological lesions.

Morphological studies document this interpretation, in that the anterior cingulate region has been shown to be part of an older evolutionary system. Braak (1980) considered the anterogenual region to be a limbic-derived or proisocortical ganglionic core zone in contact with retrosplenial cortex posteriorly, as well as amygdala and hippocampal formation. The relationship between anterior cingulate and retrosplenial cortex is consistent with clinical evidence that these regions mediate primitive, or preliminary, stages in motility and perception (Brown, 1988). On this view, an archaic stage in forebrain evolution supports or underlies an early stage in action generation.

SUPPLEMENTARY MOTOR AREA

Interest in SMA has been sparked by findings of a bilateral increase in cerebral flow during overt and covert language tasks (Larsen et al., 1978), as well as during lower extremity movements (Orgogozo et al., 1979) though it has been known for some time (Penfield and Welch, 1949; Penfield and Roberts, 1959) that the area is involved in speech production. Clinical and anatomical aspects of the SMA in relation to microgenetic theory have been reviewed in a recent target paper by Goldberg (1985).

Paroxysmal Cases

Speech arrest and iterative vocalizations have been well documented with seizure activity in left and/or right SMA (e.g., Chusid et al., 1954). According to Alajouanine et al. (1959), iterative and palilalic vocalizations point to left SMA activity while speech arrest occurs mainly with discharge in either hemisphere.   The phenomenon has strong clinical localizing importance.   However, stimulation of either SMA has been reported to give vocalization, hesitation, distortion and palilalic iterations in addition to motor speech arrest.   On the other hand, clinical deficits seem to occur primarily with left SMA lesions (Jonas, 1981).

Vocalizations induced by stimulation or spontaneous seizure activity are often rhythmic or "quasi-sinusoidal" and accompanied by limb movements, facial contractions and awareness for the speech alteration (Chauvel, 1976).   The limb movements are chiefly proximal, tonic and contralateral, mainly involving the arm with abduction and elevation. Bilateral movements may occur, but ipsilateral movements are uncommon.   Adversive movements of the head and eyes to the opposite side occur, usually as part of a postural seizure (Laplane et al., 1977).

Jonas (1981) reviewed cases with paroxysmal lesions of SMA, and described the various alterations of speech that occur; sudden vocalization is perhaps the most common effect, often a rhythmic expiratory vowel or CV sound, e.g., ah, ah or la, la.   Perseveration of the last word or word fragment, hesitation and stuttering also occur, or less commonly, word finding difficulty, paraphasia and mutism.   The majority of cases have speech arrest at the beginning or end of the attack.   Dextrals have been described with speech arrest due to paroxysmal activity to the right SMA (e.g., Caplan and Zervas, 1978).

The effects of naturally occuring seizure activity in SMA are similar to those of stimulation (Arseni and Botez, 1961).   It has been shown that the probability of eliciting speech arrest or vocalization corresponds with hemispheric dominance as determined by intracarotid Amytal (Chauvel et al., 1985).   These latter authors also describe twitches in the tongue and soft palate on single shocks to the SMA, while repetitive stimulation results in arrest or vocalization that may be accompanied by tonic or clonic contractions in the oropharyngeal musculature.   Of note, speech restitution after arrest did not show aphasic errors.   According to Chauvel et al. (1985), surgical removal of SMA can give rise to transient akinetic mutism, though extirpation in epileptic cases usually leads to few residual motor or speech impairments (Penfield and Welch, 1949; Laplane et al., 1977).

Unilateral Lesions

Although Liepmann and Maas (1890) described an aphasic patient with softening in the distribution of left anterior cerebral artery, the first case in which the left SMA has been implicated in speech appears to be that of Petit-Dutaillis, et al. (1954), a 28 year old man with a 7 year history of speech arrest and motor activity in the right arm during seizures from a left SMA arteriovenous malformation, and a brief period of mutism with rapid recovery following surgery. Arseni and Botez (1961) reviewed the literature in light of 12 personal cases of parasaggital tumor and provided excellent descriptions of paroxysmal speech disorders, transient post-operative impairments and persistent changes. Their conclusion is still valid today, that the "main function of the supplementary motor area of the dominant hemisphere is connected with the incitation to speak and the setting into motion of the mechanisms of speech".

Apart from paroxysmal speech arrest, and transient post-operative impairments of speech, cases with more extensive damage may have persistent mutism or mutism may resolve to transcortical motor aphasia (Rubens, 1975), a state in which there is little or no spontaneous speech but repetition and naming may be relatively intact, perhaps as simpler performances. Repetition may be normal or agrammatic but most often it is deliberate, not echolalic. There are cases where speech has returned to normal but writing shows agrammatism, or even paragraphia (Masdeu et al., 1978). Articulation is generally intact. With the return of spontaneous speech, there is initial dysfluency and often agrammatism. Impairments of initiation, pacing, inhibition of speech and sustaining the speech flow have also been described (see Jonas, 1981).

Although aphasic errors have been reported with left SMA lesions, this is uncommon (Ross, et al., 1986). Conceivably, aphasic errors in cases of vascular occlusion reflect the involvement of deep parietal areas by way of an interruption of penetrating branches of the anterior cerebral artery. Regarding lateral asymmetries, cases of mutism or transcortical motor aphasia with right SMA lesions are rare, though a few cases have been reported in dextrals with vascular lesions of the right SMA (e.g., Brust et al., 1982), the incidence appearing to conform to that of crossed aphasia in general (Jonas, 1981). There are few cases with bilateral SMA lesions (Ross, et al., 1986), but presumably a persistent deficit occurs since unilateral cases tend to show recovery.

With regard to transcortical motor aphasia, it is of interest that Jürgens (1985) reports that monkeys with bilateral SMA lesions show a disruption of the isolation call, a self-generated vocalization, while other stimulus-dependent vocalizations are intact. This suggests that the impairment in transcortical motor aphasia may lie in a failure to generate a vocal action (spontaneous speech) when it is independent of specific perceptual cues (repetition, reading aloud, naming).

Motor Phenomena

The patient with transcortical motor aphasia has a type of partial mutism with impaired initiation of spontaneous speech, but there is also a partial akinesia affecting predominantly the upper limbs.   There is often a marked difficulty initiating actions with the arms, especially on the contralateral side.   For example, when asked to lift or lower the arm, the patient may require initiation of the movement by the examiner.   A touch of the patient's finger in the direction of the movement often suffices for it to be completed.   The facilitation of limb movement by initiation is similar to the facilitation of speech through repetition, and points to a common basis for both disorders.   There may be an impression that the patient is uncooperative for strength and tone are usually normal and he may stare at the examiner without attempting to carry out the command.   Of interest in regard to the deficit in the initiation of proximal movement in human cases is the observation that stimulation in SMA gives rise to contralateral or bilateral movements of the proximal (shoulder) musculature (van Buren and Fedio, 1976), while hypertonia at the shoulders is reported as a consequence of ipsilateral ablations in monkey (Travis, 1955).   With regard to the role of SMA in proximal motility, the phenomenon of hemiplegic writing in left hemisphere damaged stroke patients, where the residual shoulder movement is utilized in writing with the aid of a prosthesis (Brown   et al., 1983) may represent an SMA-elicited behavior.

Motor neglect (Waltregny, 1972; Laplane and Degos, 1983) may occur after natural and surgical lesions, with difficulty initiating actions with the affected limbs.   The disorder is usually greater in the arm than the leg, and there is a predilection for right hemisphere lesions.   The condition appears in association with large ablations and is possibly related to the alien hand phenomenon, though a link to cingulate gyrus has been suggested (Chauvel, 1976).   Contralateral grasping has also been described (Penfield and Jasper, 1954; Gelmers, 1983). Perseveration (Brown and Chobar, 1989) may occur with or without grasping (Fig. 5).   Cases of limb apraxia which occur with mesial frontal lesions, particularly anterior cerebral artery occlusion (e.g., Watson   et al., 1986) have in the past been interpreted on a callosal basis but may reflect SMA involvement or, as in the case of aphasic errors with SMA lesion, the interruption of deep penetrating branches of the anterior cerebral artery.   Unusual movements of the arm may occur as part of the alien hand syndrome.   With regard to the lower extremities, ambulation is usually good, though inertia or slowness resembling Parkinsonism may occur.   Of interest, selective difficulty initiating movements with the lower extremities occurs in the so-called gait apraxia, or magnetic gait, often associated with hydrocephalus. Gerstmann and Schilder (1926) related this disorder to lesions of the medial and basal parts of the frontal lobe, and this was also found by Denny-Brown (1958; see Knutsson and Lying-Tunnell, 1985).   It is conceivable (see below) that the global action representation realized through anterior cingulate gyrus parcellates into upper and lower limb systems throught SMA and basal frontal regions respectively.

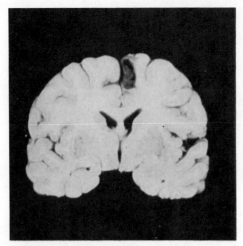

Left first frontal gyrus infarction.

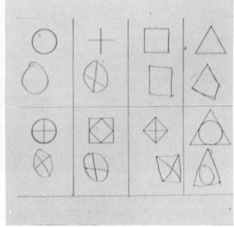

PICA Graphic test F.

Fig. 5.   Case of SMA lesion with perseveration (courtesy of J. Masdeu).

Alien   hand   syndrome

        This disorder was first described by Goldstein (1908) in a patient with
a resolving left hemiparesis, who stated that she could no longer control
her left limb.   There was diminished sensation on the left, poor object
recognition and difficulty releasing the grasp with the left hand
though objects were manipulated correctly.   Transient difficulty
relaxing the grip has been described in some callosal patients.   Brion
and Jedynak (1972) noted a feeling of estrangement for the left hand
and referred to the condition as le main etrangere.   Other features
include a tendency for the arm to drift off and assume odd postures,
especially when the eyes are closed or attention is diverted.
Intermanual conflict or competition has been noted, and patients report
that they cannot will or command the limb to act.

        The disturbance is especially marked for extensor movements
resulting in a persistent grasp or flexion posturing of the hand, and at
times wandering movements of the limb.   It may be activated by tactual
stimulation and/or mitigated by visual attention to the affected limb,
differing from a grasp reflex in the relation to attention and the
awareness of difficulty initiating the action.   Moreover, in forced
grasping the problem is not a failure of "willed relaxation" but a
persistence of stimulation (Denny-Brown, 1951).   Perhaps related is the
phenomenon of levitation described by Denny Brown et al. (1952) in
association with parietal lesions.   Their patient assumed extensor
postures of the left fingers and wrist.   When attention was directed to
her hand she could relax it and assume a normal posture.   Schilder

described a case of this type, and Hecaen and Ajuriaguerra (1954) reported patients with peculiar hand postures.

The conclusion of Brion and Jedynak (1972) that the disturbance represents a callosal syndrome is disputed by Goldberg et al. (1981), who reported two patients with lesions of left supplementary motor area involving the right hand.   The characteristic posture of such cases is illustrated in a personal case (Fig. 6) with a left mesial frontoparietal infarction, where the right hand assumed unusual flexor postures when the eyes were closed or he was distracted.   With the eyes closed and arms extended, the right hand began to clench and drift posteriorly and superiorly.   When the patient was instructed to open his eyes, he reached out with the left hand to grasp the right limb and draw it down. The left hand then forceably released the right hand grasp.   Once relaxed, the right hand remained in a normal posture so long as the eyes were open and attention was not diverted to a specific task.   In this case there were mild sensory deficits in the right hand.   I have observed other similar cases where more severe sensory deficits were thought, perhaps incorrectly, to be the basis of the disorder.   Finally, there is an unusual case of Marchiafava-Bignami disease with "crossed avoiding" of the upper limbs to visual stimuli and extensor posturing of the left arm (Lechevalier et al., 1977), which may be related to the alien hand   syndrome.

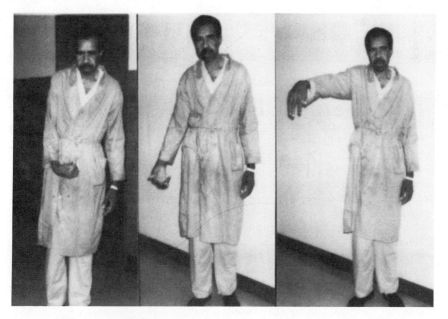

Fig. 6.   Limb posture in a case of alien hand (see text).

The Role of Supplementary Motor Area in Vocalization: An Interpretation

On the basis of the described clinical lesion effects, the SMA can be inferred to mediate preparatory stages in action generation. Lesions of this area disrupt speech, limb and body movement early in the action exposed by SMA lesions or proximal lower limb action exposed by basal frontal lesions. The lesion effects appear in disorders of initiation rather than in the selection of partial motor units or in the implementation of actions already selected. The speech disturbance is for the initiation of processing of the action, prior to conscious awareness, at a point where the motor envelope that develops through AC parcellates to separate vocal and limb motor components. Lesions expose these components prior to the specification of their constituent movement patterns. One can say that the representation of axial motility exposed by AC lesions gives way to the representation of vocal or proximal upper limb vocalization or in partial and recovering cases for spontaneous speech only with preserved repetition, a motoric not a linguistic or propositional disorder.

This interpretation, first developed by Brown (1977) and based on the study of clinical disorders, has been supported by subsequent physiological research. Kornhuber's (1974, 1985) description of the readiness potential led to its correlation in 1980 with a paralimbic midline source. These findings have been confirmed and extended by Goldberg (1985; 1987). Chauvel and Bancaud (personal communication, 1984) have observed slow wave activity from SMA preceding limb movement and motor cortex discharge in human subjects. Anatomical studies are also consistent with the view of SMA as part of an older evolutionary network (Sanides, 1969; Goldberg, 1985).

Arguing from the physiological literature, Eccles (1982) claimed that the SMA was a locus for the initiation of voluntary movement, recalling the old concept of Willenlosigkeit, a loss of the volitional impulse described in the early neuropsychological literature. On the microgenetic view, however, the sense of volition is a product of the action development; it is realized with the action and not something that gives rise to it (Brown, 1987). Volition is not a faculty that can be independently impaired. Disorders of volitional or skilled action, as in apraxia, are associated with damage to the frontal and posterior convexity, that is, to subsequent levels in the action sequence. One can say that automaticity and volition are elaborations at successive moments in the unfolding of an action, capturing stages in the outward flow of the action microgeny, not mental states triggering motor keyboards or propelling behavior.

In sum, the motor envelope, a base level or early processing stage, elaborates an archaic phase in speech and motility combining the incipient vocal and somatic elements of the action in a space centered on the body axis. The action is organized about the axial and proximal musculature, linked to respiratory, locomotor and other rhythmic automatisms, and close to motivational and drivelike states. As it develops, the action undergoes specification of its motor components with an isolation of limb, body and vocal motility. Pathology can give rise to selective impairments of vocalization (mutism) and of initiation of action involving both the upper limbs (inertia, alien hand) and the lower limbs (gait apraxia). This phase is mediated by frontal paralimbic formations, including the AC and SMA. The action system is bilaterally represented at early stages with a gradual bias to a left hemisphere representation, first apparent at the level of the SMA.

REFERENCES

Alajouanine, T., Castaigne, P., Sabouraud, O., and Contamin, F., 1959, Palilalie paroxystique et vocalisations iteratives au cours de crises epileptiques par lesion interessant l'aire motrice supplementaire, Rev. Neurol., 101:685.

Arseni, C., and Botez, M., 1961, Speech disturbances caused by tumours of the supplementary motor area, Acta Psychiat.Neurol. Scand., 36:279.

Bancaud, J., Talairach, J., Geier, S., Bonis, A., Trottier, S., and Manrique, M., 1976, Manifestations comportementales induites par la stimulation electrique de gyrus cingulaire anterieur chez l'homme, Rev. Neurol., 132:705.

Barris, R., and Schuman, H., 1953, Bilateral anterior cingulate gyrus lesions, Neurology, 3:44.

Bogen, J., 1976, Linguistic performance in the short-term following cerebral commissurotomy, in: "Studies in Neurolinguistics," H. Whitaker, ed., Academic Press, New York.

Botez, M., and Carp, N., 1968, Nouvelles donnees sur le probleme du mecanisme de declenchement de la parole, Rev. Roum. de Neurol., 5:153.

Braak, H., 1980, "Architectonics of the Human Telencephalic Cortex," Springer, Berlin.

Brion, S., and Jedynak, C.-P., 1972, Troubles du transfert interhemispherique: a propos de trois observations de tumeurs du corps calleux. Le signe de la main etrangere, Rev. Neurol., 126:257.

Brown, J. W., 1977, "Mind, Brain and Consciousness," Academic Press, New York.

Brown, J. W., 1987, The microstructure of action, in: "The Frontal Lobes Revisted," E. Perecman, ed., IRBN Press, New York.

Brown, J. W., 1988, "The Life of the Mind: Selected Papers," Erlbaum Press, New Jersey.

Brown, J. W., Blum, C., and Leader, B., 1983, Hemiplegic writing in severe aphasia, Brain and Language, 19:204.

Brown, J. W., and Chobar, K., 1989, Frontal lobes and the problem of perseveration, in: "Issue honoring A. R. Luria of the Journal of Neurolinguistics," M. Paradis, ed., in press.

Brust, J., Planck, C., Burke, A., Guobadia, M., and Healton, E., 1982, Language disorder in a right-hander after occlusion of the right anterior cerebral artery, Neurology, 32:492.

Buge, A., Escourolle, R., Rancurel, G., and Poisson, M., 1975, "Mutisme akinetique" et ramollissement bicingulaire, Rev. Neurol., 131:121.

Caplan, L., and Zervas, N., 1978, Speech arrest in a dextral with a right mesial frontal astrocytoma, Archiv. Neurol., 35:252.

Castaigne, P., Buge, A., Cambier, J., Escourolle, R., and Rancurel, G., 1971, La maladie de Marchiafava-Bignami: Etude anatomoclinique de dix observations, Rev. Neurol. 125:179.

Chauvel, P., 1976, Les stimulations de l'aire motrice supplementaire chez l'homme, Paris, These.

Chauvel, P., Bancaud, J., and Buser, P., 1985, Participation of the supplementary motor area in speech, Exper. Brain Res., 58:A14.

Chusid, J., Gutierrez-Mahoney, C., and Margules-Lavergne, M., 1954, Speech disturbances in association with parasaggital frontal lesions, J. Neurosurg. 11:193.

Corkin, S., Twitchell, T., and Sullivan, E., 1979, Safety and efficacy of cingulotomy for pain and psychiatric disorder, in: "Modern Concepts in Psychiatric Surgery," E. Hitchcock, ed., Elsevier, Amsterdam.

Denny-Brown, D., 1951, The frontal lobes and their functions, in: "Modern Trends in Neurology," A. Feiling, ed., Butterworth, London.

Denny-Brown, D., 1958, The nature of apraxia, J. Nerv. Ment. Dis., 216:9.

Denny-Brown, D., Meyer, J., and Horenstein, S., 1952, The significance of perceptual rivalry resulting from parietal lesion, Brain, 75:433.

Eccles, J., 1982, The initiation of voluntary movements by the supplementary motor area, Arch f. Psychiat. u. Nervenkr., 231:423.

Faris, A., 1969, Limbic system infarction, Neurology, 19:91.

Freemon, F., 1971, Akinetic mutism and bilateral anterior cerebral artery occlusion, J. Neurol. Neurosurg. Psychiat., 34:693.

Gelmers, H., 1983, Non-paralytic motor disturbances and speech disorders: the role of the supplementary motor area, J. Neurol. Neurosurg. Psychiat., 46:1052.

Gerstmann, J., and Schilder, P., 1926, Uber eine besondere Gangstorung bei Stirnhirnerkrankung, Wien. Med. Wochenschr. 3:97.

Goldberg, G., 1985, Supplementary motor area structure and function: review and hypotheses, Behav. Brain Sci., 8:567.

Goldberg, G., 1987, From intent to action: evolution and function of the premotor systems of the frontal lobe, in: "The Frontal Lobes Revisted," E. Perecman, ed., IRBN Press, New York.

Goldberg, G., Mayer, N., and Toglia, J., 1981, Medial frontal cortex infarction and the alien hand sign, Arch. Neurol., 38:683.

Goldstein, K., 1908, Zur Lehre von der motorischen Apraxie, Z. Physiol. Neurolog. , XI(4/5):169.

Hecaen, H., and Ajuriaguerra, J. de, 1954, Brain, 77:373.

Jonas, S., 1981, The supplementary motor region and speech emission, J. Comm. Dis., 14:349.

Jürgens, U., 1985, Implication of the SMA in phonation, Exp. Brain Res.,58:A12.

Jürgens, U., and von Cramon, D., 1982, On the role of the anterior cingulate cortex in phonation: a case report, Brain and Language 15:234.

Jürgens, U., and Pratt, R., 1979, The cingular vocalization pathway in the squirrel monkey, Exp. Brain Res., 34:499.

Knutsson, E., and Lying-Tunnell, U., 1985, Gait apraxia in normal-pressure hydrocephalus, Neurology, 35:155.

Kornhuber, H., 1974, Cerebral cortex, cerebellum and basal ganglia, in: "The Neurosciences: Third Study Program," F. Schmitt and F. Worden, eds., MIT Press, Cambridge.

Kornhuber, H., 1985, Bereitschaftspotential and the activity of the supplementary motor area preceding voluntary movement, Exp. Brain Res., 58:A10-A11.

Laplane, D., and Degos, J., 1983, Motor neglect, J. Neurol. Neurosurg.Psychiat., 46:152.

Laplane, D., Talairach, J., Meininger, V., Bancaud, J., and Bouchareine, A., 1977, Motor consequences of motor area ablations in man, J. Neurol. Sci., 31:29.

Larsen, B., Skinhoj, E., and Lassen, N., 1978, Variations in regional cortical blood flow in the right and left hemispheres during automatic speech, Brain, 101:193.

Lechavalier, B., Andersson, J., and Morin, P., 1977, Hemisphere disconnection syndrome with a "crossed avoiding" reaction in a case of Marchiafava-Bignami disease, J. Neurol. Neurosurg. Psychiat. 40:483.

Liepmann, H., and Maas, O., 1890, cited in Arseni and Botez.

Masdeu, J., Schoene, W., and Funkenstein, H., 1978, Aphasia following infarction of the left supplementary motor area, Neurology, 28:1220.

Nielsen, J., 1951, Anterior cingulate gyrus and corpus callosum, Bull. Los Angeles Neurol. Soc., 16:235.

Nielsen, J., and Jacobs, L., 1951, Bilateral lesions of the anterior cingulate gyri, Bull. Los Angeles Neurol. Soc., 16:231.

Orgogozo, J., Larsen, B., Roland, P., and Lassen, N., 1979, Activation de l'aire motrice supplementaire au cours des mouvements volontaire chez l'homme, Rev. Neurol., 135:705.

Penfield, W., and Jasper, H., 1954, "Epilepsy and the Functional Anatomy of the Human Brain", Little Brown, Boston.

Penfield, W., and Roberts, L., 1959, "Speech and Brain Mechanisms", Princeton University Press, Princeton.

Penfield, W., and Welch, K., 1949, The supplementary motor area of the cerebral cortex of man, Trans. Amer. Neurol. Assoc., 74:179.

Petit-Dutaillis, D., Guiot, G., Messimy, R., and Bourdillon, C., 1954, A propos d'une aphemie par atteinte de la zone motrice supplementaire de Penfield, au cours de l'evolution d'un aneurisme arterio-veineux guerison de l'aphemie par ablation, Rev. Neurol., 90:95.

Poeck, K., and Kerschensteiner, M., 1975, Analysis of sequential motor events in oral apraxia, in: "Cerebral Localization," K. Zulch, ed., Springer, Heidelberg.

Ross, M., Damasio, H., and Eslinger, P., 1986, The role of the supplementary motor area (SMA) and anterior cingulate (AC) in the generation of movement, Neurology, 36:346.

Rubens, A., 1975, Aphasia with infarction in the territory of the anterior cerebral artery, Cortex, 11:239.

Sanides, F., 1969, Comparative architectonics of the neocortex of mammals and their evolutionary interpretation, Ann. New York Acad. Sci., 167:404.

Segarra, J., 1970, Cerebral vascular disease and behavior, Arch. Neurol., 22:408.

Sutton, D., Samson, H., and Larson, C., 1978, Brain mechanisms in learned phonation of Macaca mulatta, in: "Recent Advances in Primatology," vol. 1, D. Chivers and J. Herbert, eds., Academic Press, New York.

Travis, A., 1955, Neurological deficiencies following supplementary motor area lesions in Macaca mulatta, Brain, 78:174.

Van Buren, J., and Fedio, P;., 1976, Functional representation on the medial aspect of the frontal lobes in man, J. Neurosurg., 44:275.

Waltregny, A., 1972, L'Epilepsie de l'aire motrice supplementaire, Med. de Hyg., 815.

Watson, R., Fleet, W., Gonzalez-Rothi, L., and Heilman, K., 1986, Apraxia and the supplementary motor area, Arch. Neurol., 43:787.

Ward, A., 1948, The anterior cingular gyrus and personality, Res. Publ. Assoc. Nerv. Ment. Dis., 27:438.

NEURAL CORRELATES OF AUDIO-VOCAL BEHAVIOR: PROPERTIES OF

ANTERIOR LIMBIC CORTEX AND RELATED AREAS

Peter Müller-Preuss

Dept. of Primate Behavior
Max-Planck-Institute for Psychiatry
Munich, Germany

INTRODUCTION

Most reports concerned with the neural mechanism of sound production in mammals have pointed out that the involvement of cortical structures is restricted to primate species (for reviews e.g. see Jürgens, 1979; Müller-Preuss and Ploog, 1983; Sutton and Jürgens, in press). Furthermore, only in man has it been shown that several neocortical areas are engaged in the generation and control of speech (Penfield and Welch, 1959), whereas in nonhuman primates mostly mesocortical regions take part. These somewhat "older" cortical structures are located mainly around the knee of the corpus callosum, an area here comprehensively described as the anterior limbic cortex (ALC); in particular it is composed of structures such as the anterior cingulate gyrus (ACG), the gyrus subcallosus, the gyrus rectus and the region around the anterior cingulate sulcus, which seems to be a transitional zone between new and older parts of the cortex. The latter is bordered dorsally by medial parts of Brodmann areas 6 and 8, known as the supplementary motor area (SMA). The involvement of the SMA in sound production even in nonhuman primates has been suggested for the squirrel monkey (Kirzinger and Jürgens, 1982) and for macaques (Sutton et al., 1985). Type and extent of involvement in man and primates is still matter of discussion, also in this volume. According to current literature, the anterior limbic cortex, from a structural as well as functional point of view, seems far from being a homogeneous brain area. It receives projections from, and sends them out to, nearly all parts of the telencephalon (cortex, basalganglia), to

many nuclei of the thalamus and there are even multiple connections with the midbrain and the brainstem. Its terminal fields
lie within brain areas related to different sensory modalities,
and within regions considered to be involved in the processing
of various motor tasks. It is assumed, therefore, that more
general or more complex abilities are controlled and processed
by the anterior limbic cortex, and that its neuronal populations
do not relate to only one particular function. However, as already indicated, one of the most prominent task often associated
with this area is the control of sound production. This has been
demonstrated by several experimental approaches, such as stimulation studies (Robinson, 1967; Jürgens and Ploog,1970; Jürgens,
1976), lesion studies (Sutton et al., 1974; Aitken, 1981; Kirzinger and Jürgens, 1982) and projection studies (Müller-Preuss
and Jürgens, 1976; Jürgens and Müller-Preuss, 1977; Jürgens,
1983). Besides other cortical areas, this area has been shown to
play a role in the production of speech in man (e.g. see Penfield and Roberts, 1969; Jürgens and v.Cramon, 1982). From the
data so far available, the conclusion has been drawn that the
anterior limbic cortex is primarily engaged in the volitional or
intentional control of vocalization rather than exerting an influence directly upon the particular motor centers in the brainstem, a functional property already quite well documented, even
on the neuronal level, for the SMA (Tanji, 1984). Astonishingly
few trials have been made to evaluate the functional properties
of this and other "vocalization structures" by neural recording
techniques: some laboratory groups recorded neural activity
within the nucleus ambiguus, which is the motor nucleus of the
laryngeal muscles, of rats and bats (Yajima and Hayashi, 1983;
Rübsamen and Betz, 1986). Larson (1985) studied the properties
of neurons in the periaqueductal grey of primates during vocal
activity. Several recording experiments (Bachman and MacLean,
1971; Robinson and Wang, 1979; Niki and Watanabe, 1979; Tanji,
1984; Stwertka, 1985) have been centered upon the anterior limbic cortex, but there is only one report in the literature regarding neuronal activity in the ALC of primates during vocal
behavior (Sutton et al., 1974). In that study,a relation was
found to exist between neuronal activity and conditioned vocalization. These authors additionally report about neurons which
responded to external auditory stimuli. This may suggest involvement of ALC neurons not only in purely vocal processing but
also in a mechanism of audio-vocal integration. The study of
Bachman and MacLean already dealt with the question of auditory,
somatic and visual input into this area in squirrel monkeys and
resulted in a negative answer with regard to all three modalities tested: explorations failed to reveal any significant
change of unit activity by this particular stimulation. Sutton
et al. explained their diverse findings as having been caused by

possible   species-specific differences between macaques and
squirrel monkeys. However, an anatomical tracing study in
squirrel monkeys disclosed a reciprocal connection between ALC
and parts of the auditory cortex, making an auditory input into
this region probable (Müller-Preuss et al., 1980). On the basis
of these results, experiments were designed for the purpose of
describing the relations of the ALC with areas known to be involved in acoustic communicative processes and evaluating the
properties of ALC neurons in squirrel monkeys during both vocal
and auditory stimulation. These relations will be explained from
a structural point of view, firstly, by showing the efferent
and/or afferent connections of the ALC within the subregions of
the area itself, secondly, their pathways to and from other
vocal as well as auditory brain areas and, thirdly, their linkage with those structures where the auditory system projects as
well. They shall be further elucidated from a more functional
point of view, by describing the results of some recording experiments carried out on those "related areas". It is hoped that
the neuroanatomical and neurophysiological data discussed here
will be considered a useful contribution to the current debate
regarding the pysiological control of mammalian vocalization.

The description of the anatomical connections of the ALC
will be based, on the one side, on a more detailed, thematically
condensed review of already published studies (Müller-Preuss and
Jürgens, 1976; Jürgens and Müller-Preuss, 1977; Müller-Preuss et
al., 1980; Jürgens, 1983; Jürgens, 1984) and, on the other side,
on unpublished data gathered in tracing experiments involving
both,auditory and vocal structures. The efferent projections of
the particular regions were exclusively evaluated by injections
of 3H-Leucine, whereas the afferents were investigated also with
the aid of injections of tritiated horseradish-peroxidase.

ANATOMICAL CONNECTIONS OF THE ANTERIOR LIMBIC CORTEX

First the connections within the area itself will be considered, because the intrinsic connections may cast some light
on the extent of involvement of the particular subregions within
audio-vocal behavior. The most dorsal part of the region, that
is, the upper part of the cingulate gyrus and the lower part of
the supplementary motorarea (SMA) within and above the cingulate
sulcus, sends its projections to all other parts except the gyrus rectus. With regard to the afferents, the connections seem
to be quite reciprocal with the exception of the gyrus rectus:
injections into the gyrus rectus cause terminal fields in the
ACG, however weak, whereas HRP injections into the ACG failed to
show any tracing in the gyrus rectus. The precallosal section of
the cingulate gyrus has terminal fields even in the dorsal re-

gions of the ACG as well as ventrally within the gyrus subcallosus and the gyrus rectus. As revealed by retrograde techniques, afferents come from all other sections of the ALC.

The gyrus subcallosus sends its fibres to the neighboring gyrus rectus and up to the whole anterior cingulate gyrus. Above the cingulate sulcus, which receives projections from all other parts of the ALC, only weak terminal fields are found. The terminal fields of the gyrus rectus reach up only to the cingulate gyrus below the sulcus and receive projections from the subcallosal and precallosal areas. Again, retrograde tracing failed to support the assumption that there exists an afferent connection from the upper part of the anterior cingulate gyrus to the gyrus rectus. Thus there seems to be a quite simple organization of the intrinsic connections of the ALC which is defined by the particular distances of the individual subregions from each other. Figure 1 illustrates the situation in a very schematically

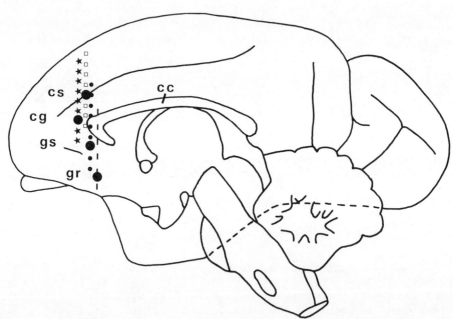

Fig. 1.   Medial view of a sagittal section through squirrel monkey's brain, where the connections between the particular subregions of the ALC are shown in their dorso-ventral extension. Injection sites are symbolized by big dots, size of extension by lines, dots, stars and squares. Abbrev.: cc - corpus callosum; cg - cingulate gyrus; cs - cingulate sulcus; gr - gyrus rectus; gs - gyrus subcallosus.

way, emphasizing the relation of decreasing density of terminal fields to distance from the injection site. Beyond that dorso-ventral organization, the particular regions seem to have far-ther reaching connections with regard to the rostro-caudal axis. The anterior cingulate gyrus, for example, receives from and yields projections to the caudalmost parts of the gyrus itself (area 23). The situation in the SMA is similar (Jürgens, 1984).

The other cortical areas to be regarded are those which, at least in man, have been shown to play a role in sound production and/or are auditory responsive. These are the homologues of Broca's area in the lateral frontal cortex (Brodmann's area 44), Wernicke's area in the posterior third of the first temporal gyrus, the already mentioned supplementary motor area in the dorsomedial frontal cortex and, finally, the auditory cortex in the superior temporal gyrus. To start with the last, all regions of the ALC project to association areas of the auditory cortex in a particular order: the more dorsal the injection within the ALC, the more ventral the terminal fields within the superior temporal gyrus. For example, the region around the cingulate gyrus projects down to the upper bank of the superior temporal sulcus, whereas the gyrus rectus has its terminal fields in those auditory association areas which are close to the primary field. As regards the projections which the ALC receives from the auditory cortex, there is a rather good reciprocal connec-tion between cortical regions subserving auditory and vocal functions (Bieser and Müller-Preuss, 1987). Besides the gyrus rectus, the ALC has connections to the medio-dorsal cortex (SMA), the reciprocity of which is not clear with regard to the afferent studies. The cortical fields homologous to the area of Wernicke failed to show any efferent or afferent connections to the ALC, while the anterior cingulate gyrus and the regions around the cingulate sulcus project heavily to those parts of area 44 which may be homologous to Broca's area in man. That there is also afferent input from area 44 has been demonstrated by retrograde tracing studies (Jürgens, 1984). It may of inter-est to note that the SMA also has terminalfields within area 44 (Jürgens, 1984), but not within the auditory cortex. Finally it should be noted that injections between the cingular sulcus and the knee of the corpus callosum reveal terminal fields in an area of the dorsolateral cortex which receives also fibers from the STG and where units have been shown to be responsive to acoustic stimulation (Newman and Lindsley, 1978).

Many parts of the basal ganglia in the telencephalon re-ceive projections from the ALC, but only one can be closely re-lated with audiovocal functions: the central nucleus of the

amygdala. It yields projections not only from all parts of the
ALC, but also from parts of the auditory association cortex. Until to now,the existence of afferents has been shown only for
the anterior cingulate gyrus (Jürgens, 1983), but not for the
remaining areas of ALC. Some convergent projections, not directly overlapping, also have been found for the nucleus basolat-
eralis of the amygdala and for the head and the tail of the caudate nucleus. Similar to the situation of the basal ganglia is
that of <u>the diencephalon</u>: the projections are manifold,but those
related to the production of vocalization and to audition are
rare. The medio-ventral belt of the medial part of the pulvinar
nucleus has efferent as well as afferent connections with both
structures. The reciprocity of the connection has been confirmed
by orthograde as well as retrograde tracing studies and, thus,
there is a rather good demonstration of convergence of both
systems at the thalamic level. It may be noteworthy that the
projections from the auditory cortex rostrally extend somewhat
to the medial thalamic nucleus, a site receiving the strongest
subcortical projection from the ALC.

Neurons of the medial geniculate body, labelled with 3H-
Leucine, send projections, in the proposed convergent sense, only to the central nucleus of the amygdala, but not to the caudate nucleus. One injection which primarily affected the medial
parts of the MGB caused also terminal fields in the medial pulvinar nucleus. One further convergent projection originating
within the cortical parts of the systems has been found in the
peripeduncular nucleus. This nucleus lies closely ventromedial
to the auditory thalamus but anatomically still belongs to the
diencephalon. The reciprocity of these connections also has been
confirmed by HRP experiments.

Although further down in the <u>midbrain</u> the distance between
the structures participating in both systems decreases more and
more, there is no increase of connections between them. There
are, of course, strong relations within the systems themselves,
as shown by projections from the ALC to the central grey or projections from the auditory cortex to the MGB or inferior colliculus. But direct connections between structures involved in
audition and vocalization are remarkably poor in the midbrain in
comparison with those at the cortical level. As a centrifugal
connection from telencephalon to midbrain, only the subcallosal
part of the ALC projects to marginal regions of the auditory
midbrain. It is a weak projection, however, and not confirmed to
be reciprocal. A reference to connections of the inferior colliculus with the auditory system itself seems trivial, but it is
worthy of note that parts of the auditory cortex send back efferents to the midbrain only as for as the marginal zones of
this nucleus. There is a small region at the border of the au-

ditory midbrain which is directly connected not only with parts
of the ALC, but additionally with cortical parts of the auditory
system. The most prominent part of the vocal system in the midbrain has been demonstrated to be the periaqueductal grey (PAG)
and the lateral adjacent parabrachial nuclei. All parts of the
anterior limbic cortex send projections to these areas. However,
the reciprocity seems to be restricted: only a few cells were
found in the central grey after HRP injections into the anterior
cingulate cortex (Jürgens, 1983), and 3H-Leu injections into the
PAG did not reveal terminalfields in the ALC. On the other hand,
all three auditory structures (AC,MGB,IC) so far studied project to the medial and/or dorsal part of the PAG. Again, with
regard to reciprocity, no terminalfields have been found within
auditory nuclei after PAG injections. However, of interest is
the fact that there are areas around the whole IC which show
heavy tracing. Thus, neurons of the midbrain level of both systems, although not intermingled, are in very close neighboring
regions.
In a synopsis, Figure 2A accentuates all direct connections of
the anterior limbic cortex with the auditory system and shows
all those areas where both systems project convergently. In 2B,
the auditory structures and the anterior limbic cortex with its
connection to the vocalization system are described. Finally,
and this cannot be emphasized too much, this report of course is
biased: of many connections it considers only those which can be
related with audio-vocal processes. There are other connections
from the ALC to structures involved in the processing of other
functions or related to other sensory modalities, such as olfaction, vision or somatosensation. But, for evaluating the neural
correlates of a particular behavior (i.e. audio-vocal), it seems
reasonable to exclude all connections not directly involved.

PROPERTIES OF NEURONS OF THE ANTERIOR LIMBIC CORTEX

One major tool in the evaluation of relationships between
particular brain structures and underlying functions is to record neuronal activity by electrophysiological methods. Therefore, to gain such information in addition to the data obtained
by stimulation, lesion and tracing studies, the activity of
neurons of the ALC was recorded. The neuronal discharges have
been studied during three testing procedures: firstly, white
noise, clicks, tones and tape recorded species-specific vocalizations were presented via a loudspeaker to examine the acoustic properties of the neurons in general. Secondly, to test the
neurons' involvement in the production of vocalizations, the
neuronal activity was recorded during the utterance of electrically elicited vocalizations. And thirdly, to avoid possible
consequences due to artifacts caused by the electrical brain

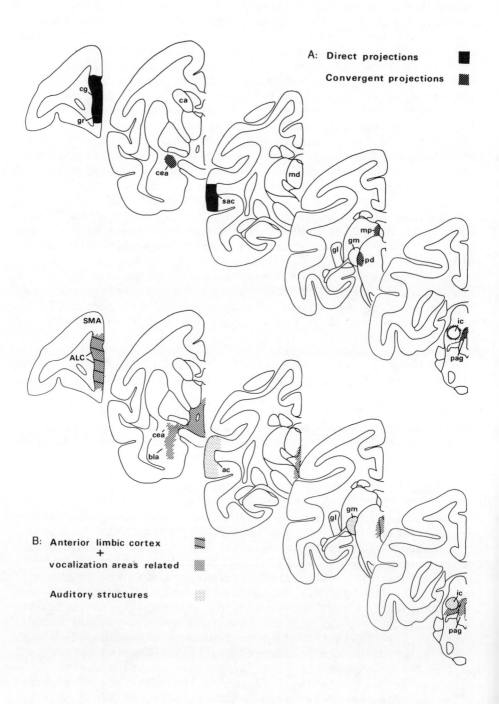

stimulation, attempts were made to obtain recordings of neural activity during spontaneously uttered calls. In the recording experiments (which were carried out on unanaesthetized, awake squirrel monkeys), tungsten microelectrodes (2-10 MOhm) were used. With the aid of a stereotactic device mounted on an epi-durally implanted plastic chamber, the microelectrodes were gui-ded dorso-ventrally through the ALC. The single- and multi-unit recordings were carried out extracellularly, applying the tra-ditional window and amplifier techniques for storing the neural activity. The usual PSTHs were calculated with a LSI computer. Location of electrode penetrations within the ALC was recon-structed along the stereotactic protocol with the aid of several tracks, histologically verified through lesions. They are indi-cated schematically in the medial view of a sagittal section through the squirrel monkey's brain shown in Figure 3A.

Vocalizations were elicited by electrical stimulation of the central grey matter. Only those points within the central grey where electrical activation also caused vocalization when the actual stimulation was over were selected. This was done so as to avoid the effects of the stimulus artifact which complicate the analysis of neural recording. Further details of stimulation and recording techniques have been described elsewhere (Müller-Preuss and Ploog, 1981).

The activity of about 220 neurons from both hemispheres in two animals were recorded. Almost every neuron was tested during the utterance of electrically elicited vocalizations as well as du-ring the presentation of an external acoustic stimulus. During the utterance of spontaneous vocalizations, only 44 neurons could be tested. This relatively small number is due to the fact, that squirrel monkeys in the experimental setup necessary

Fig. 2.   Part A: Frontal sections through the squirrel monkey's brain showing direct (black) connections of ALC and auditory structures and convergent (crosshatching) projections of ALC, other vocalization structures and auditory structures, as specified in part B. Abbrev.: ac - auditory cortex; ALC - anterior limbic cortex; bla - basolateral nucleus of amygdala; ca - caudate nucleus; cg - cingulate gyrus; cea - central nucleus of amygdala; gl - lateral geniculate body; gm - medial geniculate body; gr - gyrus rectus; ic - inferior col-liculus; md - dorsomedial nucleus of thalamus; mp - medial nucleus of thalamus; pag - periaqueductal grey pd - peripeduncular nucleus; sac - secondary auditory cortex; SMA - supplementary motor area.

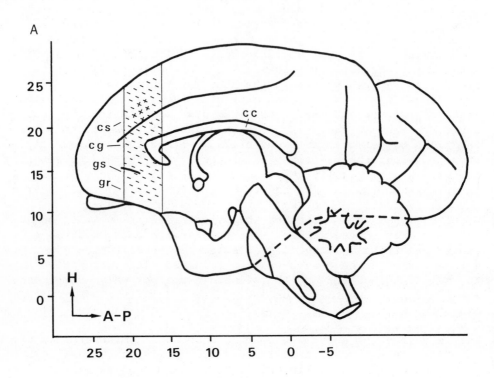

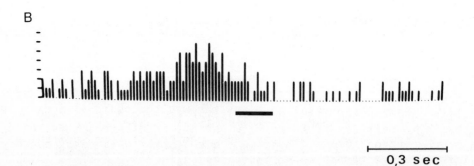

0,3 sec

Fig. 3.   Part A: Location of recording area in medial view of a
          sagittal   section   through the squirrel monkey's brain.
          Stippled hatching from upper left to lower right indi-
          cates regions of auditory units, crosses show area of
          units responsive during vocalization. Part B: PSTH of
          a unit reacting before and during vocalization; Bin
          width 6 msec.

for recording, do not often vocalize spontaneously; even vocal conditioning tests conducted elsewhere failed in this species (Symmes, D., pers. communication).

Responses to _electrically_ elicited vocalizations: of 221 cells recorded within the area shown by stippled lines, none responded in a clear relation to the uttered vocalizations. As already pointed out, only those vocalizations uttered after termination of the electrical stimulus were related to the neuronal activity. In 16 neurons, a decrease of activity was observed after stimulation but a synchronization with vocal activity could not be established. In the same way, an increase of activity was detected for 3 units. Thus, there seems to be a mainly inhibitory effect on the activity of some neurons after electrical stimulation of the PAG, but no influence seems to be exerted by these self-produced vocalizations. The histological inspection of the electrode tracks displayed no concentration of responsive units within a particular area of the ALC.

Responses to _acoustic_ stimulation: 226 neurons were tested by loudspeaker-transmitted stimuli and only in a few cases was a response detected. Nine units showed a reaction to simple, artificial stimuli, such as noise, tone or click. In the case of reactions to clicks, the latency was 10 to 100 msec. The response patterns were always of a simple "on"-type. Such a simple kind of reaction has also been observed in responses to species-specific vocalizations (5 cases): on-responses and no selectivity between different types of vocalizations. Acoustically responsive neurons were detected within the whole recording area.

Responses to _spontaneous_ vocalization: of the 44 neurons tested during vocal activity not caused by electrical stimulation, 7 displayed an activity which could be related to the vocalization. The response latencies clearly showed that these cells are engaged in motor activity rather than in sensory processing: Stimulus related action potentials were measured to occur up to 100msec before the beginning of a call and they lasted only for a few milliseconds during the call. An example of such a unit is shown in figure 3, part B. Histological localization of such units showed that they are found only above the cingulate sulcus. Thus, these units probably belong to the transition zone between the upper most part of ALC and lower part of SMA. Unfortunately, due to the small number of units found and the limited histologal findings, a more precise localization was not possible.

NEURAL RESPONSES WITHIN AUDITORY AREAS RELATED TO ALC

In searching for the neural correlates of audio-vocal behavior, the studies were at the beginning concentrated primarily
on the anterior limbic cortex, but of course they should - and
partly do - include all those brain structures connected with
the ALC and having demonstrated to play a role in acoustic communication. Of those areas which have been indicated above as
beeing involved, only structures of the auditory pathway, including closely adjacent regions, were investigated so far, at
least as far as the squirrel monkey is concerned. A stimulation
study has been carried out in squirrel monkeys to test the properties of the connection between the ALC and the secondary auditory cortex (Müller-Preuss et al., 1980). It has been shown
that activation of neural populations within the ALC can cause a
decrease of the spike rate of auditory neurons, suggesting an
inhibitory influence by this cortical vocalization area on the
auditory system. However, the observed effect was the consequence of an artificial activation of one particular part of the
vocalization system. To clarify whether such an inhibitory influence is exerted in general on auditory input or indicative of
a specific mechanism for the auditory representation of an individuals own vocal activity, the activity of auditory neurons has
been studied during vocalization, for calls can only uttered after the activation of a fairly large number of the structures
involved. An analysis of neural responses evoked through vocalization and, for comparative purposes, during playback of vocalization as well as simultaneous presentation of both vocalization and playback, revealed that the auditory input itself (in
general) is not inhibited during vocal activity. This was demonstrated by the fact that the response pattern of most units of
the auditory midbrain and numerous cells of auditory thalamus
and cortex to the particular stimuli was similar (Müller-Preuss,
1983). An example of such a unit is given in Figure 4B; this
type of unit has been considered to be of a purely "auditory"
nature. Attention is invited to the different latency of responses which mainly is caused by the differing distances of the
particular sound sources to the ear. However, other units, found
mostly within the auditory thalamus and cortex (but also within
the midbrain), had response pattern indicative of interactions
between the auditory system and structures involved in sound
production: a relatively large number of units within the
superior temporal gyrus and the medial geniculate body and some
from the marginal regions of the inferior colliculus reacted
weakly, not at all or with decreased discharge to emitted vocalizations, but exhibited a clear response to the same vocalization as a playback stimulus. It was concluded that an inhibitory
effect is exercised by activated vocalization-producing struc-

tures on auditory neurons and may represent a neural correlate with a certain self-monitoring function regarding self-produced vocal activities. Such a unit has been considered to be the "audio-vocal" type, and an example from the midbrain is shown in the middle of figure 4B. Histological examination of the electrode penetrations displayed no favoured location of those units within the STG and MGB, but in the IC such units have been recorded either at the beginning and the end of tracks or those which passed marginal regions of the IC. Their location is demonstrated in Figure 4A. In exploring the auditory midbrain, the electrodes occasionally also passed regions which either border immediately ventral to the IC or lie deeper within the reticular formation. Most units recorded there were unresponsive to any acoustic stimulus. Nevertheless, some neurons have been found in the closest neighbourhood of the IC, clearly not belonging to it, displaying response patterns never seen in recordings within the auditory pathway: the increase of activity began up to 80 msec before the utterance of the vocalization. The example shown in the lower third of figure 4B demonstrates this and indicates furthermore that there was no response to stimuli presented via a loudspeaker. It should be mentioned that the vocal activity during these recordings was elicited electrically. As regards their response pattern, such units seem to belong only to structures involved in the production of vocalization and have been defined therefore as being of the "vocal" type. That only a very few units of this type were detected may be due to the fact that the experiments on the midbrain were focussed on auditory structures and the units of the vocal system were encountered more or less accidentally. An other explanation may be that, in contrast to a sensory structure like the inferior colliculus, areas shown to participate in a definite motor function need not necessarily be densely packed with neurons related to a specific function. The latter consideration is supported by the observations of Larson (1986), who carefully investigated the dorsal part of the periaqueductal grey: He reported that the "vast majority" of units did not display a relation to the uttered calls. And even more noteworthy, in this area only a very few units were found which responded to acoustic stimulation.

CONCLUSIONS

The purposes of this chapter are twofold: Firstly, to contribute results of tracing and recording experiments carried out on the anterior limbic cortex of squirrel monkeys relevant to the theme of this volume; secondly, in consequence of the results of the ALC tracing experiments, to introduce the interrelations between the ALC and other structures involved in vocalization and the auditory system into this topic. That is why the

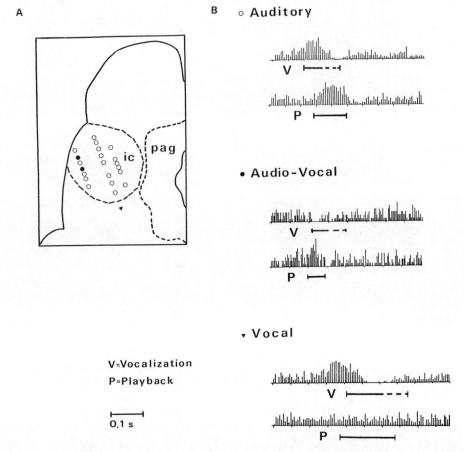

Fig. 4.   Location of several of the three different types of
           neurons within the midbrain are shown in part A. In
           part B the types of different response patterns,
           evoked during the utterance of a vocalization (V) as
           well as during playback (P), of 3 representative
           neurons are demonstrated. Bars indicate duration of
           stimuli, stippled parts point to variable length of
           (V). Bin width of PSTH: 3 and 6 msec. Abbrev.: ic -
           inferior colliculus; pag - periaqueductal grey.

results of tracing and recording experiments undertaken within the auditory pathway were included.

With regard to the connections of the ALC, several aspects may cast light on its role within audio-vocal behavior. Most of all, the evident cortical (SMA, area 44) and subcortical connections (amygdala, hypothalamus, PAG) of the ALC with structures playing a role in sound production are indicative, from a structural point of view, of its involvement in vocal processes. Nevertheless, on cortical level there are relations with the auditory system (connection with the superior temporal gyrus) which point on possible ALC participation in integrative processes between audition and sound production. The assumption that such participation in audio-vocal interactions is possible is further substantiated by the demonstrated common convergent projections of ALC and auditory cortex (Nucl. centralis amygdalae, Nucl. peripeduncularis, Nucl. pulvinaris medialis, region immediately bordering around inferior colliculus). Additionally, there are connections of the auditory midbrain, thalamus and also cortex with the periaqueductal grey. In turn, the PAG projects to areas very narrowly related to the auditory midbrain and thalamus (Area surrounding IC; Nucl. peripeduncularis). The PAG is one of the most important vocalization structures in the midbrain to which the ALC is strongly related. Thus, there are locations at different levels within the brain likely to be involved, from a structural point of view, in interactions between both systems,and the cortical level is the most conspicious one.

As regards the particular subregions of ALC and their connections within the audio-vocal systems, it seems that the more dorsal parts (area around cingulate sulcus, cingulate gyrus) are "more" related to vocalization, whereas its ventral parts (gyrus subcallosus, gyrus rectus) are "more" connected with the auditory system. This view, however, is only partially supported by the recording study of ALC: auditory neurons are found evenly distributed over the whole area, whereas "vocal" units have been recorded only in the dorsal-most part of ALC (CS). Thus, structurally the units appear to be mingled, at least in the dorsal part of the ALC, whereas functionally they are separated, either triggered by the auditory input or by instructions of the vocalization system. Concerning the latency, auditory input varies in time from a very short latency, which provides direct input, to a more lasting one hinting at indirect connections with the auditory pathway. The duration of the prestimulus activity of "vocal" neurons points on a participation on the initiation of vocalization rather than exertion of a direct influence on the periphery. One of the main findings reported here is a negative

one: no neuronal responses were detected in the ALC during vocalizations evoked by electrical stimulation elsewhere in the
brain. There is one explanation for this finding which would fit
quite well with the suggestions evaluated so far over the role
of the ALC in sound production: a call evoked by force through
artificial activation of a structure lying more caudally (PAG)
does not necesssarily include activation of a structure which is
supposed to be related more indirectly (volitional) with sound
production. In turn, a call which is uttered from a monkey more
volitionally may need for its production advance activation of a
structure like the ALC.

Concerning the properties of those areas defined here as
related to the ALC, only information about involvement of structures of the auditory pathway in audio-vocal behavior has been
supplied so far. The recording studies during vocalization disclosed one type of neural response pattern indicative for interactions between auditory and vocal structures. The nonrespon-
siveness to, or inhibition during, vocalization of some auditory
neurons may be caused by structures active during vocalization.
Although precise localization of such neurons is still lacking
for the thalamus and the cortex, for the midbrain they are found
only within the marginal regions. Hence they lie just in or
close to those areas which have been shown to be connected with
vocalization structures (gyrus subcallosus, PAG). And in the
immediate vicinity of the collicular margins, units have been
found which clearly belong to the vocal system (see fig.4). The
latency of prestimulus activity of these neurons is rather long
and, therefore, units of this part of the vocal system are not
likely to be involved directly in motor coordinating processes.
On the other hand, these neurons responded before and during
electrically evoked vocalizations, a fact showing that they may
be linked closer with vocal processes than units of the ALC.

In general, the ALC, together with the areas considered
here to be related, may partly serve as a neural correlate for
mechanism controlling audio-vocal behavior. Such a correlate
seems to be organized at various levels within the brain and one
of the highest level within this organization would be the axis
of STG and ALC.

ACKNOWLEDGMENTS

The author wishes to thank Mrs. E. Rösner for her help in
translating the manuscript and Dr. A. Bieser and Prof. D. Ploog
for comments.

Supported by Deutsche Forschungsgemeinschaft SFB 204.

REFERENCES

Aitken, P. G., 1981, Cortical control of conditioned and spon-
    taneous vocal behavior in rhesus monkeys, Brain and
    Language, 13:171.
Bachman, D. S., and MacLean, P. D., 1971, Unit analysis of in-
    puts to cingulate cortex in awake sitting Squirrel mon-
    keys. I. Exteroceptive systems, Intern. J. Neuroscience,
    2:109.
Bieser, A., and Müller-Preuss, P., 1987, Efferent projections
    from the auditory cortex in the Squirrel monkey, in: New
    Frontiers in Brain Research, N. Elsner and O. D. Creutz-
    feldt, eds., Thieme, Stuttgart and New York.
Jürgens, U., 1976, Reinforcing concomitants of electrically
    elicited vocalizations, Exp. Brain Res., 26:203.
Jürgens, U., and Müller-Preuss, P., 1977, Convergent projections
    of different limbic vocalization areas in the Squirrel
    monkey, Exp. Brain Res., 29:75.
Jürgens, U., and v.Cramon, D., 1982, On the role of the anterior
    cingulate cortex in phonation: a case report, Brain and
    Language, 15:234.
Jürgens, U., 1983, Afferent fibers to the cingular vocalization
    region in the Squirrel monkey, Exp. Neurol. 80:395.
Jürgens, U., 1984, The efferent and afferent connections of the
    supplementary motor area, Brain Res., 300:63.
Jürgens, U., and Richter, K., 1986, Glutamate-induced vocaliza-
    tion in the Squirrel monkey, Brain Res., 373:349.
Kirzinger, A., and Jürgens, U., 1982, Cortical lesion effects
    and vocalization in the Squirrel monkey, Brain Res.,
    233:299.
Larson, C. R., 1985, The midbrain periaqueductal gray: a brain-
    stem structure involved in vocalization, J. of Speech and
    Hearing Res., 28:241.
Müller-Preuss, P., and Jürgens, U., 1976, Projections from the
    "cingular" vocalization area in the Squirrel monkey,
    Brain Res., 103:29.
Müller-Preuss, P., Newman, J. D., and Jürgens, U., 1980, Anato-
    mical and physiological evidence for a relationship bet-
    ween the "cingular" vocalization area and the auditory
    cortex in the Squirrel monkey, Brain Res., 202:307.
Müller-Preuss, P., and Ploog, D., 1981, Inhibition of auditory
    cortical neurons during phonation, Brain Res., 215:61.
Müller-Preuss, P., 1981, Acoustic properties of central auditory
    pathway neurons during phonation in the Squirrel monkey,
    in: "Neuronal Mechanisms of Hearing", J.Syka and L.
    Aitkin, eds., Plenum Publishing Corporation, New York.
Müller-Preuss, P., and Ploog, D., 1983, Central control of sound

production in mammals, in: "Bioacoustic", B. Lewis, ed., Academic Press, London.

Newman, J. D., and Lindsley, D. F., 1976, Single unit analysis of auditory processing in Squirrel monkey frontal cortex, Exp. Brain Res., 25:169.

Niki, H., and Watanabe, M., 1979, Prefrontal and cingulate unit activity during timing behavior in the monkey, Brain Res., 171: 213.

Penfield, W., and Roberts, L., 1969, "Speech and Brain Mechanisms", Princeton University Press, Princeton, N. J.

Robinson, B. W., 1967, Vocalization evoked from forebrain in Macaca mulatta, Physiology and Behavior, 2:345.

Robinson, J. H., and Wang, S. C., 1979, Unit activity of limbic system neurons: Effects of morphine, diazepam and neuroleptic agents, Brain Res., 166:149.

Rübsamen, R., and Betz, M., 1986, Control of echolocation pulses by neurons of the nucleus ambiguus in the rufous horseshoe bat, Rhinolophus rouxi I. Single unit recordings in the ventral motor nucleus of the laryngeal nerves in spontaneously vocalizing bats, J. Comp. Physiol. A, 159: 675.

Stwertka, S. A., 1985, Visually driven units in the anterior limbic cortex of the cat, Exp.Neurol., 89:269.

Sutton, D., Samson, H. H., and Larson, C. R., 1978, Brain mechanisms in learned phonation of Macaca mulatta, in: "Recent advances in primatology, Vol. I, D. J. Chivers and J. Herbert, eds., Academic Press, London.

Sutton, D., Larson, C. R., and Lindeman, R. C., 1974, Neocortical and limbic lesion effects on primate phonation, Brain Res. 16:61.

Sutton, D., Trachy, R. E., and Lindeman, R. C., 1985, Discriminative phonation in macaques:effects of anterior mesial cortex damage, Exp. Brain Res., 59:410.

Sutton, D., and Jürgens, U., in press, Neural control of vocalization, in: Comparative Primate Biology, Vol. 2, Part A, G. Mitchell and J. Erwin, eds., Alan R. Liss, New York.

Tanji, J., 1984, The neuronal activity in the supplementary motor area of primates, Trends in Neurosciences, 7:282.

Yashima, Y., and Hayashi, Y., 1983, Ambiguous motorneurons discharging synchronously with ultrasonic vocalizations in rats, Exp. Brain Res., 50:359.

NEURAL AND NEUROCHEMICAL CONTROL OF THE SEPARATION DISTRESS CALL

Jaak Panksepp[1], Larry Normansell[1], Barbara Herman[2]
Paul Bishop[3] and Loring Crepeau[1]

[1]Department of Psychology, Bowling Green State Univ.
   Bowling Green, OH 43403
[2]Brain Research Center and Departments of Psychiatry
   and Neurosurgery, Children's Hospital National
   Medical Center, George Washington Univ. School of
   Medicine, Washington, D.C.
[3]Computer Center, Washington College, Chestertown, MD

INTRODUCTION

Our work in the area of separation-induced distress
vocalizations (DVs) was precipitated by the discovery of brain
opioid systems in the early 1970's. The discovery of these systems
led to diverse lines of research to identify the psychobehavioral
functions of endogenous opioid systems. Many ideas have been
generated, including hypotheses related to neurochemical mechanisms
of reward-pleasure, stress-induced analgesia, and memory (for an
overview see, Davis, 1984). Our own perspective was that this
system may constitute a major neurochemical underpinning of social
bonding. To put it simply, we reasoned that social attachments may
reflect an opioid mediated addictive process in the brain. As
summarized in Table 1, there are many reasons to believe that this
might be the case. Accordingly, we decided to evaluate the
putative emotional dynamics underlying social interactions
(including social bonding and closely related social processes,
such as gregariousness, play and dominance) by determining how
opiates and other neuroactive drugs modulate DVs arising from
social separation.

From the outset of the research program, we decided that the
most straightforward way to evaluate the underlying emotional
dynamics of social bonding was to study isolation calls. The

assumption was that there is at least one basic emotional circuit
in the brain which elaborates social cohesion (Panksepp, 1982), and
that the best objective indicator of the status of that system is
the frequency and intensity of separation-induced DVs.
Accordingly, not only did we initially employ that measure to
evaluate the opioid hypothesis of social bonding (Table 1), but our
work rapidly broadened to an overall analysis of neural control of
prosocial behaviors (Table 2).

Table 1

SIMILARITIES BETWEEN

&

OPIATE ADDICTION	SOCIAL DEPENDENCE
DRUG DEPENDENCE	ATTACHMENT
TOLERANCE	ESTRANGEMENT
WITHDRAWAL	SEPARATION
PSYCHIC PAIN	LONELINESS
LACRIMATION	CRYING
ANOREXIA	LOSS OF APPETITE
DEPRESSION	DESPONDENCY
INSOMNIA	SLEEPLESSNESS
AGGRESSIVENESS	IRRITABILITY

At the beginning of our research, separation DVs had yet to be
systematically studied from a neurological perspective. Our
colleague John Paul Scott, however, had already embarked on an
extensive research program analyzing the environmental causes and
behavioral correlates of separation distress in various canine
breeds (Scott, Stewart & DeGhett, 1973). With Scott's backing, we
conducted some initial experiments in 1974 on young Beagle and
Telomian puppies which were being bred for his research program.
It soon became evident that opiates had very powerful effect in
ameliorating separation distress (Panksepp, Herman, Conner, Bishop
& Scott, 1978). After many unsuccessful attempts to obtain
extramural funding for our expanding research efforts in this new
area (the most common criticisms of our proposed work being that we
were working on a "fragile hypothesis" with additional
recommendations, to our chagrin, that this work should be done on

rats since there was more known about their brains), we had to close down our dog laboratory. We then moved on to study less expensive species--first to guinea pigs, which exhibited similar behavioral effects to opiates (Herman & Panksepp, 1978). When that work became financially unfeasible without extramural support, we then shifted to domestic chicks, whose separation distress was also quelled with opiates (Panksepp, Meeker & Bean, 1980). Rats, as it

Table 2

EVIDENCE FOR BRAIN OPIOID
HYPOTHESIS OF SOCIAL AFFECT
OPIATE AGONISTS | OPIATE ANTAGONISTS

OPIATE AGONISTS	OPIATE ANTAGONISTS
1. REDUCE SEPARATION DISTRESS (DOGS, GUINEA PIGS, CHICKS)	INCREASE SEPARATION DISTRESS (GUINEA PIGS, CHICKS, CATS)

(BRAIN CRYING CIRCUITS ARE LOCATED IN OPIOID RICH BRAIN AREAS)

2. DECREASE TAIL-WAGGING IN DOGS	INCREASE TAIL-WAGGING IN DOGS
3. DECREASE GREGARIOUSNESS IN RATS	INCREASE SEEKING OF SOCIAL CUES
4. INCREASE PLAY FIGHTING	DECREASE PLAY FIGHTING
5. INCREASE DOMINANCE	REDUCE DOMINANCE
6. NO EFFECT ON PUP RETRIEVAL	DISRUPT PUP RETRIEVAL
7. REDUCE MATERNAL AGGRESSION	INCREASE MATERNAL AGGRESSION

ADDITIONAL EVIDENCE BY OTHERS:

1. NALOXONE INCREASES SOCIAL GROOMING IN MONKEY (MELLER ET AL., (1980)
2. NALOXONE INCREASES SEXUAL SOLICITATION (GESSA ET AL., 1979)
3. SOCIAL VARIABLES MODIFY BRAIN OPIATE RECEPTOR DENSITIES (BONNET ET AL., 1976)
4. SOCIAL CROWDING INCREASES THE POTENCY OF NALOXONE AS AVERSIVE STIMULUS FOR CONDITIONED TASTE AVERSIONS (PILCHER & JONES, (1981)
5. SOCIAL ISOLATION INCREASES VOLUNTARY OPIATE CONSUMPTION (ALEXANDER ET AL., 1978)
6. NALOXONE DISRUPTS SCHOOLING BEHAVIOR IN FISH (KAVALIERS, 1981)

turns out, are not an ideal species for working on such issues; not only do they vocalize in the ultrasonic range when isolated, but they also exhibit a clear separation response for only a very short period of early life (Noirot, 1968).

Twelve years of research on isolation-induced distress calling in a number of vertebrate species has now been completed in our lab. We can therefore report with certainty that opioids in the brain do modulate activity in separation distress circuitry--a finding which we believe constitutes a preliminary understanding of how social bonding and related social processes are elaborated in the brain (for review see Table 2 and Panksepp, Herman, Vilberg, Bishop & DeEskinazi, 1980; Panksepp, 1981; Panksepp, Siviy & Normansell, 1985; Panksepp, 1986). We have a reasonable idea of the specific parts of the brain that the separation circuit traverses (Bishop, 1984; Herman, 1979; Herman & Panksepp, 1981). We know a great deal about which brain chemistries are important in elaborating the response to separation, as well as other social behaviors, especially juvenile play (Panksepp, Siviy & Normansell, 1984). Although the importance of such lines of inquiry for understanding a variety of psychiatric disorders seems evident (Klein, 1981; Panksepp, 1979, 1981; Panksepp & Sahley, 1987; van der Kolk, 1987), the difficulty of obtaining support for this type of work is perhaps understandable within the present scientific climate, which is not enamoured with indirect neuro-theoretical approaches to understanding ancient affective functions of the brain.

Thus, the analysis of the separation/panic system remains a "cottage industry"--it is a small area of research that has not reached a stage where vigorous advocacy exists for proliferation of work in the area. Partially, also, we suspect that the notion that brain opioid systems--the substrates for narcotic drug dependence--might participate in one of the most valued aspects of our society, the familial bond (of "mom and apple pie" so to speak), is not a congenial notion. An editor for Science turned down our first paper on the topic, after it was accepted by both reviewers, because, as he put it to us over the phone in 1976; "it was too hot to handle." Finally, this work broaches a topic which has long been anethema for experimental psychology--the largely neglected topic of how the brain controls emotions (Panksepp, 1982). Neophobic biases against such research are gradually diminishing, and the present volume constitutes perhaps the first compendium of basic research on this fundamental emotional system of the brain. Now that a foundation is being established, it is to be hoped that the psychobiology/neuroscience community will begin to study such important brain systems in earnest. It is hard to imagine that we can have a credible understanding of the sources of behavior until we begin to address the neural underpinnings of emotions. Fortunately, the separation-call objectively reflects activity in a robust neuro-affective system, which is exquisitely amenable to rigorous empirical analysis. This circuit, it seems, may be the primal substrate for social motivation (MacLean, 1985).

THE STUDY OF SOCIAL ATTACHMENT SYSTEMS

A broad ranging review of work in this area, as it relates to both human and animal research, has recently been edited by Reite & Field (1985). Historically, the basic experimental analysis of social attachment processes during the middle part of this century appears attributable to 1) the recognition of the devastating effect caused by the absence of social support in human infants (Bowlby, 1973; Spitz, 1946), and 2) the systematic analysis of the consequences of separation for the social development of dogs (Scott & Fuller, 1965) and primates (Harlow, 1971, 1986). From a psychobiological perspective, the major consequence of this work is the recognition that the key brain system which mediates these effects may be the circuitry which elaborates the separation call.

This system appears to constitute a (perhaps *the*) key genetically ordained operating system to sustain social cohesion and social-emotional homeostasis, which is essential for the adequate growth and maturation of young animals who must depend on elders for safety, shelter, nourishment, and acquisition of knowledge about themselves and their surroundings. Although several other brain emotional processes may also help achieve these ends (especially juvenile play circuitry), the most primitive substrate appears to be the one which leads a young animal to experience "panic" and emit persistent distress signals when it is separated from social support.

We hypothesize that both the affective distress and the separation-related behaviors are concurrently triggered by this ancient emotional command system which courses between paleocortical areas such as cingulate gyrus, which elaborates social perceptions, and brain stem areas which control pertinent autonomic and behavioral outputs. Although subjective experiences of animals cannot be measured directly, we believe it is reasonable to utilize human subjective insights concerning the functions of such primitive emotive systems to derive hypotheses concerning the actions of homologous circuits in the brains of other mammals.

We believe that activity within this brain system is a major force behind social motivation and social intent, and thereby a critical vector in all forms of social learning. The analysis of the neural circuitry which underlies the separation response is presently *the* most workable psychobiological problem in the area of social emotions. Although our work was initiated within the specific theoretical context outlined above (Table 1), most of that

work has been summarized several times   (Panksepp, Herman, Vilberg,
Bishop & DeEskinazi, 1980; Panksepp, 1981; Panksepp, Siviy &
Normansell, 1985; Panksepp, 1986), and hence, except for the
overall summary found in Table 2, will not be repeated here.   The
aim of this chapter is simply to focus on existing empirical
knowledge concerning the neuroanatomies and diverse
neurochemistries which control the separation-distress response,
without a focus on the opioid hypothesis.

The general picture which has emerged is that separation-induced
distress calling is elaborated by a primitive brain stem circuit
whose general organization is substantially similar in all mammals
and birds.   The system is hierarchically organized, as are other
emotional circuits (Panksepp, 1982), with the functions of higher
areas being dependent on the integrity of lower ones.   A variety of
higher perceptual processes can apparently modulate the intensity
of activity in the lower representations of distress circuitry,
although the functional nature of no higher modulatory influence
has been adequately elucidated at the present time.   Whether
pertinent paleocortical areas, such as cingulate, have intrinsic
abilities to elaborate subtle aspects of social emotions such as
shame, guilt, and jealousy, or whether such higher functions emerge
merely as social constructions based on the motivation impact of
separation distress, remains unknown.   Still, it is certain that
all emotional systems, including the one that mediates social
separation distress, are controlled by a variety of sensory and
perceptual inputs.   For instance, in our chick work, if we simply
hang a washcloth from the ceiling of the test chamber so the animal
can "hide" or "find comfort" in its folds, distress vocalization
diminishes dramatically (as found with Harlow's "terry-cloth"
mothers).   Presumably, the effect in chicks is due to the cloth
being able to provoke perceptions of safety and contact comfort,
even though the stimulus itself cannot logically be considered a
social stimulus.   Likewise, a variety of other basic homeostatic
processes can control the vigor of protest: Hungry animals vocalize
more than satiated ones; animals placed in cold test chambers cry
more than those in warm chambers; pain, of course, is a powerful
trigger for crying, while warmth and contact alleviate distress
(see Oswalt & Meier, 1974; Pettijohn, Wong, Ebert & Scott, 1977).
At present, the manner in which such processes interact with the
separation distress circuit remains unknown, yet it is quite
capable of being answered with existing neuroscience technologies.

We believe that the separation call is the emotional system of
the brain which is presently most capable of being analyzed at the
neuronal level, and we also believe that the full understanding of
this system may have more important consequences for understanding
the nature of human psychopathologies than the study of any other
primal emotional circuit in the mammalian brain.

LOCATIONS OF NEURAL CIRCUITS WHICH CONTROL SEPARATION DISTRESS
VOCALIZATIONS

The aim of the following section is to summarize the
organization of distress vocalization circuitry in the brains of
guinea pigs and domestic chicks. The usefulness of these species
over most other common laboratory creatures is evident because they
cry in response to separation at around the same audible frequency
range as humans, which greatly simplifies the experimental
analysis. More complex creatures such as dogs, cats, and primates
provide additional advantages, especially for the analysis of
higher modulatory processes, but there is presently very little
evidence that they will provide any decisive advantage in
understanding the basic neurology of the underlying systems.
     Although the neural details of organization will surely
differ, especially when it comes to the higher nervous system
modulatory processes which control activity in the lower zones of
the separation distress system, the basic command circuitry for
this response exhibits remarkable evolutionary conservation. In
the following sections, we restrict our coverage to work done on
brains of guinea pigs and domestic chicks. Summaries of work done
on primates can be found in Jürgens (1979) and Ploog (1986).

Guinea Pigs

Using acute electrical stimulation of the brain (ESB) we have
mapped the adult guinea pig brain for emotional vocalization loci
while the animals were anesthetized. The success of this acute
exploratory study in guinea pigs is indicated by follow-up
investigations in which reliable DV sites were examined using
chronic indwelling electrodes (Herman, 1979; Herman & Panksepp,
1981; Panksepp et al., 1980). The advantage of this acute ESB
method is that it provides an overview of the organization of a
response in the brain in a very short time while using few animals.
     In this study, a total of 10 adult guinea pigs were used as
subjects. Each animal was anesthetized with chloral hydrate (400
mg/kg, i.p.) and the head was positioned in a cat-monkey
stereotaxic instrument. Using supplemental chloral hydrate,
animals were maintained at a level of anesthesia where pinching did
not produce vocalization. Pre-determined coordinates based upon
the atlas of Luparello (1967) were marked off and drilled along the
right skull top. Using a monopolar electrode (250 μA sine-wave
current, pulse frequency of 1 pulse per 5 sec, total stimulation
time of 30 sec), a total of 33 pre-determined sites were
stimulated. The number of vocalizations produced during the 30 sec
stimulation period and the interstimulus-off period, were recorded.
Other stimulus-bound (S-B) responses were also noted. Following
the initial screening, the electrode was once again lowered into

each tract, and brain tissue within each column was stimulated at 1 mm intervals until the base of the brain was reached.

For five guinea pigs, sites were explored in an anterior-posterior (A-P), lateral-medial, dorsal-ventral direction, and for the remaining five subjects, sites were stimulated in a posterior-anterior (P-A) direction. The reason for this division of subjects was that pilot studies revealed that in some animals it was not possible to obtain vocalizations by stimulating posterior sites after extensive anterior brain screening, and similar problems were encountered if screening proceeded in a P-A direction. The reason for this difficulty is not known, although it may reflect the inadvertent stimulation of sites inhibitory to vocalization or neural shock from the preceding damage. The five A-P subjects were used to determine vocalization sites in the first three anterior planes (A 15.0, 13.0, 9.0), and all ten guinea pigs were used to assess sites in the two remaining planes (A (5.0), (3.0)). Tracts that were explored included the following:

A (15.0)   L (1.5)
A (13.0)   L (6.0, 1.5, 0.2)
A (9.0)   L (6.8, 3.5, 0.8)
A (5.0)   L (6.0, 2.0, 0.3)
A (3.0)   L (3.5, 2.0, 0.5)

Positive vocalization areas are indicated below only if at least 80% of the animals tested showed the same response. Most of these sites were chosen based upon research by other investigators on brain substrates mediating vocalization (Bernston, 1972; de Molina & Hunsperger, 1959; Jürgens, 1976; Jürgens et al., 1967; Jürgens & Ploog, 1970; Kanai & Wang, 1952; Martin, 1976; Peek & Phillips, 1971; Robinson, 1967), and brain research on social cohesion (Dalhouse, 1976; Enloe, 1975; Johnson et al., 1972; Jonason & Enloe, 1971; Jonason et al., 1973). Results of these trials are summarized in Figures 1a & 1b, with anterior vocalization sites shown in Figure 1a and posterior vocalization sites shown in Figure 1b. At every plane, the cortex was free of vocalization sites, including the proximate dorsal structure (corpus callosum, CC) and the ventral cortex (pyriform cortex, PIR). Other large structures free of vocalization sites included the hippocampus and the cerebellum. At the most anterior plane (A (15.0), not shown), low amplitude DVs and increases in respiration accompanied stimulation of the nucleus accumbens (NA) and the medial forebrain bundle (MFB). Mouth movements were associated with MFB but not NA stimulation. At A (13.0) (Panel A), high amplitude, high frequency DVs and increases in respiration accompanied stimulation of the medial septal (MS) and preoptic (POA) region.

Two types of vocalizations--DVs and "pain-like" screams--were

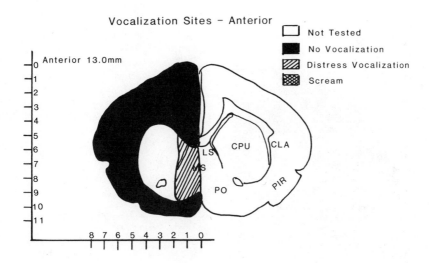

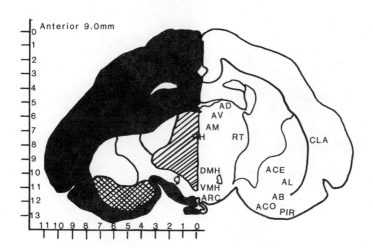

Figure 1a.   Anterior vocalization sites (13.0 mm and 9.0 mm
              from earbar zero) in anesthetized guinea pigs
              receiving ESB.

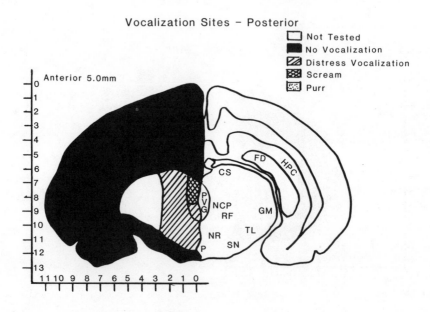

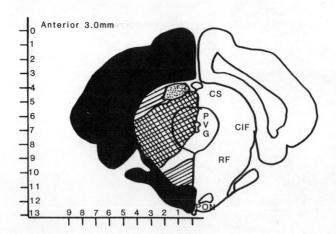

Figure 1b.   Posterior vocalization sites (5.0 mm and 3.0 mm
             from earbar zero) in anesthetized guinea pigs
             receiving ESB.

ABBREVIATIONS

AB	Nucleus amygdaloideus basalis
ACE	Nucleus amygdaloideus centralis
ACO	Nucleus amygdaloideus corticalis
AD	Nucleus anterior dorsalis thalami
AL	Nucleus amygdaloideus lateralis
AM	Nucleus anterior medialis thalami
AME	Nucleus amygdaloideus medialis
ARC	Nucleus arcuatus
AV	Nucleus anterior ventralis thalami
CC	Corpus callosum
CI	Capsula interna
CIF	Colliculus inferior
CLA	Claustrum
CPU	Nucleus caudatus putamen
CS	Colliculus superior
DBB	Tractus diagonalis (Broca)
DMH	Nucleus dorsomedialis (hypothalami)
GM	Corpus geniculatum mediale
HPC	Hippocampus
LH	Lateral hypothalamus
LM	Lemniscus medialis
LS	Nucleus septi lateralis
MFB	Fasciculus medialis prosencephali
NA	Nucleus accumbens
NCP	Nucleus commissurae posterioris
NR	Nucleus ruber
P	Nucleus Paraventricularis (thalami)
PIR	Cortex piriformis
PO	Nucleus preopticus
PON	Pons
PVG	Substantia grisea periverntricularis
RF	Formatio reticularis
RH	Nucleus rhomboideus
RT	Nucleus reticularis thalami
SN	Substantia nigra
TL	Nucleus lateralis tegmenti

recorded from the A (9.0) plane. Stimulation of the anterior
medial thalamic nucleus (AM), the most reliable DV site in this
plane, was associated with low to moderate amplitude DVs and limb
movements. Very low amplitude DVs, limb movements, and respiratory
changes were associated with dorsomedial hypothalamic (DMH)
stimulation. Stimulation of two amygdaloid nuclei--lateral
amygdaloid nucleus (AL) and medial amygdaloid nucleus (AME)--was
accompanied by stimulus-bound screams and mouth movements.

Surprisingly, sites related to pain perception and response,
including the internal capsule (CI) and the reticular thalamic
nucleus (RT), were not associated with any vocalization
response.

Both DV and screaming sites were also detected at A (5.0) (panel
B). Stimulation of the dorsal PVG at this A-P level was associated
with either screams or low amplitude DVs and with respiration
increases, and mouth and limb movements. Stimulation of the
posterior commissure (NCP)/reticular formation (RF) area was
associated with DVs and "escape-like" limb movements. As mentioned
above, no vocalizations were elicited by stimulation of any
hippocampal site.

In the final plane (A (3.0), panel B) three distinct
vocalization types--purr, DV and scream--were noted. The new
vocalization type encountered in this plane, the purr or coo
response, is a sound generally made by adult male guinea pigs when
they obtain lateral body contact with a female immediately prior to
copulation.

Stimulation of a very discrete region in proximity to the
superior colliculus (CS) was associated with a purr response and
limb movements. At this level, screams, accompanied by respiratory
increases, mouth movements, and "escape-like" limb movements, were
associated with stimulation of many sites including the ventral CS,
the inferior colliculus (CIF), and the dorsal-lateral PVG. DVs
accompanied stimulation of some sites in the lateral CS region and
in the RF.

These acute ESB studies suggest the following about the
organization of emotional vocalization in the adult guinea pig
brain. First, the cortex appears to be free of vocalization sites.
In agreement with these results, other researchers have not found
vocalization sites in the cortex of rhesus or squirrel monkey brain
(Jürgens, 1976; Jürgens & Ploog, 1970; McCullough, 1944; Myers,
1972; Robinson, 1967; Sutton et al., 1974). Similarly, stimulation
of cortex in humans is not associated with emotional vocalization,
although phonetic and speech sounds have been obtained (Leyton &
Sherrington, 1917; Penfield & Roberts, 1959). Thus, these data
suggest that emotional vocalization is subcortically organized in
guinea pigs, as well as in higher-order mammals.

Second, five response modalities characterize ESB vocalizations
in guinea pigs. (1) Stimulation of some subcortical sites (NA,
MFB, POA, MS, DBB) was consistently associated with DVs in the

absence of limb movement. Since locomotion is not correlated with separation DVs in infant guinea pigs (Herman & Panksepp, 1978), these sites may participate in separation distress. Subsequent research based upon chronic ESB studies has revealed that the POA and AM regions (see reference to AM below) are the most reliable DV areas in guinea pig brain, and appear to be modulated by opioid systems (Herman & Panksepp, 1981). (2) Stimulation of a second set of subcortical sites (AM, DMH, VMH, NCD, anterior RF and DV (ventral tegmental tract)) was associated with DVs and limb movements. For two of these areas (NCP, anterior RF), ESB may have activated some component of a pain circuit, since the powerful limb movements associated with ESB made the animal appear as if it were attempting to escape. (3) Stimulation of a third set of subcortical areas (AL, AME, anterior dorsal and posterior ventral PVG, posterior RF) was associated with stimulus-bound "pain screams" followed by low amplitude DVs, and was frequently accompanied by "escape-like" limb movements. These sites are probably a component of some pain pathway. (4) There were other "pain" sites (CIF, posterior dorsal PVG) where ESB was associated with only "pain-like" screams and "escape-like" motor movements. (5) Finally, the CS was the single site where stimulation elicited a purr response typically observed in guinea pigs during sexual encounters.

In comparing guinea pigs with other species, there appear to be numerous similarities in the central organization of emotional vocalizations. First, as described above, the cortex is free of emotional vocalization sites in guinea pig, monkey, and human brain. Second, two additional areas (HPC, SC) are free of vocalization sites in guinea pig as well as rhesus monkey brain (Robinson, 1967). Third and most important, guinea pigs, in common with monkeys, cats, and birds, possess several common brain vocalization loci including the amygdala, POA, hypothalamus, PVG, and ventral-lateral tegmental area (cf. de Molina & Hunsperger, 1959; Jürgens & Ploog, 1970; Kanai & Wang, 1962; Martin, 1976; Peek & Phillips, 1971). Fourth, similar with cats (Testerman, 1970) there is a striking overlap between vocalization and respiratory zones in guinea pig brain.

A striking difference between guinea pigs and some other species exists in the role of the LM region. In guinea pigs, the LM proved to be an ambiguous DV site. In contrast, the LM region has been demonstrated to be a highly reliable vocalization site in the brains of monkeys (Jürgens & Ploog, 1970) and cats (de Molina & Hunsperger, 1959; Kanai & Wang, 1962). The role of the LM region in separation distress vocalization in the guinea pig is an important question to answer, since LM stimulation in cats has been reported to induce "distress-type" mewing (de Molina & Hunsperger, 1959; Kanai & Wang, 1962).

Further research in guinea pigs and other species will be needed to clarify how the brain organizes emotional, perceptual, and motor components of vocalization. Moreover, although our initial studies have implicated opioid systems in the regulation of vocalization in guinea pigs (Herman & Panksepp, 1978, 1981), other research will be needed to elaborate the chemistry of brain sites which modulate vocalization in this species. Most of our neuropharmacological work to date has been done on the domestic chick (vide infra). The studies described above may provide a preliminary map for conducting such investigations in guinea pigs.

Domestic Chickens

An extensive map of the brain areas yielding stimulation-bound vocalizations has been published for both awake (Phillips, Youngren, & Peek, 1972) and anesthetized (Peek & Phillips, 1971) chickens. Active sites appear to be centered in two regions, one medial and the other lateral. The medial region extends from the pre-optic region of the hypothalamus caudally through a region ventral to n. ovoidalis which coincides with tractus occipitomesencephalicus (OM) at that point. More caudally, the system was reported to descend along a path just medial to n. isthmi, pars parvocellularis.

The lateral region from which vocalizations can be elicited appears to be centered ventral and medial to n. mesencephalicus lateralis, pars dorsalis (MLd), in n. mesencephalicus lateralis, pars ventralis (MLv), n. reticularis lateralis, and n. intercollicularis (ICo). Stimulation within this region elicits calls with the lowest current thresholds, and is associated least with other behaviors. Other midbrain areas yielding calls during stimulation, but generally at higher thresholds, include n. isthmi pars parvocellularis, n. semilunaris, and the pars compacta of the pedunculo-pontine nucleus.

From the midbrain, the vocalization circuit descends to the medulla. Phillips and Youngren (1976) stimulated midbrain call areas and reported bursting activity from neurons located in the region of the obex, including much of n. intermedius and parts of the vagal nucleus, as well as n. centralis medullae oblongatae, pars dorsalis and ventralis.

Lesion techniques have also been used extensively in the study of avian vocalization circuitry. In general, lesions in brain regions from which vocalizations can be elicited by electrical stimulation produce a loss in calling capability. Lesions restricted to the anterior or medial aspects of the ICo result in almost complete muting (Bishop, 1984; de Lanerolle & Andrew, 1974; Normansell, Bishop & Panksepp, 1985). Damage to MLv (Area C) in conjunction with destruction of ICo, however, has been reported to spare calling associated with locomotion (de Lanerolle & Andrew, 1974).

In addition to being mute, chicks with lesions of the ICo also behave abnormally. Behaviors associated with calling, or which

when performed generally occur in conjunction with calling, are
also reduced or eliminated (Andrew & de Lanerolle, 1974). When
presented with food after mild deprivation, for instance, intact
chicks twitter excitedly as they engage in a period of frenzied
feeding. Chicks with ICo lesions neither twitter nor exhibit the
excited feeding bout. When presented with novel objects or small
moving targets, normal chicks vocalize, visually track the objects,
and attempt to peck them. Lesioned chicks, on the other hand, do
not vocalize.

They also fail to track or peck at the objects (Andrew, 1974;
Andrew & de Lanerolle, 1974). Further, when normal chicks are
placed into a large open field, they continually scan the
environment and emit peep-type distress vocalizations, while
inhibiting other behaviors like pecking, preening, and locomotion.
Lesioned animals do not peep; nor do they scan or inhibit other
behaviors (Andrew & de Lanerolle, 1974).

By using stimulation/lesion techniques, we attempted to
distinguish those brain areas which might directly control call
production from those areas which may indirectly modulate
vocalization frequency by altering the sensory or social
capabilities of the animals (Figure 2). Three-day old domestic
chicks were administered bilateral electrolytic lesions to either
the ventral archistriatum (Av), dorsomedial thalamus (DMT), ICo, or
Area C.

Two days after surgery, the number of calls emitted during 10
min of social isolation was assessed (Figure 2). ICo lesions
reduced DVs to less than 5% of unoperated controls, while DMT and
Area C lesions reduced calling to about 30% and 50%, respectively.
Av-lesioned chicks were the least affected. They emitted about
one-third less vocalizations than control animals.

Following isolation testing, like-lesioned animals were paired
in an open field for 3 minutes, during which time control animals
emitted an average of 220 calls. Animals with lesions of the ICo,
DMT, or Area C had DV reductions (compared to control birds)
similar to those recorded when they were tested in isolation.
Chicks with Av lesions, on the other hand, completely suppressed
calling in the presence of another bird.

On the following day, animals were tested in isolation in a cold
(15°C) environment, which generally increases the number of calls
emitted (Kaufman & Hinde, 1961). Under these conditions, the
vocalization of DMT-lesioned animals more than doubled, reaching
the level at which control birds were calling. All other groups
were essentially unaffected by the cold. In sum, while the dramatic
reduction of DVs following ICo and Area C lesions were not affected
by climatic or social conditions, birds with more rostral lesions
exhibited DV modulation by these variables. This suggests that ICo
and Area C are directly involved with call organization or
production, whereas DMT and Av exert an influence on vocalizations
by relaying sensory or emotional information into critical call
regions.

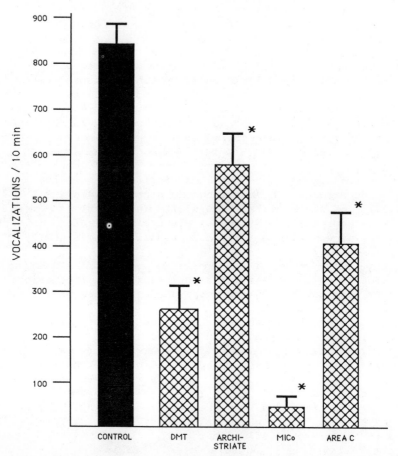

Figure 2. Effects of brain lesions on distress vocalizations in
         isolated chicks (Bishop, 1984).

   * Reliably different from non-lesioned controls, p < .01

THE NEUROCHEMISTRY OF VOCALIZATION CONTROL

Initial pharmacological work on the separation call was conducted by Scott (1974), who concluded that the major tranquilizers chlorpromazine and reserpine, and the minor tranquilizers meprobamate, diazepam, and alcohol, are essentially ineffective in alleviating separation distress. Sodium pentobarbital and d-amphetamine yielded modest increases in vocalization. The only drug tested which appeared to exert a specific anti-distress effect was the tricyclic imipramine which at 8 mg/kg reduced DVs of Beagles essentially to zero for two hours, and had more modest effects in Australian Terrier X Beagle hybrids. Other breeds, such as Telomians, Telomian X Beagle hybrids, and Telomian X Sheltie hybrids, exhibited very little sensitivity to the drug. Subsequent work by Suomi and colleagues (1978) also demonstrated the effectiveness of imipramine in alleviating separation distress in rhesus monkeys, but this effect was not replicated by Porsolt, Roux & Jalfre, 1984). We have also found imipramine to be without effect in domestic chicks (Panksepp, Meeker & Bean, 1980), and we have since analyzed the drug from a large number of perspectives (chronic administration, interaction with social cues which alleviate DVs, interaction with drugs that increase DVs), and we simply have observed no specific effect of imipramine in that species. To the contrary, we have found the drug to be reasonably effective in reducing DVs in guinea pigs at doses above 10 mg/kg.

There is presently no credible explanation for these breed and species differences, but it should be noted that this drug is especially efficacious in quelling panic attacks in humans (Klein, 1981), but again it is not uniformly effective. Some agoraphobic individuals are not helped at all by imipramine treatment. This diversity of results suggests that imipramine modulates higher-order perceptual processes which control the separation distress system, as opposed to directly influencing the primary-process emotional response itself. Surely a variety of inputs can modulate the basic distress/panic circuitry, and some species, breeds, and perhaps selected individuals of a breed are especially influenced by an imipramine-sensitive control.

Opiate and non-opiate inhibition of DV circuitry

Our own experience with a very diverse set of psychopharmaceuticals is comparable to Scott's. Practically none of the traditional classes of drugs used in psychiatric practice alleviate this type of distress (Panksepp, Meeker & Bean, 1980), even though facilitation of serotonin activity can reduce DVs, and blockade of muscarinic cholinergic and serotonergic activity can increase DVs (Panksepp, Bean, Bishop, Vilberg & Sahley, 1980).

Several neurochemical systems seem to exert powerful inhibitory effects on DVs. Indeed, the first system we explored, namely the opioid system, was found to exert powerful and specific effects on DVs in dogs (Panksepp, Herman, Conner, Bishop & Scott, 1978), guinea pigs (Herman & Panksepp, 1978), and domestic chicks (Panksepp, Meeker & Bean, 1980) (see Table 2). Opioid peptides, administered intracerebrally so they perfused the mesencephalon, were also highly effective (Panksepp, Vilberg, Bean, Coy & Kastin, 1978; Panksepp, Normansell, Siviy, Rossi & Zolovick, 1984; Vilberg, Panksepp, Kastin & Coy, 1984). These effects clearly seemed to be due to modulation of brain-stem circuits, since the harvesting of opiate receptors in the brain-stem with ß-chlornaltrexamine not only increased spontaneous vocalizations, but completely blocked the ability of intracerebral opiates to reduce DVs (Panksepp, Siviy, Normansell, White & Bishop, 1982).

Although we have yet to accomplish a thorough analysis of receptor types due to limited resources, the strong implication of the data is that mu receptor stimulation is critical to the effects observed, not only because of naloxone reversibility of all the effects we have observed, but also by the relative weakness of some fairly specific delta agonists such as $D-Ala^2-D-Leu^5$-Enkephalin to reduce DVs. Also, tritiated diprenorphine binding is high in all brain areas which have been implicated in vocalizations in guinea pigs, chicks, and rats (unpublished observations), as are enkephalin and endorphin systems visualized by immunocytochemistry (de Lanerolle, Elde, Sparber & Frick, 1981).

Several other systems have also been found to exert strong inhibitory control over DVs. Perhaps the most powerful non-opiate effect has been observed with the alpha-2-norepinephrine receptor agonist, clonidine (Panksepp, Meeker & Bean, 1980), but this effect does not appear to be due to pre-synaptic effects, since it survives total depletion of brain NE in chicks (Rossi, Sahley & Panksepp, 1983). Nicotine also has a reasonably powerful effect on DVs, but the effect may ultimately be due to brain ACh release, since muscarinic antagonists can suppress this effect (Sahley, Panksepp & Zolovick, 1981).

Benzodiazepine Influences on DVs

Although minor tranquilizers can certainly produce modest reductions in DVs, Scott's (1984) work on dogs and our initial work on chicks (Panksepp, Meeker & Bean, 1980) suggested that this was neither a powerful nor a behaviorally specific effect. However, Insel and colleagues (1986), have recently reported a much more potent effect on the ultrasonic DVs of rat pups than previously reported for other species. Since Insel's animals were tested at a time in life when the pups are poikilothermic (and animals were tested at room temperature), it is possible that the benzodiazepines (BZs) are more efficacious in alleviating the stress caused by reduced body temperature than the stress produced by the perception of social separation. In any event, we have not seen robust and specific effects in chicks or dogs, even though statistically reliable reductions were uniformly observed, as with many other drugs. Also, since the fear circuitry of the brain may operate synergistically with separation distress circuitry (Panksepp, 1982), some effect on DVs might be expected simply from such cross-talk. Accordingly, we have evaluated several benzodiazepine related anxiogenic manipulations with the DV measure.

First, in order to determine whether the separation distress system would be able to detect benzodiazepine withdrawal symptoms, we have conducted extensive work in chicks using high doses of chlordiazepoxide (CDP). In a series of experiments, animals were injected twice each day with either 20 mg/kg CDP or distilled water (1 cc/kg) and tested 20 minutes after the first injection each day. In experiment 1, drug testing was conducted for 7 consecutive days, followed by 5 drug-free test days. DVs were collected from animals alternately while alone and in pairs. In experiment 2, drug testing was conducted for 14 days, followed by 6 drug-free days of testing. These animals were tested for three trials per condition alternately in plain boxes or in boxes where the chicks were surrounded by mirrors, which also has been shown to reduce separation-induced DVs (Kaufman & Hinde, 1961; Montevecchi, Gallup and Dunlap, 1973; Panksepp et al., 1980).

In both experiments, CDP reliably reduced vocalizations. In experiment 1, CDP animals exhibited DV reductions of 61% and 53% when tested alone and in pairs, respectively, compared to water-injected controls. In experiment 2, CDP reduced again vocalizations by 61% in the plain boxes, but by only 22% in the mirrored condition (see Figure 3). DV rates increased sharply to, but did not exceed, control levels following drug withdrawal. Although the DV reductions in this experiment were quite large, the animals were also clearly sedated, so we would not argue that the effect on DVs is specific. The failure to see any withdrawal symptoms in DVs suggests that the vocalization measure may not be especially sensitive to anxiogenic states.

Because there was no evidence for withdrawal in either of the previous studies, the following experiment attempted to precipitate the syndrome using the BZ inverse agonists ethyl-ß-carboline-3-carboxylate (ß-CCE) and methyl-ß-carboline-3-carboxylate (ß-CCM). Another BZ antagonist drug (CGS 8216, a pyrazoloquinoline) has been reported to precipitate withdrawal symptoms in diazepam-dependent dogs (McNicholas, Martin and Cherian, 1983), as well as rats which have received chronic CDP for 5 days (File and Pellow, 1985). Chicks were injected with either CDP (20 mg/kg) or vehicle twice a day for

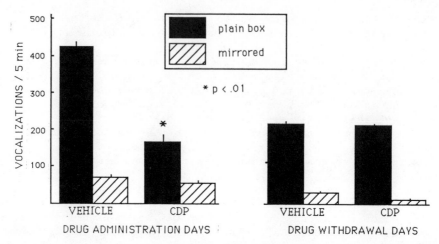

Figure 3. DVs among birds treated with CDP (20 mg/kg) or vehicle
during 14 days of drug administration, and 6 days of
drug withdrawal.

10 days. Birds were tested for DVs in plain boxes during a single
10-minute trial on days 1, 3, 5, 7, and 10. Across all days,
chronic CDP reduced DVs by about half.

On day 11, half the animals in each group were injected i.p. with
ß-CCE (10 mg/kg) or vehicle. All animals were tested 20 minutes
later for 10 min in plain testing chambers, then injected with 20
mg/kg CDP, and tested 20 minutes later for an additional 10 minute
trial. In control animals, ß-CCE reduced DVs by 27%. CDP further
reduced vocalization levels in both ß-CCE and water-injected
animals by 58% and 57%, respectively. Those animals chronically
treated with CDP vocalized at about half the level of the control
animals. ß-CCE did not reduce this level further, nor did acute
CDP administration have any effect.

On test day 12, those animals which did not receive ß-CCE on test
day 11 received 10 mg/kg of ß-CCM, while the other animals received
1 cc/kg vehicle. All animals were then tested 20 minutes after
injection for a single 10 minute trial, then injected with 20 mg/kg
CDP, and were tested for an additional 10 minutes beginning 20
minutes later. Among vehicle group animals, ß-CCM reduced
vocalization rates by a third. CDP further reduced DVs in these
animals by 92%. ß-CCM reduced vocalizations in the chronic CDP
animals by 89%. Acute CDP had no additional DV-reducing effect.
Once again, we could find no evidence that manipulations which
should have been anxiogenic promoted DVs.

In summary, in two studies involving longitudinal CDP administration (7 and 14 days, respectively), DVs were reliably reduced, although this reduction appeared to be secondary to a persistent sedation effect of the drug at this dose. Abrupt abstinence from the drug failed to produce a withdrawal syndrome in these animals, as indicated by DV rates, which increased to, but failed to exceed those of vehicle-treated animals. Attempts to precipitate a withdrawal syndrome using the BZ inverse agonists ß-CCE and ß-CCM also failed. ß-CCE reduced DV rates in animals naive to CDP; ß-CCM reduced DVs both in animals experienced with and naive to chronic CDP treatment. CDP continued to reliably reduce DVs in vehicle group animals, even following administration of either form of ß-carboline. CDP failed to affect DV rates in CDP-experienced animals following treatment with vehicle or either form of ß-carboline.

It appears, then, that the BZ system does not play a behaviorally specific role in the mediation of distress vocalizations in domestic chicks. CDP appears to reduce DVs by producing a persistent sedation in these animals, rather than via some mode of affective relief. Therefore, separation-induced DVs do not seem to reflect distress which can be considered analogous to anxiety as experienced by humans, but might rather indicate a qualitatively different emotional state of trepidation, perhaps one more akin to panic attacks in humans (Klein, 1981; Panksepp, 1982).

Neurochemistries Which Facilitate Separation Distress

All of the following work is based on work with domestic chicks. Although blockade of opiate receptor systems with naloxone, serotonergic systems with methysergide, and muscarinic cholinergic systems with atropine or scopolamine can increase DVs under some testing conditions (Panksepp, Bean, Bishop, Vilberg & Sahley, 1980) these effects are not especially striking, since the animals do not continue to vocalize when they are returned to the flock. Indeed, the naloxone effect is quite variable from experiment to experiment and across species, and some pertinent variables remain to be identified. Accordingly, we suspect that those studies have nothing to tell us about the major throughput chemistries--the "command" transmitters, of the separation distress system. However, we have now identified three separate neurochemical systems which can activate separation type vocalizations unconditionally, as if the fixed-action pattern substrates had been tonically activated. These are, in the order of their discovery 1) curariform drugs, 2) glutamate receptor agonists, and 3) corticotropin-releasing factor (CRF), all administered directly into the brain (between cerebellum and cerebral hemispheres into the vicinity of the fourth ventricle as in all of our intracerebral studies to date). We will discuss each of these discoveries separately.

Curariform Activation of Panic and Flight

Curare administered into the brain yields as striking an
emotional display as any manipulation that presently exists.
Although we were ignorant of similar Eastern European work (Decsi &
Varszegi, 1969) at the beginning of our studies, our results
completely corroborate that earlier work. Chicks given several
micrograms of curare into the ventricular system rapidly begin to
exhibit a striking "panic" attack (Panksepp, Normansell, Siviy,
Buchanan, Zolovick, Rossi & Conner, 1983). Under specific
conditions, the rate of vocalization can double or triple, and
mirrored environments become totally ineffective in alleviating the
distress.

The vocalization appears driven, and nothing seems to markedly
alleviate the apparently intense distress response. The birds
vocalize persistently, even if they are in a flock. They run
around wildly, disregarding other nearby animals, apparently
getting no comfort from their companionship. Sometimes they freeze
against the side of their home cages in seeming terror. At higher
doses, isolated animals, although in apparent terror, may actually
vocalize less than controls, but when paired with a similarly
treated companion, their vocalization greatly exceeds that of the
controls (Figure 4).

At still higher doses, the chicks lose all muscular
coordination, flail wildly, and convulse. We have yet to find a
manipulation, opioid, cholinergic (agonist or antagonist),
anticonvulsant (dilantin or chlordiazepoxide) or otherwise, that
alleviates this distress. Although informal observations suggest
that the animal's visual processing may be disrupted (they do not
readily avert approaching objects), it appears that the panic
response is not simply due to blindness, since the birds exhibit
increased vocalization even when tested in complete darkness. We
simply do not have a clear idea of what receptor might be causing
this dramatic effect, and for lack of any other clear possibility,
would agree with the suggestion (Myers, 1974) that it is mediated
by a unique curarinic receptor that has yet to be adequately
characterized.

Although vocalization is a prominent aspect of the "panic"
attack that is induced, the animal also appears to be in an intense
fear state, and presently we suspect that these are separable
aspect of the syndrome. Muscarinic agonists such as curare are
capable of producing the fear/flight state without the stereotyped
vocalizations. Thus, the curare-induced emotional storm appears to
be a mixture of several distinct emotions, and probably is not a
manipulation which can be claimed to induce a pure form of the
separation response.

In a subsequent study, we assessed the capability of curare to
induce vocalizations in ICo-lesioned chicks. If muting occurs

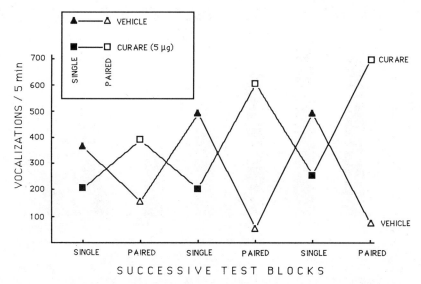

Figure 4. Mean DVs emitted by chicks tested individually or
in pairs after ICV injections of 5 µg curare or
vehicle.

following destruction to ICo because emotional information can no
longer gain access to call regions, then curare might be expected
to remain effective. On the other hand, if the ICo is an essential
component of the vocalization machinery, then after its
destruction, no chemical stimulation should be capable of
reinstating vocal behavior. In brief, curare was totally incapable
of resurrecting vocalizations in the lesioned animals, but all
animals still exhibited the other aspects of their panic attacks,
namely, flight, crouching, and freezing. They simply no longer
vocalized, suggesting that the final vocal motor command circuitry
upon which curare may act was no longer operative.

Glutaminergic system

Localized infusions of the excitatory amino acid glutamate has
been shown to induce vocalizations in both cats (Bandler, 1982) and
squirrel monkeys (Jürgens and Richter, 1986), presumably by
activating synaptic fields where vocalization pathways are relayed.
We have investigated the effects in chicks of intracerebroventricular
administration of glutamate, as well as several glutamate receptor
agonists and antagonists.

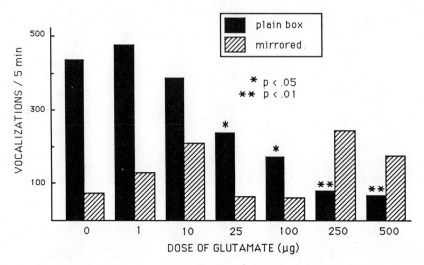

Figure 5. Mean DVs emitted by animals tested in plain test boxes
and in mirrored boxes following ICV injections of
glutamate, in doses as indicated.

When animals were tested in isolation, centrally injected
monosodium glutamate (at doses from 25 to 500 μg) decreased calling
in a dose-dependent manner (see Figure 5). Because administration
of glutamate simultaneously activates several varieties of
receptors (Fagg, 1985; Watkins & Evans, 1981) which may subserve
interacting or reciprocal functions in the brain, we further
investigated the role of glutaminergic systems using
receptor-specific agonists.

In plain testing boxes, administration of N-methyl-D-aspartate
(NMDA) had no effect on the number of vocalizations emitted at any
of the doses tested (.1, .25, .5, & 1.0 μg). On the other hand, in
mirrored boxes (which reduce baseline levels of calling), the two
highest doses produced dramatic increases in calling frequency
(437% and 456%, respectively). In contrast, quisqualate (QA)
produced a dose-dependent decrease in the number of calls, except
at the highest dose (1.0 μg) where calling frequency increased to
control levels. The effect of kainate (KA) administration was
similar to that of NMDA. No changes in vocalization frequency were
detected in the plain boxes at any dose tested, but dose-dependent
increases occurred in the mirrored boxes (see Fig. 6). The kainic
acid effect was reminiscent of the curare effect, in that

vocalization seemed driven, and typically continued when animals
were returned to the flock. Although we have been unable to
conduct a sonographic analysis yet, to the human ear the kainic
acid-promoted vocalizations appear to be qualitatively different
than typical DVs (being shorter and often being emitted at a faster
momentary rate).

The finding that NMDA and KA seem to affect vocalization
frequency in one direction, whereas QA shifts the propensity to
call in the other, may partially explain the vocalization reduction
observed following glutamate administration. If NMDA or KA systems
serve activational roles for separation distress, while a QA system
acts in a counteracting manner, relative density of the receptor
subtype in the area perfused by drug administration may lead to
either an increase or decrease in calling. The finding that all
three agonists had behavioral effects suggests that all receptor
subtypes are present near the area of the 4th ventricle (the target
site for the injections). Additionally, that the highest dose of QA
produced an increase in vocalizations would seem to suggest that
the specificity of agonists for a particular receptor occurs within
a limited concentration range.

The effects on vocalization of glutamate receptor antagonists
have also been assessed. Both D-2-amino-5-phosphonovalerate (APV),
a selective NMDA receptor antagonist, and gamma-D-glutamylglycine
(DGG), a broad spectrum/QA-KA receptor antagonist (Fagg, 1985),
produced dose-dependent decreases in calling. Administration of
either NMDA (1 µg) or KA (.25 µg) completely reversed the
suppression of calling that followed APV (.1 µg) treatment. KA
partially reversed the DGG-induced suppression of calling, whereas
NMDA did not.

Although glutaminergic participation in vocalization control
appears to be quite robust, in that vocal output often appears
driven as opposed to modulated, much more work is needed to
determine what functional role this system serves in the normal
separation distress syndrome.

Corticotropin Releasing Factor

After many years of waiting for the price of this peptide to
come down to levels we could afford, we have now completed a series
of preliminary studies to determine whether separation type DVs
could be provoked by this agent. Our suspicion that it might was
piqued by Swanson et al's (1983) initial immunocytochemical
analysis which demonstrated the anatomy of this system in the rat
brain. It was essentially confluent with our maps of separation
distress circuitry in the guinea pig brain (as reviewed in Figures
1a and 1b). Concentrations of cell bodies were located around the
horns of the anterior commissure, in the bed nuclei of the stria
terminalis, with axons descending through the dorsomedial thalamus,
through the vicinity of the central gray. These were the "hottest"

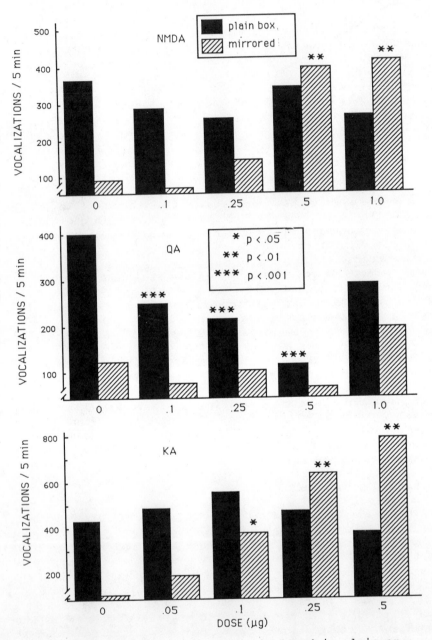

Figure 6. Mean DVs emitted by chicks isolated in plain or mirrored boxes following ICV administration of NMDA, QA or KA.

sites for induction of DVs with localized electrical stimulation of the guinea pig brain. Accordingly, we anticipated that administration of this peptide into the brain would promote DVs.

By the time we started our work, the ability of CRF to promote vocalizations in rhesus monkeys had already been demonstrated (Kalin et al., 1983). The first bird we injected intracerebrally with 1 μg of CRF exhibited an unambiguous intensification of vocalization, and our initial study analyzed the dose response characteristics of the effect in plain and mirrored boxes (Panksepp, Crepeau & Clynes, 1987). Four day old chicks were isolated from their flock and administered 0.04, 0.2, 1.0 or 5.0 μg CRF to the fourth ventricle region, and were promptly tested for four 5-minute trials. The first and third trials were in our plain boxes, and for the second and fourth, all animals were transferred to mirrored chambers. The results, summarized in Figure 7, suggest a dose-dependent, albeit modest increase of DVs in the plain boxes, with a very dramatic effect again in the mirrored conditions. At CRF doses above 0.2 μg, the ability of mirrors to reduce DVs was almost totally attenuated, and these animals, especially at the two highest doses, also continued to vocalize when returned to their flocks. The vision of the animals did not appear to be impaired in any obvious way. They effectively avoided obstacles, and retracted their heads from approaching objects.

The effect was long-lasting (at least six hours at the two highest doses), and did not appear to exhibit any tolerance with repeated testing. To evaluate whether only visual inhibition of DVs was attenuated by CRF, we also determined that music (as well as various other noises) could reduce DVs. CRF was as effective in negating these inhibitory effects as it was with visual cues (see Figure 7).

We presently feel that the CRF effect is as close to a pure unconditional potentiation of DVs as we have seen. Chicks treated with CRF simply vocalized more, and appeared to actively seek social companionship and support without the massive agitation and fear-like states evoked especially by curare and kainic acid. The anatomy of the CRF system is highly suggestive of what we might presently envision separation distress command circuitry to look like. Whether a subset of the CRF system is devoted uniquely to separation related processes, or whether this system is merely one that mediates a generalized stress which is synergistic with separation processes needs to be determined by additional research.

We have also found that intracerebral injections of alpha-Melanocyte Stimulating Hormone (alpha-MSH) can increase vocalizations (Vilberg et al., 1984), but in subsequent work we found this to be an extremely short-lived effect, lasting no more than 15 minutes. Indeed, the short period of DV facilitation is followed by a prolonged period of DV inhibition, which is accompanied by a stereotyped squatting freezing/immobility

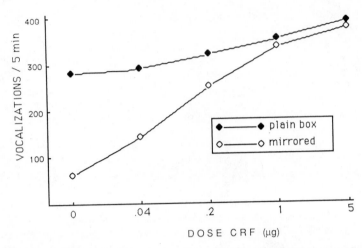

Figure 7. Effect of CRF on DVs in plain test boxes and in
          mirrored boxes. CRF increased DVs in the mirrored
          boxes in a substantial, dose-dependent manner.

response, which may indicate heightened fear (Panksepp & Abbott,
1987, Unpublished data). Thus, it is possible that the alpha-MSH
effect on DVs reflects a synergism of fear and separation distress
processes in the brain.

DRUG AND BRAIN LESION INTERACTIONS

   Aside from new techniques such as *in vivo* voltammetry, dialysis,
push-pull perfusion and PET scans, the traditional ways to
determine where in the brain various neurochemicals are exerting
their effects is via direct intracerebral administration of
neurochemical agents or an analysis of how the effects of such
agents, peripherally administered, are modified by
previously-inflicted brain damage. These approaches remain to be
implemented in the analysis of distress vocalizations. Although
much of our work with drugs and peptides has utilized central
administration, the injections have typically been into the
ventricular system. Since at least part of the DV circuitry is
situated quite close to the ventricles, it will be difficult to
determine whether the effects of tissue injections are due to local
effects, or to ventricularly-transmitted diffusion. We did conduct
one series of studies using tissue injections of morphine in chicks
in an attempt to specify the sites of action for morphine effects,
and the active sites were invariably close to the ventricles
(Vilberg, 1979). Subsequent unpublished studies with radioactive

morphine indicated that the injections led to very widespread diffusion of that lipophilic substance in the newborn chick brain. Whether clearer results can be obtained with less lipid soluble substances needs to be determined. The lesion-drug interaction method is another approach to this question.

Although there is a substantial literature evaluating the effects of brain lesions on DVs in chicks (Andrew and de Lanerolle, 1974; Bishop, 1984; Figure 2), and some work in rhesus monkeys (Newman and MacLean, 1982), the interaction of pharmacological agents which specifically modulate vocalizations and drug effects should be able to provide a general overview of which areas of the brain are especially important in the various modulatory control of DVs. The obvious shortcoming of such an approach is the possibility that lesions of key DV areas in the brain will compromise the vocalization response to such an extent that the sensitivity of the behavioral measure will be lost. In any event, we have tried to utilize this approach to help better localize the opiate effects. The lesioned animals described in Figure 2 were tested following intraperitoneal injections of saline vehicle, naloxone (5 mg/kg) and morphine (1 mg/kg) in counterbalanced manner (Bishop, 1984). The results, as percent of baseline scores, are summarized in Table 3. Neither the vehicle nor the naloxone had any clear effects on DV frequencies, although it is noteworthy that the greatest increases following naloxone were seen in animals with the lowest baselines, namely the Medial ICo and Area C lesioned animals. Morphine effects appeared to be intact (even amplified, at least in relative terms) in all lesioned groups, suggesting that the lesion-drug interaction approach is unlikely to be profitable in elucidating central sites of action.

An alternative to the surgical lesion approach would be the utilization of neurochemical lesions. For instance, one could temporarily harvest opiate receptors with alkylating agents in localized areas of the brain (autoradiographically confirmed) and determine how subsequent drug effects are modulated. We have done preliminary work with this approach, and have found that central administration of ß-chlornaltrexamine, which essentially eliminated lower brain-stem diprenorphine sensitive opiate receptors, completely attenuated the DV reducing effects of morphine (Panksepp et al., 1982). Using a similar strategy, we have evaluated the effects of clonidine and morphine following depletion of central norepinephrine with 6-hydroxydopamine in chicks, and found that the effects of neither agent is attenuated by such brain damage (Rossi et al., 1983). In sum, the actual analysis of where in the brain various neurochemical influences operate remains essentially virgin territory. Although various approaches are available for addressing such issues, the lesion approach does not yet appear to hold much promise. Even the more modern techniques will probably have serious limitations, and clearly such question will require convergent approaches. Probably such issues can not really likely

Table 3. Drug effects for the various lesion groups of
         Figure 2 on isolation-induced distress vocalizations

Group	Saline	Naloxone	Morphine
Controls	8.9%↓	19.8%↓	50.9%↓ ***
DMT	0%	26%↓	62.7%↓ **
Archistriate	6.5%↑	21.4%↓	79.9%↓ ***
Medial ICo	4%↓	41.1%↑	96.2%↓ **
Area C	17.9%↓	53.7%↑	65.8%↓ *

* p<.025
** p<.05
*** p<.01

to be addressed in a cogent fashion until the actual command
circuitry for separation distress is outlined more conclusively.
Perhaps the CRF system will prove to be the core anatomy as
suggested above, and that issue may be capable of being resolved
using antibody approaches to selectively inactivate that system.
    When we have a solid neuroanatomical base, then the application
of single-unit approaches, along with the newer *in vivo*
neurochemical technologies, may be able to definitively address the
detailed nature of the many neurochemical interactions which
control and modulate the various behavioral and physiological
functions of this primal emotive system.

CONCLUDING REMARKS

    Some basic properties of brain mechanisms which mediate
separation distress have now been elucidated. Although our
knowledge in the area remains at a very preliminary stage, we are
finally beginning to determine, in detail, how the brain mediates
this basic emotional process. It might be fair to say that at the
present time more is known about the underlying brain mechanisms of
the separation distress emotion than any other emotive system of

the brain, except perhaps for the anger/rage/affective attack system. A more vigorous analysis of such emotional systems by the neuroscience community appears to be indicated. Not only do such systems constitute major adaptive systems for mediating key psychologically-mediated survival needs of organisms, but imbalances in such brain systems are probably major causes for psychiatric disorders.

Although it is not yet clear which emotional disorders emerge from imbalances of separation distress circuitry, the most evident possibilities for syndromes which may reflect overactivity or oversensitivity of the system are panic attacks, obsessive-compulsive disorders, and other post-traumatic stress syndromes (Klein, 1981; Panksepp, 1982; van der Kolk, 1987). Long-term consequences of overactivity also probably lead to anaclitic depression (Spitz, 1946) and other melancholic syndromes. As we have discussed elsewhere, a disorder which may reflect underactivity or undersensitivity of the system may be early childhood autism. We have considered the possibility that such unresponsivity of this system may be due to excess brain opioid activity which inhibits the normal development of social intent (for recent review, see Panksepp and Sahley, 1987), and some preliminary clinical trials now indicate that opiate receptor blockade with naltrexone does reduce some symptoms of the disorder (Herman et al., 1986). The further elucidation of the biochemical and functional properties of the brain systems which mediate separation distress and the separation call should provide further insight into the genesis of a variety of psychiatric disorders, as well as providing a rigorous analysis of the underling neurobiological causes of social emotions and social bonding.

REFERENCES

Alexander, B.K., Coambs, R.B., and Hadaway, P.F., 1978, The effect of housing and gender on morphine self-administration in rats, Psychopharmacol, 58: 175.

Andrew, R.J., 1974, Changes in visual responsiveness following intercollicular lesions and their effects on avoidance and attack, Brain Behav Evol, 10: 400.

Andrew, R.J. and de Lanerolle, N., 1974, The effects of muting lesions on emotional behaviour and behaviour normally associated with calling, Brain Behav Evol, 10: 377.

Bandler, R., 1982, Induction of 'rage' following microinjections of glutamate into midbrain but not hypothalamus of cats, Neurosci Lett, 30: 183.

Bernston, G.G., 1972, Blockade and release of hypothalamically and naturally elicited aggressive behviours in cats following midbrain lesions, J Comp Physiol Psych, 81: 541.

Bishop, P., 1984, Brain and opiate modulation of avian affective

vocalizations, Unpublished doctoral dissertation, Bowling Green
State Univ., Bowling Green, Ohio.

Bonnet, K.S., Miller, J.M., and Simon, E.J., 1976, The effects of
chronic opiate treatment and social isolation on opiate
receptors in the rodent brain, in: "Opiate and Endogenous Opioid
Peptides," H.W. Kosterlitz, ed., Elsevier, Amsterdam.

Bowlby, 1973, "Attachment and Loss, Vol. II Separation," Basic
Books, New York.

Dalhouse, A.D., 1976, Social cohesiveness, hypersexuality and
irritability induced by p-CPA in the rat, Physiol Behav, 17:
697.

Decsi, L. and Varszegi, M.K., 1969, Fear and escape reaction evoked
by the intrahypothalamic injection of D-tubocurarine in
unrestrained cats, Acta Physiol Acad Sci Hung, 36: 95.

de Lanerolle, N. and Andrew, R.J., 1974, Midbrain structures
controlling vocalization in the domestic chick, Brain Behav
Evol, 10: 354.

de Lanerolle, N., Elde, R.P., Sparber, S.B. and Frick, M., 1981,
Distribution of methionine-enkephalin immunoreactivity in the
chick brain: an immunohistochemical study, J Comp Neurol, 199:
513.

de Molina, A.F. and Hunsperger, R.W., 1959, Central representation
of affective reactions in forebrain and brain stem: Electrical
stimulation of amygdala, stria terminalis, and adjacent
structures, J Physiol, 145: 251.

Enloe, L.J., 1975, Extra mediation of emotionality and social
cohesiveness effects, Physiol Behav, 15: 271.

Fagg, G.E., 1985, L-glutamate, excitatory amino acid receptors and
brain function, Trend Neurosci, 8: 207.

File, S.E., and Pellow, S,, 1985, Chlordiazepoxide enhances the
anxiogenic action of CGS 8216 in the social interaction test:
Evidence for benzodiazepine withdrawal?, Pharmacol Biochem
Behav, 23: 33.

Gessa, G., Paglietti, E, and Pellegrini Quarantotti, B., 1979,
Induction of copulatory behavior in sexually inactive rats by
naloxone, Science, 204: 203.

Harlow, H.F., 1971, "Learning to Love," Albion Pub. Co., San
Francisco.

Harlow, C.M. (ed.) 1986, "From Learning to Love: The Selected
Papers of H.F. Harlow," Praeger, New York.

Herman, B.H., 1979, An exploration of brain social attachment
substrates in guinea pigs, Unpublished doctoral dissertation,
Bowling Green State Univ., Bowling Green, Ohio.

Herman, B.H., Hammock, M.K., Arthur-Smith, A., Egan, J., Chatoor,
I., Zelnik, N., Corradine, M., Appelgate, K., Boeckx, R.L. and
Sharp, S.D., 1986, Role of opioid peptides in autism: Effects of
acute administration of naltrexone. Neuroscience Abs, 12: 1172.

Herman, B.H. and Panksepp, J., 1978, Effects of morphine and
naloxone on social attachment in infant guinea pigs, Pharmacol
Biochem Behav, 9: 213.

Herman, B.H. and Panksepp, J., 1981, Ascending endorphin inhibition of distress vocalizations, Science, 221: 1060.

Insel, T.R., Hill, J.L., and Mayor, R.B., 1986, Rat pup ultrasonic isolation calls: Possible mediation by the benzodiazepine receptor complex, Pharmacol Biochem Behav, 24: 1263.

Johnson, D.A., Poplawsky, A., and Bieliauskas, L., 1972, Alterations of social behavior in rats and hamsters following lesions of the septal forebrain, Psychonom Sci, 26: 19.

Jonason, K.R., and Enloe, L.J., 1971, Alterations in social behavior following septal and amygdaloid lesions in the rat. J Comp Physiol Psych, 75: 286.

Jonason, K.R., Enloe, L.J., Contrucci, J. and Meyer, P.M., 1973, Effects of simultaneous and successive septal and amygdaloid lesions on social behavior in the rat, J Comp Physiol Psych, 83: 54.

Jürgens, U., 1976, Reinforcing concomitants of electrically elicited vocalizations, Exp Brain Res, 26: 203.

Jürgens, U., 1979, Vocalization as an emotional indicator: A neuroethological study in the squirrel monkey, Behaviour, 69: 88.

Jürgens, U., Maurcus, M., Ploog, D. and Winter, P., 1967, Vocalization in the squirrel monkey (Saimiri sciureus) elicited by brain stimulation, Exp Brain Res, 4: 114.

Jürgens, U. and Ploog, D., 1970, Cerebral representation of vocalization in the squirrel monkey, Exp Brain Res, 10: 532.

Jürgens, U. and Richter, K., 1986, Glutamate-induced vocalization in the squirrel monkey, Brain Res, 373: 349.

Kalin, N.H., Shelton, S.E., Kraemer, G.W., and McKinney, W.T., 1983, Associated endocrine, physiological and behavioral changes in rhesus monkeys after intravenous corticotropin-releasing factor administration, Peptides, 4: 211.

Kanai, T. and Wang, S.C., 1952, Localization of the central vocalization mechanism in the brain stem of the cat, Exp Neurol, 6: 426.

Kaufman, I.C. and Hinde, R.A., 1961, Factors influencing distress calling in chicks, with special reference to temperature changes and social isolation, Anim Behav, 9: 197.

Kavaliers, M., 1981, Schooling behavior of fish: An opiate-dependent activity, Behav Neur Biol, 33: 379.

Klein, D.F., 1981, Anxiety reconceptualized, in "Anxiety: New Research and Changing Concepts," D.F. Klein and J. Rabkin, eds, Raven Press, New York.

Leyton, A.S.F. and Sherrington, C.S., 1917, Observations on the excitable cortex of the champanzee, orangutan and gorilla, Q J Exp Physiol, 11: 135.

Luparello, T.J., 1967, "Stereotaxic Atlas of the Forebrain of the Guinea Pig," S. Karger AG, Basel.

MacLean, P.D., 1985, Brain evolution relating to family, play, and the separation call, Arch Gen Psychiat, 42: 405.

Martin, J.R., 1976, Motivated behaviors elicited from hypothalamus, midbrain and pons of the guinea pig (*Cavia porcellus*), J Comp Physiol Psych, 90: 1011.

McCullough, W.S., 1944, The functional organization of the cerebral cortex, Physiol Rev, 24: 390.

McNicholas, L.F., Martin, W.R., and Cherian, S., 1983, Physical dependence on diazepam and lorazepam in the dog, J Pharmacol Exp Ther, 226: 783.

Meller, R.E., Keverne, E.B., and Herbert, J., 1980, Behavioral and endocrine effects of naltrexone in male talapoin monkeys, Pharmacol Biochem Behav, 13: 435.

Montevecchi, W.A., Gallup, G.G., Jr., and Dunlap, W.P., 1973, The peep vocalization in group reared chicks (*Gallus domesticus*) in relation to fear. Anim Behav, 21: 116.

Myers, R.E., 1972, Role of prefrontal and anterior temporal cortex in social behavior and affect in monkeys, Acta Neurobiol Exp, 32: 567.

Myers, R.E., 1974, "Handbook of drug and chemical stimulation of the brain," Van Nostrand Reinhold, New York.

Newman, J.D., and MacLean, P. D., 1982, Effects of tegmental lesions on the isolation call of squirrel monkeys, Brain Res, 232: 317.

Newman, J.D., Smith, H.J., and Talmage-Riggs, G., 1983, Structural variability in primate vocalizations and its functional significance: An analysis of squirrel monkey chuck calls, Folia Primatol, 40: 114.

Noirot, E., 1968, Ultrasounds in young rodents. II. Changes with age in albino rats, Anim Behav, 16: 129.

Normansell, L., Bishop, P. and Panksepp, J., 1985, Anatomy of affective vocalizations in chicks, Soc Neurosci Abstr, 11: 1171.

Oswalt, G.L. and Meier, G.W., 1975, Olfactory, thermal, and tactual influences on infantile ultrasonic vocalization in rats, Devel Psychobiol, 8: 129.

Panksepp, J., 1979, A neurochemical theory of autism, Trends Neurosci, 2: 174.

Panksepp, J., 1981, Brain opioids—A neurochemical substrate for narcotic and social dependence, in: "Theory in psychopharmacology," S. Cooper, ed., Academic Press, London, p. 149.

Panksepp, J., 1982, Toward a general psychobiological theory of emotions, Behav Brain Sci, 5: 407.

Panksepp, J., 1986, The psychobiology of prosocial behaviors: Separation distress, play and altruism. in: "Altruism and Aggression: Biological and Social Origins," C. Zahn-Waxler, E.M. Cummings & R. Iannotti, eds., Cambridge Univ. Press, Cambridge.

Panksepp, J., Bean, N.J., Bishop, P., Vilberg, T., and Sahley, T,L., 1980, Opioid blockade and social comfort in chicks, Pharm Biochem Behav, 13: 673.

Panksepp, J., Crepeau, L., and Clynes, M., 1987, Effects of CRF on separation distress and juvenile play. Neurosci Abst, 13: In Press.

Panksepp, J., Herman, B., Conner, R., Bishop, P. and Scott, J.P., 1978, The biology of social attachments: Opiates alleviate separation distress, Biol Psychiat, 13: 607.

Panksepp, J., Herman, B.H., Vilberg, T., Bishop, P., and DeEskinazi, F.G., 1980, Endogenous opioids and social behavior, Neurosci Biobehav Rev, 4: 473.

Panksepp, J., Meeker, R. and Bean, N.J., 1980, The neurochemical control of crying, Pharmacol Biochem Behav, 12: 437.

Panksepp, J., Normansell, L., Siviy, S., Buchanan, A., Zolovick, A., Rossi, J. and Conner, R., 1983, A cholinergic command circuit for separation distress?, Soc Neurosci Abstr, 9: 979.

Panksepp, J., Normansell, L., Siviy, S., Rossi, J. and Zolovick, A., 1984, Casomorphins reduce separation distress in chicks, Peptides, 5: 829.

Panksepp, J. and Sahley, T.L., 1987, Possible brain opioid involvement in disrupted social intent and language development of autism, in: "Neurobiological Issues in Autism," E. Schopler, and G.B. Mesibov, eds., Plenum, New York.

Panksepp, J., Siviy, S. and Normansell, L., 1984, The psychobiology of play: Theoretical and methodological perspectives, Neurosci Biobehav Rev, 8: 465.

Panksepp, J., Siviy, S.M. and Normansell, L.A., 1985, Brain opioids and social emotions, in: "The psychobiology of attachment and separation," M. Reite, and T. Field, eds., Academic Press, New York, p. 3.

Panksepp, J., Siviy, S., Normansell, L., White, K. and Bishop, P., 1982, Effects of ß-chlornaltrexamine on separation distress in chicks, Life Sci, 31: 2387.

Panksepp, J., Vilberg, T., Bean, N.J., Coy, D.H., and Kastin, A.J., 1978, Reduction of distress vocalizations in chicks by opiate-like peptides, Brain Res Bull, 3: 663.

Peek, F.W., and Phillips, R.E., 1971, Repetitive vocalizations evoked by local electrical stimulation of avian brains. II. Anesthetized chickens (Gallus gallus), Brain Behav Evol, 4: 417.

Penfield, W., and Roberts, L., 1959, "Speech and Brain Mechanisms," Princeton University Press, Princeton.

Pettijohn, T.F., Wong, T.W., Ebert, P.D. and Scott, J.P., 1977, Alleviation of separation distress in 3 breeds of young dogs. Devel Psychobiol, 10: 373.

Phillips, R.E. and Youngren, O.M., 1976, Pattern generator for repetitive avian vocalization: Preliminary localization and functional characterization, Brain Behav Evol, 13: 165.

Phillips, R.E., Youngren, O.M. and Peek, F.W., 1972, Repetitive vocalizations evoked by electrical stimulation of avian brains. I. Awake chickens (Gallus gallus), Anim Behav, 20: 689.

Pilcher, C.W.T., and Jones, S.M., 1981, Social crowding enhances
    aversiveness of naloxone in rats, Pharmacol Biochem Behav, 14:
    299.
Ploog, D., 1986, Biological foundations of the vocal expressions of
    emotions, in: "Emotion: Theory, Research, and Experience, Vol.
    3, Biological Foundations of Emotion," R. Plutchik & H.
    Kellerman, eds., Academic Press, New York.
Porsolt, R.D., Roux, S, and Jalfre, M., 1984, Effects of
    imipramine on separation-induced vocalizations in young rhesus
    monkeys, Pharmacol Biochem Behav, 20: 979.
Reite, M. and T. Field, eds., 1985, "The psychobiology of
    attachment and separation," Academic Press, New York.
Robinson, B.W., 1967, Vocalization evoked from forebrain in Macaca
    mulatta, Physiol Behav, 2: 345.
Rossi, J., Sahley, T.L., and Panksepp, J., 1983, The role of brain
    norepinephrine in clonidine suppression of isolation-induced
    distress in the domestic chick, Psychopharm, 79: 338.
Sahley, T.L., Panksepp, J. and Zolovick, A.J., 1981, Cholinergic
    modulation of separation distress in the domestic chick, Eur J
    Pharmacol, 72: 261.
Scott, J.P., 1974, Effects of psychotropic drugs on separation
    distress in dogs, Proc IX Neuropsychopharmacol (Paris), Ex Med
    Int Con Ser 359: 735.
Scott, J.P. and Fuller, J.L., 1965, "Genetics and the Social
    Behavior of the Dog," University of Chicago Press, Chicago.
Scott, J.P., Stewart, J.M., and DeGhett, V.J., 1973, Separation in
    infant dogs, in: "Separation and Depression: Clinical and
    Research Aspects," E. C. Senay & J.P. Scott, eds., (Publication
    94), American Association for the Advancement of Science,
    Washington, D.C.
Spitz, R.A., 1946, Anaclitic depression, Psychoanal Study Child, 2:
    313.
Suomi,S.J., Seaman, S.F., Lewis, J.K., DeLizio, R.D. and McKinney,
    Jr., W.T., 1978, Effects of imipramine treatment on separation
    induced disorders in rhesus monkeys, Arch Gen Psychiat, 35: 321.
Sutton, D., Larson, C., and Lindeman, R.C., 1974, Neocortical and
    limbic lesion effects on primate phonation, Brain Res, 71: 61.
Swanson, L.W., Sawchenko, P.E., Rivier, J., and Vale, W.W., 1983,
    Organization of ovine corticotropin-releasing factor
    immunoreactive cells and fibers in the rat brain: An
    immunohistochemical study, Neuroendocrin, 36: 165.
Testerman, R.L., 1970, Modulation of laryngeal activity by
    pulmonary changes during vocalization in cats, Exp Neurol, 29:
    281.
van der Kolk, B.A., 1987, The separation cry and the trauma
    response: Developmental issues in the psychobiology of
    attachment and separation. in: "Psychological Trauma," B.A. van
    der Kolk, ed., American Psychiatric Press, Washington, D.C.
Vilberg, T.R., 1979, Endorphine modulation of chick distress

    vocalization, Unpublished doctoral dissertation, Bowling Green
    State Univ., Bowling Green, Ohio.
Vilberg, T.R., Panksepp, J., Kastin, A.J. and Coy, D.H., 1984, The
    pharmacology of endorphin modulation of chick distress
    vocalization, Peptides, 5: 823.
Watkins, J.C. and Evans, R.H., 1981, Excitatory amino acid
    transmitters, Ann R Pharmacol Toxicol, 21: 165.

ONTOGENY OF ADRENERGIC AND OPIOID EFFECTS ON SEPARATION
VOCALIZATIONS IN RATS

Priscilla Kehoe

Trinity College
Hartford, CT

INTRODUCTION

Altricial mammals are capable of forming a variety of
associations and relationships which allow the infant to recognize
home and caretaker (Brake, 1981; Johanson & Hall, 1979; Kehoe &
Blass, 1986a, 1986b; Pedersen, Williams, & Blass, 1982; Rudy &
Cheatle, 1979; Smith & Spear, 1978). These learned affectional
relationships are of great significance to the infant's survival
and perhaps for adult motivated behaviors, as seen, for example, in
males' reproductive behavior depending on postnatal olfactory
experience (Fillion & Blass, 1986). Recent studies have
investigated the central mechanisms that might underlie the
development of such important relationships and emotions (Kehoe &
Blass, 1986b, 1986c, 1986d, 1986e; Panksepp, 1981; Panksepp, Siviy,
& Normansell, 1985; Spear, Enters, Aswad, & Louzan, 1985).
Exploration of the neurobiology mediating the ontogeny of affective
behavior may lead to an understanding of infant responsivity, adult
motivated behaviors and possibly anxiety disorders.
Mammalian infant separation from parents and siblings evokes a
quantifiable emotional response, namely, vocalizations. Neonatal
rats under various social and thermal conditions emit ultrasonic
cries in the range of 30-50 KHz which is well beyond the range of
human hearing (Allin & Banks, 1972; Noirot, 1972). Short-term
individual isolation of rat pups seems to be a severe biosocial
stress as judged by these ultrasonic vocalizations which are a
potent stimulus for maternal retrieval (Smotherman, Bell, Starzec,
Elias, & Zachman, 1974). Isolated rat pups, then, offer a model for
the study of an important emotional response, namely, separation
distress.

Neonatal rats' ultrasonic vocalizations can be demonstrated soon after birth and become most intense from postnatal days 5 to 12 (Noirot, 1972), decreasing rapidly after eye opening occurs. Distress vocalizations can be pharmacologically manipulated by several neurochemical agents. The neuropharmacology of vocalizations in various species has been studied presenting data that is interesting and complex. Specifically, opiates and opiate antagonists modulate emitted cries in neonatal chicks, young guinea pigs, and adult squirrel monkeys; morphine decreases and naloxone increases vocalizations (Herman & Panksepp, 1978; Harris & Newman, 1986; Panksepp, Vilberg, Bean, Cay, & Kastin, 1978). The Gaba system may also be involved in mediating vocalizations as the anxiolytic agent, diazepam, decreases rat pup vocalizations while the anxiogenic agent, pentylenetetrazol, increases them (Insel, Hill, & Mayor, 1986). Furthermore, clonidine, an alpha-2 adrenergic agonist, decreases distress calls in chicks (Panksepp, Meeker & Bean, 1980) and adult squirrel monkeys (Harris & Newman, 1985), an effect that is reversed with yohimbine, an alpha-2 adrenergic antagonist.

The possibility exists that the pharmaceuticals modulating separation vocalizations may actually affect the neural systems by which natural stimuli work. The opioid and noradrenergic systems are importantly implicated in the neurochemical control of crying (Panksepp, et al. 1980). In short, these systems might influence the general stress response to naturally occurring maternal separation during development. To further explore this psychobiology and its development, the neonatal albino rat isolated for a short time under thermal nest conditions was the paradigm used.

Opioid Mediation of Separation Distress

Behavioral properties of opioid systems have recently been evaluated in neonatal rats (Kehoe & Blass, 1986b, 1986c, 1986d, 1986e) because these systems are present centrally as early as fetal day 16 (Bayon, Shoemaker, Bloom, Mauss & Guillemin, 1979; Clendeninn, Petraitis, & Simon, 1976; Coyle & Pert, 1976; Khachaturian, Alessi, Munfakh, & Watson, 1983). Furthermore, opiates have been implicated in adult motivation (Beluzzi & Stein, 1977; Hunter & Reid, 1983; Stein, 1978). In fact, it appears that a behaviorally positive opioid system exists in neonatal rats as early as 5 days of age, resulting in a preferred olfactory or gustatory stimulus at 10 days of age (Kehoe & Blass, 1986b, 1986d). As in adult rats, endogenous opioid systems also appear to be involved in mediating pain and stress in neonates. Group housing away from the dam, a seemingly mild social stress, slightly increased analgesic responses to heat (Kehoe & Blass, 1986b). Moreover, individual isolation, a more severe stress, produced a marked analgesia that was blocked by pretreatment with an opioid antagonist (Kehoe & Blass, 1986d, 1986e; Spear et al., 1985).

To further elucidate the role of opioids during maternal separation it was necessary to establish the relationship between distress vocalizations, response to nociception and opioids in isolated infant rats (Kehoe & Blass, 1986d, 1986e). Ten day old rats were individually isolated for 5 minutes in a cup with clean pine bedding in an environment maintained at nest temperature (32 C). Prior to the isolation the pups were treated with either 0.5mg/kg of intraperitoneal morphine, 0.5mg/kg of naltrexone, saline or nothing. During the isolation the pup's ultrasonic vocalizations were made audible through a Bat Detector (QMC), counted and recorded. At the end of the 5 minutes the pups were tested on a hot-plate (46 C) for a paw withdrawal response. During the 5 minutes of isolation the pups not pretreated emitted a mean of 300 ultrasonic vocalizations, a response virtually identical to that of rats pretreated with saline (Figure 1). Naltrexone-treated rats emitted a high number of calls while the morphine-treated pups were fairly quiet (mean values of 630 and 105, respectively).

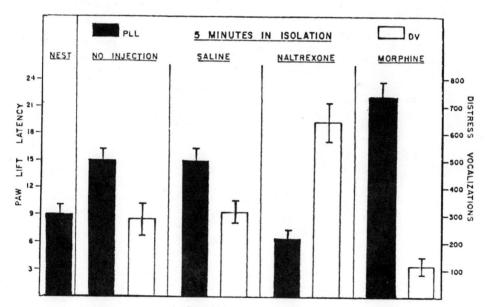

Fig. 1. Paw lift latency (black bars) to a hot plate for pups removed directly from the nest or isolated for 5 min after pretreatment with no injection, saline, naltrexone or morphine (ip). White bars represent the number of separation vocalizations during the 5 min isolation period for each group of pups.

The paw-lift latencies reflected the treatment of each group of pups. Isolated rat pups, either non-injected or pretreated with saline demonstrated a decreased heat sensitivity (15 sec) in comparison to the non-isolated pups (9 sec). Naltrexone-treated pups had an extremely short mean latency of 6 seconds as opposed to morphine-treated pups with a mean latency of 22 seconds. Thus, an exogenous opioid significantly increased paw withdrawal latency and markedly decreased the number of distress vocalizations in isolated neonatal rats. These pups were not cataleptic, righting appeared normal, and they occasionally locomoted in the cup. To further rule out sedation as a cause of reduced cries, morphine at the low dose of 0.25mg/kg was administered yielding a similar decrease in vocalizations. In contrast, an opioid antagonist reduced paw-lift latency and increased vocalizations. Analgesia and neonatal cries are both obviously influenced by opioids, suggesting that the level of distress calls in isolated pups is reduced by release of endogenous opioids. In short, it appears that the endogenous opioid systems are recruited in the coping process of isolation distress in neonatal rats.

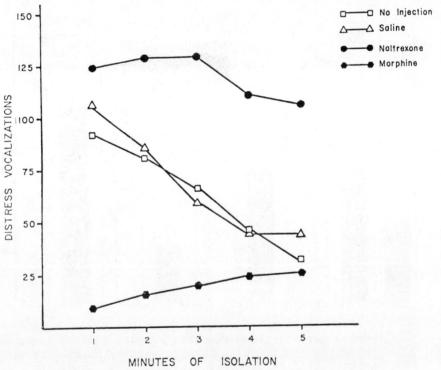

Fig. 2. Number of separation vocalizations for each minute of the 5 minute isolation period emitted by the pups in each group.

Perhaps the biological relevance of the infant vocalizations can be better emphasized when analyzed on a minute by minute basis (Kehoe & Blass, 1986e). Pups that had received the opiate or its antagonist did not change in their levels of vocalizations over the isolation period, but maintained them over the 5 minutes, that is low levels for the morphine-treated pups and high levels for the naltrexone-treated ones (Figure 2). The most informative group, however, were the untreated or saline-treated pups. These rats demonstrated a significant linear decrease in their vocalizations over time. By the third minute of isolation the cries had significantly decreased compared to the first minute. Possibly, such a change in behavior could reflect alterations in endogenous opioid activity, producing a quiet state in the pup. In fact, there was a significant negative correlation between heat withdrawal responses and vocalizations at the third minute (-.69), and even greater at the fifth minute (-.83). In other words, the fewer the calls the greater the latency to withdraw from heat. Thus, a commonality exists over time between these two behaviors perhaps due to the release and processing of opioids affecting crying and pain sensitivity.

The pattern of vocalizations of the isolated rat pup may prove to be an adaptive response for the rodent. The pups treated pharmacologically may demonstrate the limitations of the crying response. Specifically, naltrexone causes continuous high levels of vocalizations and morphine causes continuous low levels. The undrugged pup cries mostly during the first few minutes and then becomes almost quiet. Dams achieve fairly reliable pup retrieval when she perceives their ultrasonic calls (Hennessey, Kaplan, Mendoza, Lowe & Levine, 1979). If she has not responded to their calls during the first few minutes then it becomes potentially dangerous for the pup to advertise its position to nearby predators.

The further investigation of opioid recruitment during neonatal stress involved the events that apparently comfort the isolate, their influence on vocalizations and pain sensitivity. At issue, therefore, is the alleviation of isolation-induced stress by various stimuli that are meaningful to the infant rat. In a counter experiment, analgesia and ultrasonic vocalizations were evaluated after returning the dam or her component features to the isolated pup (Kehoe & Blass, 1986e).

After the initial 5 minutes of isolation in a cup with clean pine bedding, each pup was transferred to a second condition for 1, 3, or 5 minutes during which their vocalizations were counted and after which they were tested for paw withdrawal from the hot-plate. They were placed on the ventrum of an anesthetized dam, or an anesthetized virgin, in a cup of soiled home bedding, or in one with clean bedding. Proximity and nipple attachment to the

anesthetized dam caused responses that most closely resembled those
of the non-isolated sibling (Figure 3), with short paw-lift
latencies. The presence of the virgin female, however, was equally
effective in relieving isolation stress.

Isolated pups placed in the familiar odor of soiled bedding
demonstrated a profile over the 5 minutes that, although less
dramatic than that of rats returned to a female, differed
noticeably from that of pups placed in clean bedding. The salient
odors found in the home-bedding, through their familiarity, served
to reduce the separation-induced stress but not with the speed that
the female could. In fact, the distress vocalizations of the pups
put in the various conditions greatly paralleled the profiles of
pain sensitivity (Figure 4). While, in general, all levels of
crying were reduced, female contact was successful in producing
almost virtual quiet, and the familiar odors of the nest caused a
reduction of vocalizations compared to pups remaining in the clean
bedding.

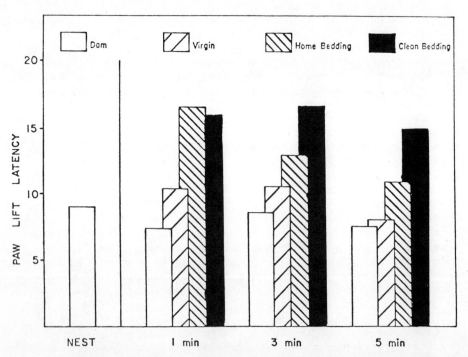

Fig. 3.   Paw lift latency of pups taken directly from the nest or
          isolated for 5 min and then placed for 1, 3, or 5 min on
          either clean bedding, home-bedding, anesthetized virgin,
          or anesthetized dam.

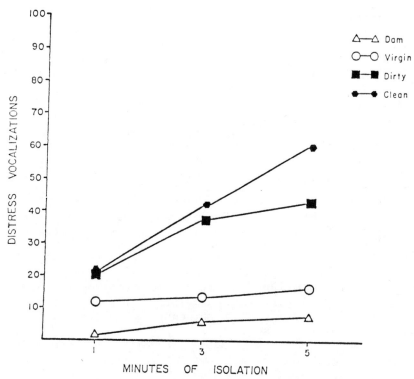

Fig. 4.   Number of separation vocalizations for pups during the 1,
          3, or 5 min period on either clean bedding, home-bedding,
          anesthetized virgin, or anesthetized dam.

     If maternal separation caused an opioid response, then
reversing the stress with maternal stimuli should reverse the
biochemical profile. The pain sensitivity seemed to normalize with
an absence of the analgesic response seen during isolation. The
ultrasonic vocalizations which were already at a low level towards
the latter part of the isolation period, now were virtually absent
when contact was made with the female. Pups in the nest are also
fairly quiet, usually only vocalizing when tread on by the dam.
Furthermore, opioid antagonism does not initiate ultrasonic
vocalizations in pups remaining in the nest. Thus, it appears that
although isolation can activate the opioid system in neonates,
comforting events are probably not acting through the same system,
or, at least, the opioid systems may be inhibited through another
mechanism. Since many of the responses were graded, it is possible
that the biochemical systems are likewise functioning in an
incremental fashion, perhaps through harmonious interaction of
several systems.

Noradrenergic effects on separation distress

Postnatally, the central nervous system undergoes remarkable anatomical and neurochemical changes (Hartley & Seeman, 1983; Lanier, Dunn, & VanHartesveldt, 1976; Morris, Dausse, Devynick & Meyer, 1980) which is most significantly demonstrated by changes in behavioral responsivity to neuropharmaceuticals (Barrett, Caza, Spear, & Spear, 1982; Cambell & Mabry, 1977; Kellogg & Lundborg, 1972; Nomura, Oki, Segawa, 1980; Reinstein, McClearn & Isaacson, 1978; Spear & Brick, 1979). The ontogeny of the noradrenergic system presents a dramatic scenario in terms of neurochemically induced behavioral changes. Specifically, clonidine, an alpha-2 adrenergic agonist, produces a dose-dependent hyperactivity in the rat pup during the first two weeks postnatally (Nomura et.al., 1980; Nomura & Segawa, 1979; Reinstein & Isaacson, 1977; Spear & Brick, 1979). This increase in locomotor activity includes a sterotypic wall-climbing when a vertical edge is encountered. Between 15 and 20 days of age, a change in clonidine effects are seen, with a dramatic shift to hypoactivity, an effect delayed in malnourished rats (Goodlett, Valentino, Resnick & Morgane, 1985). Both the clonidine-induced hyperactivity in infants and the sedation in adult rats have been antagonized by drugs such as yohimbine, phentolamine and piperoxan, strongly suggesting an alpha-2 adrenergic mediation (Anden, Grabowska, & Strombom, 1976; Drew, Gower & Marriott, 1979; Nomura et al., 1980).

The levels of catecholamines in most parts of the chick brain have reached adult levels (Kobayashi & Eiduson, 1970). Thus, it is not surprising that clonidine (0.56 mg/kg) produced sedation in chicks and significantly reduced their distress vocalizations during isolation (Panksepp, et al., 1980). Moreover, clonidine (0.1mg/kg) significantly decreased the isolation calls of adult squirrel monkeys, an effect that is reversed with yohimbine (0.2mg/kg), (Harris & Newman, 1985). In an effort to obtain an ontological profile of the adrenergic system in terms of separation distress, rat pups from postnatal days 10 to 18 were psychopharmacologically analyzed during isolation (Kehoe & Harris, 1986).

Pups ten days of age were removed from the nest, injected with intraperitoneal clonidine (.005mg/kg, .05mg/kg, or .5mg/kg) or saline and replaced in the nest for 15 minutes. The pup was then placed in a cup with clean bedding in a warm environment (32°C) for 25 minutes, during which time ultrasonic vocalizations and activity levels were monitored and recorded. At the sixth minute of isolation the pup was removed from the cup, injected intraperitoneally with either yohimbine (.05mg/kg, .1 mg/kg) or saline. At the end of the session the pup's axillary temperature was monitored, and showed no significant difference between groups.

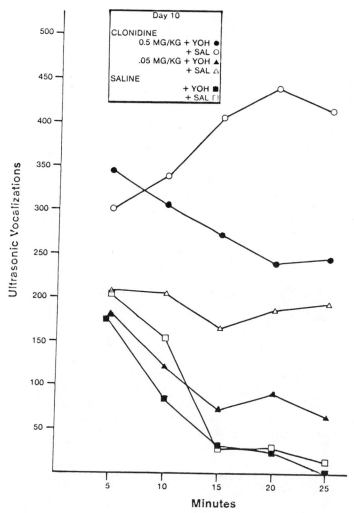

Fig. 5. Day 10 pups' number of separation vocalizations for each 5 min period of isolation. The pups were injected with the first drug 15 min before isolation and the second drug at the 6th minute of isolation.

The profile of adrenergic effects on separation vocalizations in 10-day-old rats is shown in Figure 5. Control pups injected with saline emitted 210 cries in the first 5 minutes. Over the course of the next 20 minutes these pups significantly reduced their vocalizing, replicating our previous results and suggesting a possible endogenous opioid release in response to the separation stress. Pups receiving clonidine at .005mg/kg (not shown on the

graph) were not different from controls. Clonidine at .05mg/kg,
however, caused a significantly different profile compared to the
saline controls, one very similar to that produced by naltrexone.
Thus, the first 5 minute period of isolation after low dose
clonidine did not cause a change in behavior compared to saline
controls, however, the pups continued to cry at high levels whereas
the controls became quiet. Clonidine produced a dose-response
increase in activity levels in the day-10 pups.

Yohimbine at both doses produced a profile very similar to
that of the control-saline pups that were crying at very low levels
after the first 10 minutes. Furthermore, yohimbine (0.1mg/kg) most
effectively reduced the clonidine-induced (.05mg/kg) vocalizations
to the level of controls.

Clonidine in a high dose, 0.5mg/kg, significantly increased
emitted cries for the first 5 minutes (300) and, in fact, caused a
continued almost linear increase over the 25 minute test period,
reaching a calling rate of over 400 in the last 5 minutes. This
dose did cause remarkable wall-climbing, treading and turning
stereotypy as has been previously reported (Reinstein & Isaacson,
1977). Yohimbine (0.1mg/kg), given after the high dose of
clonidine, was able to reduce the high level of calling and
significantly attenuate the hyperactivity (Nomura et al., 1980).
These pups, however, still produced vocalizations above the levels
of the control pups.

The profile of adrenergic effects on separation vocalizations
in 15-day-old rat pups is similar in many respects to that of the
10-day-old rats (Figure 6). Day 15 pups after saline injections
cried less than the younger pups, 100 vocalizations in the first 5
minutes. Moreover, the number of cries remained at a steady level
over the 25 minutes, perhaps demonstrating less of an opioid effect
resulting from separation. This change in isolation behavior may
well be a result of eye opening which occurred on Day 14. Yohimbine
(0.1mg/kg) given after saline caused a significant decrease in
vocalizations compared to saline-saline control pups, such that in
the last 5 minutes the yohimbine-treated rats cried 25 times and
controls 112.

Low dose clonidine (.05mg/kg) significantly increased calling
immediately and produced a fairly constant level of vocalizations
throughout the 25 minutes. Yohimbine caused a reduction in crying
but not until the 20th minute, demonstrating a slower effect of the
adrenergic antagonist than that seen in day-10 pups.

Day-15 pups administered clonidine (.5mg/kg) emitted more than
four times the number of cries (445) than the saline controls
(100). Yohimbine reversed the high level of calling produced by the
clonidine but not until the 20th minute. Moreover, naltrexone, an

opioid antagonist, given subsequent to the higher dose of clonidine caused an increase in calls 6 to 7 times those of the saline controls. Naltrexone alone causes a significant increase in vocalizations in 15 to 18 day old pups (unpublished observations), but the combination of clonidine and naltrexone raised the frequency considerably in the 15-day-old pups.

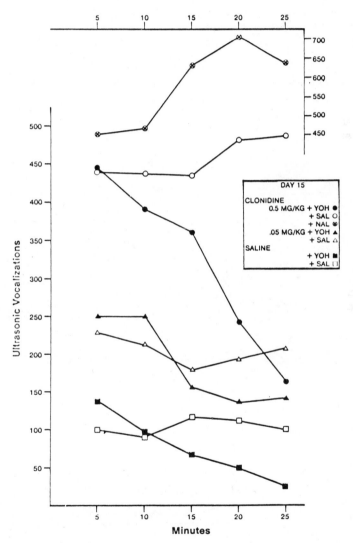

Fig. 6. Day 15 pups' number of separation vocalizations for each 5 min period of isolation. The pups were injected with the first drug 15 min before isolation and the second drug at the 6th minute of isolation.

It appears that adrenergic effects on maternally separated day 15 rat pups are qualitatively similar to those seen in 10-day-old rats. Clonidine caused a dose-response increase in ultrasonic vocalizations while yohimbine, an adrenergic antagonist, caused a significant reversal. Naltrexone administration caused a remarkable increase in emitted cries in pups 10 and 15 days of age.

Pups 17 days of age demonstrated a profile of adrenergic effects on separation vocalizations quite different from the younger pups (Figure 7). Control pups injected with saline and then isolated emitted substantially fewer cries than younger pups. They vocalized about 25 times for each 5 minute period steadily across the 25 minutes. Yohimbine given to the saline controls reduced the crying almost completely. Furthermore, yohimbine 0.1mg/kg given prior to isolation reduced pups' separation vocalizations significantly below that seen in saline control pups (not seen in graph).

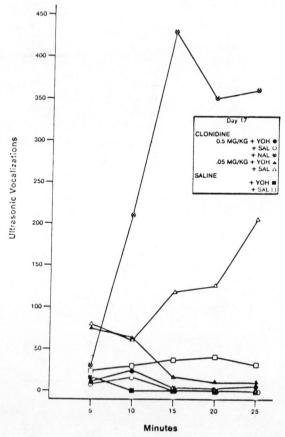

Fig. 7.   Day 17 pups' number of separation vocalizations for each 5 min period of isolation. The pups were injected with the first drug 15 min before isolation and the second drug at the 6th minute of isolation.

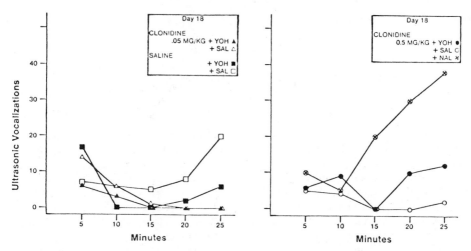

Fig. 8. Day 18 pups' number of separation vocalizations for each 5 min period of isolation. The pups were injected with the first drug 15 min before isolation and the second drug at the 6th minute of isolation.

The low dose of clonidine (.05mg/kg) significantly raised the number of emitted vocalizations with a remarkably linear increase over time. In the last 5 minutes of isolation, these Day-17 pups cried over 200 times, a response which was completely reversed with yohimbine. In short, yohimbine given subsequent to the clonidine produced a decrease in vocalizing to the saline-control level.

In the 17-day-old rat the high dose of clonidine (.5mg/kg) for the first time ontologically did not increase separation vocalizations but kept them at an even lower level than the saline controls. Yohimbine given after the high dose of clonidine did not reverse the silence. Naltrexone, however, given after the clonidine produced an extremely high level of calling which continued over the 25 minutes.

It appears, then, that the adrenergic drug, clonidine, has a dose-specific reverse effect on the day 17 pups' ultrasonic vocalizations from that seen in day 10 and day 15 pups. Specifically, high doses of clonidine now have a quieting effect, perhaps similar to that seen in adult clonidine sedation; however, a moderately low dose still produces an increase in vocalizations. Opioid antagonists cause an effective increase in crying similar to profiles seen in younger pups.

The profile of adrenergic effects on ultrasonic vocalizations in 18-day-old rats appears quite different than the younger pups, even those just 24 hours younger (Figure 8). Saline-control rats emit cries at very low levels during the entire 25 minutes, between 5 and 20 cries emitted during each 5 minutes of isolation. Yohimbine did not change this control profile, nor did any dose of clonidine given prior to isolation. In contrast, naltrexone after clonidine or given alone (not shown on the graph) remarkably increases the separation vocalizations of even these older pups to a level of 250 in the last 5 minutes of isolation.

From these data it appears that adrenergic pharmaceuticals influence ultrasonic vocalizations of neonatal pups with important ontogenic changes between day 15 and day 18. To begin with, during isolation in a warm environment 10-day-old rat pups emit cries at a very high level which decreases linearly to virtual silence by 20 days of age. Clonidine, an alpha-2 adrenergic agonist causes a direct dose-response increase in calling in Day 10 and Day 15 pups. It seems unlikely, however, that these vocalizations are specifically separation vocalizations since the pups were continuing to vocalize when returned to their nest, dam and siblings.

Yohimbine, an alpha-2 adrenergic antagonist, did reverse the high level of clonidine-induced calling in these pups while they were isolated. Moreover, yohimbine given prior to Day 10 isolation significantly decreased the number of separation vocalizations normally emitted (Figure 9). These data suggest that yohimbine may be suppressing cries via the immediately deployed mechanism under the stress of isolation, namely the noradrenergic system. While this system does seem to influence ultrasonic vocalizations in neonatal rats, stimulation by clonidine does not seem to do so in response to situational and environmental input, perhaps inducing an anxiogenic state.

The most remarkable data resulting from these studies are the ontological changes in vocalizations in response to adrenergic stimulation. From day 10 to day 15 clonidine stimulates ultrasonic vocalizing in a linear dose-response manner, whereas on day 17, a dissociation is seen. That is, a high dose of clonidine decreases emitted calls while the low dose increases them as it did in the younger pups. On day 18 all doses of clonidine tested show no sign of increasing vocalizations and in fact seem to show a trend in decreasing the already low level of calling. Yohimbine did not reverse the pups' silence. These pups, however, can be induced to vocalize at high levels with an opioid antagonist only during isolation.

The ontogenetic changes in behavioral responsivity to clonidine may be due to a number of neurobiological mechanisms. The presynaptic regulation of noradrenergic transmission may be undergoing maturational changes particularly in those brain systems regulating locomotor activity and ultrasonic vocalizations. It appears, though, that presynaptic receptor-mediated inhibition of norepinephrine transmission is functional as early as 4 days of age, since clonidine pretreatment did prevent noradrenergic loss from certain brain areas following tyrosine hydroxylase inhibition (Kellogg & Wennerstrom, 1974). It is possible that clonidine may work on alpha-2 receptors located on other neurons, such as serotonergic, which may be undergoing maturation (Raiteri, Maura & Versace, 1983; Zebrowska-Lupina, Przegalinski, Sloniec & Kleinrok, 1977). It may be that other systems mature which exert inhibitory control over noradrenergic activity, particularly cholinergic systems (Campbell, Lytle & Fibiger, 1969; Carlton, 1969). Whatever the precise mechanism for the developmental changes in clonidine-induced activity, it seems that ultrasonic vocalizing may be similarly mediated.

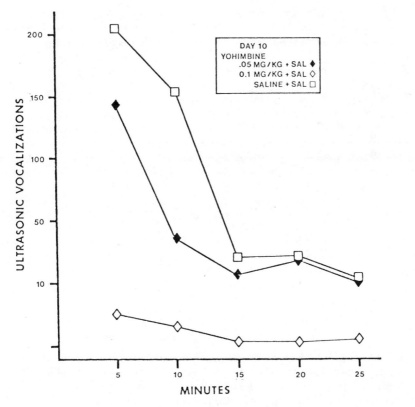

Fig. 9.   Day 10 pups' number of separation vocalizations for each 5 min period after administration of yohimbine (.05mg/kg, 0.1mg/kg) or saline 15 min prior to isolation.

CONCLUSIONS

These studies indicate that rat pups' ultrasonic vocalizations are modulated by both the adrenergic and opioid systems. Importantly, it appears that the adrenergic system influences vocalizations in rat pups, often without the necessary stimulation of isolation. In other words, the clonidine-injected pups were heard vocalizing in the home nest before they were isolated. The clonidine mediation of vocalizations closely paralleled that seen in clonidine-induced locomotor and activity levels during ontogeny. Furthermore, isolation-induced as well as clonidine-induced vocalizing behavior is reversed with yohimbine, similar to that seen with activity levels. Some psychoneurobiological event occurs on approximately day 16 to drastically change the effects of clonidine administration, interacting with changes in natural behavioral patterns, such as isolation-induced vocalizations.

The opioid system seems to be more directly and specifically involved with the ultrasonic vocalizations induced by separation from nest, dam and siblings. Thus, pups given naltrexone did not vocalize in the nest or when placed with siblings, but vocalized at an extremely high level when isolated, suggesting an important role for endogenous opioid release during neonatal stress. Furthermore, there seems to be no developmental change in response to opioid antagonism as pups from day 10 to day 18 were shown to increase their emitted cries during isolation after naltrexone administration. Even though 18-day-old rats cry very little when isolated (10 to 15 cries in 5 minutes), naltrexone increased their calling over 20 times (250 cries). Moreover, opioid antagonism reversed the clonidine depression in the older pups. The above studies suggest that the noradrenergic system may play a role in the anxiogenic state of the neonate, resulting in the infant response of crying, while the opioid system may indeed produce a quiet state. It is possible that there is an interacting modulation of isolation-induced vocalizations between the opioid and adrenergic systems in infant rats. Such information can advance our knowledge on the psychobiology of emotional responsivity of the infant, development of neural systems mediating affectional relationships and anxiety disorders.

REFERENCES

Allin, J. T., and Banks, E. M., 1972, Functional aspects of ultrasound production by infant albino rats (Rattus norvegicus). Animal Behaviour, 20:175.
Anden, N. E., Grabowska, M., and Strombom, U., 1976, Different alpha-adrenoreceptor in the central nervous system mediating

biochemical and functional effects of clonidine and receptor blocking agents. Naunyn Schmiedebergs Arch Pharmacologia, 292:43.

Barrett, B. A., Caza, P., Spear, N. E., and Spear, L., 1982, Wall climbing, odors from the home nest and catecholaminergic activity in rat pups. Physiology & Behavior, 29:501.

Bayon, A., Shoemaker, W. J., Bloom, F. E., Mauss, A., and Guillemin, R., 1979, Perinatal development of the endorphin- and enkephalin- containing systems in the rat brain. Brain Research, 179:93.

Belluzzi, J. D., and Stein, L., 1977, Enkephalin may mediate euphoria and drive reduction reward. Nature, 266:556.

Brake, S. C., 1981, Suckling infant rats learn a preference for a novel olfactory stimulus paired with milk delivery. Science, 211:506.

Campbell, B. A., Lytle, L. D., and Fibiger, H. C., 1969, Ontogeny of adrenergic arousal and cholinergic inhibitory mechanisms in the rat. Science, 166:635.

Campbell, B. A., and Mabry, P. D., 1977, The role of catecholamines in behavioral arousal during ontogenesis. Psychopharmacologia, 31:253.

Carlton, P. L., 1969, Brain acetylcholine and inhibition, in: "Reinforcement and Behavior," J.T. Tapp, ed., Academic Press, New York.

Clendeninn, N. J., Petraitis, M., and Simon, E. J., 1976, Ontological development of opiate receptors in rodent brain. Brain Research, 118: 157.

Coyle, J. T., and Pert, C. B., 1976, Ontogenetic development of 3H-naloxone binding in rat brain. Neuropharmacology, 15:550.

Drew, G. M., Gower, A. J., and Marriott, A. S., 1979, Alpha2-adrenoceptors mediate clonidine-induced sedation in the rat. British Journal of Pharmacology, 67:133.

Fillion, T., and Blass, E. M., 1986, Infantile experience with suckling odors determines adult sexual behavior in male rats. Science, 231: 729.

Goodlett, C. R., Valentino, M. L., Resnick, O., and Morgane, P. J., 1985, Altered development of responsiveness to clonidine in severely malnourished rats. Pharmacology Biochemistry & Behavior, 23:567.

Harris, J. C., and Newman, J. D., 1985, Alpha-2 adrenergic receptor involvement in adult male squirrel monkey vocal behavior. Society for Neuroscience Abstracts, 11:5.

Harris, J. C., and Newman, J. D., 1986, Synergistic effects of alpha2 adrenergic and opiate receptor blockade on vocalizations in adult squirrel monkeys. Society for Neuroscience Abstracts, 12:1133.

Hartley, E. J., and Seeman, P., 1983, Development of receptors for dopamine and noradrenaline in rat brain. European Journal Pharmacology, 91:391.

Hennessy, M. B., Kaplan, J. N., Mendoza, S. P., Lowe, E. L., and
    Levine, S., 1979, Separation distress and attachment in
    surrogate-reared squirrel monkeys. Physiology and Behavior,
    23:1017.
Herman, B. H., and Panksepp, J., 1978, Effects of morphine and
    naloxone on separation distress and at attachment: Evidence
    for opiate mediation of social effect. Pharmacology
    Biochemistry Behavior, 9:213.
Hunter Jr., G. A., and Reid, L. D., 1983, Assaying addiction
    liability of opioids. Life Sciences, 33:393.
Insel, T. R., Hill, J. L., and Mayor, R. B., 1986, Rat pup
    ultrasonic isolation calls: Possible mediation by the
    benzodiazepine receptor complex. Pharmacology Biochemistry &
    Behavior, 24:1263.
Johanson, I. B., and Hall, W. G., 1979, Appetitive learning in 1-
    day-old rat pups. Science, 205:419.
Kehoe, P., and Blass, E. M., 1986a, Conditioned aversions and their
    memories in 5-day-old rats during suckling. Journal of
    Experimental Psychology: Animal Behavior Processes, 12:40.
Kehoe, P., and Blass, E. M., 1986b, Behaviorally functional opioid
    systems in infant rats: I. Evidence for olfactory and
    gustatory classical conditioning. Behavioral Neuroscience,
    100:359.
Kehoe, P., and Blass, E. M., 1986c, Behaviorally functional opioid
    system in infant rats: II. Evidence for pharmacological,
    physiological and psychological mediation of pain and stress.
    Behavioral Neuroscience, 100:624.
Kehoe, P., and Blass, E. M., 1986d, Central nervous system
    mediation of positive and negative reinforcement in neonatal
    albino rats. Developmental Brain Research, 27:69.
Kehoe, P., and Blass, E.M., 1986e, Opioid-mediation of separation
    distress in 10-day-old rats: Reversal of stress with maternal
    stimuli. Developmental Psychobiology, 19:385.
Kehoe, P., and Harris, J. C., 1986, Separation vocalizations:
    Ontogeny of adrenergic effects in rat pups. Society for
    Neuroscience Abstracts, 12:1144.
Kellogg, C., and Lundborg, P., 1972, Ontogenetic variations in
    responses to L-DOPA and monoamine receptor-stimulating agents.
    Psychopharmacologia, 23:187.
Kellogg, C., and Wennerstrom, G., 1974, An ontogenic study on the
    effect of catecholamine receptor-stimulating agents on the
    turnover of noradrenaline and dopamine in the brain. Brain
    Research, 79:451.
Khachaturian, H., Alessi, N. E., Munfakh, N., and Watson, S. J.,
    1983, Ontogeny of opioid and related peptides in the rat CNS
    and pituitary: An immunocytochemical study. Life Sciences,
    33:61.
Kobayashi, K., and Eiduson, S., 1970, Norepinephrine and dopamine
    in the developing chick brain. Developmental Psychobiology,
    3:13.

Lanier, L. P., Dunn, A. J., and Van Hartesveldt, C., 1976, Development of neurotransmitters and their function in brain, in: "Reviews of Neuroscience, Vol. II," S. Ehrenpresis & I. J. Copin, eds., Raven Press, New York.

Morris, M. J., Dausse, J. P., Devynck, M. A., and Meyer, P., 1980, Ontogeny of alpha1 and alpha2-adrenoceptors in rat brain. Brain Research, 190:268.

Noirot, E., 1972, Ultrasounds and maternal behavior in small rodents. Developmental Psychobiology, 5:371.

Nomura, Y., Oki, K., Segawa, T., 1980, Pharmacological characterization of central alpha-adrenoceptors which mediate clonidine-induced locomotor hypoactivity in the developing rat. Naunyn Schmiedebergs Arch Pharmacologia, 311:41.

Nomura, Y., and Segawa, T., 1979, The effects of alpha-adrenoceptor antagonists and metamide on clonidine-induced locomotor stimulation in the infant rat. British Journal of Pharmacology, 66:531.

Panksepp, J., 1981, Brain opioids - a neurochemical substrate for narcotic and social dependence, in: "Theory in Psychopharmacology, 1," S.J. Cooper. ed., Academic Press, London.

Panksepp, J., Meeker, R., and Bean, D. H., 1980, The neurochemical control of crying. Pharmacology Biology and Behavior, 12:437.

Panksepp, J., Siviy, S., and Normansell, L. A., 1985, Brain opioids and social emotions, in: "Biology of social attachments," M. Reite & T. Fields, eds., Academic Press, New York.

Panksepp, J., Vilberg, T., Bean, N. J., Coy, D. H., and Kastin, A. J., 1978, Reduction of distress vocalization in chicks by opiate-like peptides. Brain Research Bulletin, 3:663.

Pedersen, P. E., Williams, C. L., and Blass, E. M., 1982, Activation and odor conditioning of suckling behavior in 3-day-old albino rats. Journal of Experimental Psychology: Animal Behavior Processes, 8: 329.

Raiteri, M., Maura, G., and Versace, P., 1983, Functional evidence for two stereochemically different alpha2 adrenoceptors regulating central norepinephrine and serotonin release. Journal of Pharmacology and Experimental Therapy, 224:679.

Reinstein, D. K., and Isaacson, R. L., 1977, Clonidine sensitivity in the developing rat. Brain Research, 135:378.

Reinstein, D. K., McClearn, D., and Isaacson, R. L., 1978, The development of responsivity to dopaminergic agents. Brain Research, 150:216.

Rudy, J. W., and Cheatle, M. D., 1979, Ontogeny of association learning: Acquisition of odor aversions by neonatal rats, in: "Ontogeny of learning and memory," N. E. Spear and B. A. Campbell, eds., Erlbaum, Hillsdale, NJ.

Smith, G. J., and Spear, N. E., 1978, Effects of the home environment on withholding behaviors and conditioning in infant and neonatal rats. Science, 202:327.

Smotherman, W. P., Bell, R. W., Starzec, J., Elias, J., and
    Zachman, T. A., 1974, Maternal responses to infant
    vocalizations and olfactory cues in rats and mice. Behavioral
    Biology, 12:55.
Spear, L. P., and Brick, J., 1979, Cocaine-induced behavior in the
    developing rat. Behavioral and Neural Biology, 26:401.
Spear, L. P., Enters, E. K., Aswad, M. A., and Louzan, M., 1985,
    Drug and environmentally-induced manipulations of the opiate
    and serotonergic alter nociception in neonatal rat pups.
    Behavioral and Neural Biology, 44:1.
Stein, L., 1978, Reward transmitters: Catecholamines and opioid
    peptides, in: "Psychopharmacology: A Generation of Progress,"
    M. A. Lipton, A. DiMascio and K. F. Killam, eds., Raven, New
    York.
Zebrowska-Lupina, I., Przegalinski, M., Sloniec, M., Kleinrok, Z.,
    1977, Clonidine-induced locomotor hyperactivity in rats. The
    role of central postsynaptic alpha-adrenoceptors. Naunyn-
    Schmiedeberg's Arch Pharmacologia, 297:227.

PRIMATE MODELS FOR THE MANAGEMENT OF SEPARATION ANXIETY

James C. Harris
Division of Child Psychiatry
Johns Hopkins University
Baltimore, MD 21205

John D. Newman
Laboratory of Comparative Ethology
NICHD, NIH
Bethesda, MD 20892

INTRODUCTION

Clinical Anxiety Disorders in Human Psychopathology

The clinical problem of anxiety has been the subject of extensive research in both child and adult psychopathology--one that has been highlighted with the increased emphasis on phenomenology in psychiatric diagnosis during the past decade. The current diagnostic and statistical manual of the American Psychiatric Association (1987) includes several forms of anxiety disorders. In adults these include the categories of generalized anxiety disorders and panic attacks as well as phobic anxiety. Panic attacks are further subdivided and may occur with or without agoraphobia. In childhood there is an additional classification with designations for separation anxiety, separation anxiety disorder, and anticipatory anxiety, the overanxious disorder of childhood. Phobias may occur at all ages but the diagnoses of generalized anxiety and panic attacks ordinarily do not present until late adolescence and early adult life. The childhood forms present as the persistence and exaggeration of a normal developmental response to separation from the caregiver. When the response becomes maladaptive leading to personal distress or failure in adaptation, e.g. inability to attend school, a disorder is designated.

Although Klein (1962,1964) suggested that panic attacks which are commonly seen in agoraphobic patients might be a variant of childhood separation anxiety, the separation anxiety beginning in childhood may be different from panic disorder in that it is not paroxysmal. It is defined by excessive anxiety on separation from major attachment figures. When separation anxiety occurs some children may show panic like behavior. However, this is different from a panic disorder where there are recurrent attacks of severe anxiety (panic) which are not restricted to any particular situation or set of circumstances. Separation anxiety disorder in preschool and early school aged children may be an exaggeration and dysfunction of a normal response that is terminated by human contact. That is, it is on a continuum and quantitatively different rather than qualitatively different from usual behavior, and in this way differs from a spontaneous panic attack. It may be the earliest experienced form of human anxiety and knowledge about its brain mechanisms and treatment might be useful in understanding the biological basis of its emergence as a behavioral disorder. A relationship between separation protest in animal species and separation anxiety in children is suggested by the view that separation anxiety has an evolutionary history different from other forms of anxiety, having its origin in the behavior of infants when separated from their mothers (Klein, 1981). Therefore, treatments effective in reducing separation protest in animals might also be effective in treating separation anxiety disorder in children.

Pharmacological Approaches To Eliciting And Treating Anxiety Disorders

In an attempt to better understand the brain mechanisms involved in the production of separation anxiety symptoms, two approaches have been taken. One is a pharmacological approach to the alleviation of symptoms and the other is an attempt to elicit anxiety symptoms through the administration of pharmacological agents. These approaches assume that there are biological mechanisms underlying normal emotional expression and that pathological deviations in these mechanisms occur in some individuals. Redmond's (1985) use of pharmacological probes to investigate anxiety reactions provided new understanding regarding the similarities and differences between these agents. For example, both epinephrine and lactate have been used to elicit anxiety and benzodiazepines, tricyclic antidepressants and MAO inhibitors have been used to reduce anxiety symptoms. Klein's observation (1962) that panic anxiety responded to tricyclic antidepressants but not to benzodiazepines suggested a pharmacological distinction between treatments for generalized anxiety and for panic anxiety. However, a recent study using a benzodiazepine to treat panic anxiety has failed to confirm this distinction (Ballenger, 1987).

A role for imipramine in the treatment of separation anxiety in children was suggested by Gittelman-Klein and Klein (1971). While improvement was noted in that study; the mechanism of action has remained unclear. Since imipramine may indirectly effect presynaptic adrenergic receptors, a possible mechanism for its action may be on presynaptic sites. Redmond (1985) has suggested parallel, congruent , and linear models to describe the action of such pharmacological agents. These models could be tested if animal models of separation symptoms were available.

Primate Models of Anxiety

Establishing the homology between separation distress in mammals and separation anxiety in children requires establishing similarity of etiologies and their treatment. Since the literature on the expression and control of separation distress in mammals and birds is extensive, the present review is restricted to the vocal component of separation distress, its pharmacological manipulation, and the use of nonhuman primates as models for separation distress symptoms.

In his pioneering investigations, Scott et al (1973, Scott, 1974) recognized that the most consistent and readily measureable behavior of puppies following separation from their litter mates was repetitive vocalization. Since these "distress calls," Scott's term for these vocalizations, occurred for long periods of time only stopping when the pup was returned to its litter, Scott reasoned that they were a vocal manifestation of separation distress. He suggested that drugs capable of reducing the number of calls would also be effective in reducing other symptoms associated with separation. Scott (1974) tested a variety of psychotropic drugs on separation-induced vocalizations in dogs. Puppies 3-8 weeks old were separated from their home compound and litter-mates, placed in a walled test enclosure, and the rate of vocalization recorded over a 10 minute period. Diazepam, a drug commonly used clinically to treat anxiety symptoms, had no specific effect on separation distress, leading Scott to conclude that separation distress is not physiologically equivalent to the emotion of anxiety. Chlorpromazine, a major neuroleptic, had a sedative effect at higher doses but the sedated puppies would immediately start vocalizing when separated. He also concluded that this drug was ineffective in alleviating symptoms of separation distress. Imipramine, a tricyclic antidepressant, was tested on the grounds that depression can be experimentally induced in animals with a history of previous separation from a familiar environment or familiar individuals. Reduction in the calling rate induced by social separation was proportional to the dosage of the drug (2-8 mg/kg). The maximum effect was evident at a dose of 8 mg/kg when testing was carried out 1 to 2 hours after drug administration. A similar vocal response to separation is exhibited by domestic chicks. Panksepp et al. (1980) found that imipramine was ineffective in reducing separation-induced vocalizations in chicks but that both clonidine and morphine significantly reduced the rate of distress calls. Therefore, two endogenous neurochemical systems have been implicated in mediating social bond formation, the noradrenergic and the opiate receptor systems. Rossi, et al. (1983) have also provided experimental evidence implicating the noradrenergic receptor system in the control of "separation distress."

Primate models have been used for the study of the behavioral, physiological, and pharmacological correlates of social separation. Suomi, et al. (1978) tested the effectiveness of imipramine on ameliorating the behavioral disturbances immediately following social separation in young rhesus monkeys, and found that imipramine treated animals demonstrated significant behavioral improvement similar to that seen following drug treatment in human subjects with depressive disorder. The results of these experiments suggested that imipramine treatment influenced the monkeys' behavior during and immediately following peer separation, but symptoms reemerged once treatment was withdrawn. In a follow-up analysis of anxiety symptoms in juvenile rhesus monkeys Suomi, et al., (1981) described some of the most characteristic aspects of anxiety in this species. They found that behavioral agitation is one of the most characteristic features of anxiety in rhesus adults, while increased agitation in juveniles takes the form of idiosyncratic stereotypies and behavioral regression. As is typical for other primate species, maternal separation produces, in the infant rhesus macaque, immediate agitation and protest, shown by frantic and frenzied behavior and a significant increase in vocalization over pre-separation levels. After repeated separations, peer-reared adolescent monkeys begin to exhibit increased anxious behavior as the time for the next separation draws near perhaps analogous to "anticipatory anxiety" seen in humans. Suomi (1986) has recently reviewed the expression of anxious-like behavior in young nonhuman primates. It presents in a variety of ways including fear like behavior in the absence of external triggers, behavioral regression, and behavioral and physiological activation. Physiological changes following social separation have been documented by Reite and Capitanio (1985) in the pigtailed macaque (Macaca nemestrina). When a mother is separated from the infant with the infant remaining in the group, the initial period of behavioral agitation exhibited by the infant is accompanied by marked increases in both heart rate and body temperature. Breese, et al. (1973) have demonstrated increased adrenal catecholamine synthesizing enzymes in infant rhesus following maternal separation. In the brain, the significant change in amine levels was an elevation of serotonin in the hypothalamus. Comparative studies of the biochemical changes accompanying maternal separation in the infants of rhesus and squirrel monkeys have been reviewed by Coe, et al. (1985). Separation of infant squirrel monkeys from their mothers revealed a progressive decrease of vocalizations and progressive increase in cortisol levels over the first 6 hours after separation. This progressive increase in cortisol is not significantly correlated with changing levels of activity, which are highest in the first hour after separation. These authors view the vocal component of separation distress as an adaptive attempt to elicit caregiving behavior and a decline of vocalizations in the absence of reinforcement as part of an adaptational process (in contrast to the view that the decline in vocal rate is an indication of the onset of a depressive state). With repeated weekly separations, the rate of calling decreases and both activity and cortisol levels remain high. These same authors attempted to pharmacologically manipulate the vocal response to separation in yearling squirrel monkeys. They found a significant reduction in calling following pretreatment with dexamethasone, which blocks ACTH secretion. The effect of dexamethasone was less dramatic when the study was repeated with 3-month old infants.

Mineka (1985) attempted to integrate a variety of conditioning phenomena studied in primates that might bear on the etiology, maintenance, and therapy of anxiety-based disorders in humans. Mineka reviewed the results of studies directed at extinguishing an intense fear of snakes in wild-reared rhesus monkeys. While all subjects showed significant decreases in behavioral avoidance over 12 sessions, they continued to show the initial behavioral disturbance component of fear. Mineka (in press a) cites studies showing that while wild-reared rhesus and squirrel monkeys demonstrate a fear of snakes, lab-reared individuals do not, suggesting that the fear reactions of the wild monkeys had been acquired through observational learning. Mineka (in press b) considers the symptomatology of monkeys' fear responses to be a model of phobic fears in humans. Pharmacological manipulation of snake-induced fear responses does not appear to have been attempted. However, Glowa and Newman (1986), using a fur-covered puppet as a fear-inducing stimulus, found enhancement of alarm vocalization rates in squirrel monkeys following treatment with benactyzine, a centrally active anticholinergic drug.

This review demonstrates the preliminary nature of our understanding of the neurochemical mechanisms mediating separation induced vocalizations in primates. Therefore, we have initiated a series of experiments directed at testing the role of adrenergic and opiate mechanisms in this behavior in squirrel monkeys.

REVIEW OF OUR RECENT RESEARCH ON THE SEPARATION CALL

First Experiment: Adrenergic Effects

As has been discussed above, a reliable indicator of the response to separation in mammals, including human infants (Rheingold, 1969), is the isolation call. This vocal component of separation distress has a specific and measurable sonographic pattern (Wolff,1969; Newman, 1985). In the squirrel monkey, <u>Saimiri sciureus,</u> isolation calls are reliably produced in the laboratory by infants and adults upon separation from conspecifics (Newman and MacLean, 1982, Symmes et al, 1979, Winter et al, 1966). This behavioral response permits us to test the effectiveness of drugs that act on specific neuronal receptors that may be involved in separation distress in this species.

In the absence of drug, adult subjects typically produced one type of vocalization, the isolation peep, for periods of up to one hour when separated from conspecifics. Our attempts to pharmacologically manipulate the production of these separation induced vocalizations were originally based on the findings of Scott (1974) regarding the effectiveness of imipramine in reducing separation induced

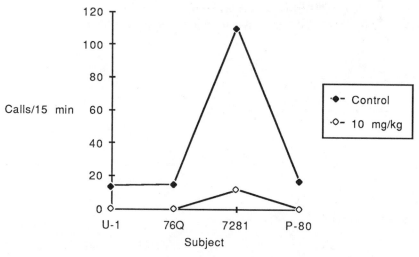

Figure 1: Imipramine Supression of Squirrel Monkey Isolation Calls (from Harris and Newman, 1987, by permission from Elsevier Science Publishers).

vocalization in puppies. In agreement with Scott's findings, acute administration of imipramine at a dose of 10mg /kg reduced or eliminated isolation call production when testing occurred one hour following drug administration. (Figure 1).

As a follow up to these findings, we tested the hypothesis that imipramine exerts its effects on separation related behavioral disturbance indirectly through feedback inhibition of $\partial 2$ adrenergic receptors. We used clonidine hydrochloride, a specific $\partial 2$ adrenergic agonist for demonstrating direct adrenergic involvement in the vocal expression of separation distress. Subjects were given a graded series of doses, testing the effect of each dose on isolation call rate (Table 1). Complete suppression was demonstrated in all subjects at the highest dose tested (0.15 mg/kg). Control injections were carried out with sterile water and nembutal was also administered to control for the sedating effects of clonidine using the same procedure.

A direct test of an $\partial 2$ mechanism in isolation call production would come from demonstrating that an $\partial 2$ but not an $\partial 1$ antagonist reversed the clonidine induced suppression of isolation calls. We found that 0.2 mg/kg yohimbine, an $\partial 2$ antagonist, when administered concurrently with clonidine in a dose which did not increase isolation call production over controls (0.2 mg/kg) blocked or reversed the vocal suppression in three of four animals. A similar experiment carried out with the $\partial 1$ antagonist prazosin was completely ineffective in reversing clonidine suppression of calling (Table 2). In a subsequent experiment the clonidine suppression was reversed in four subjects when yohimbine was given 15 minutes after the clonidine injection.

To further support the hypothesis we demonstrated that yohimbine produced an increase in calling for all subjects at a dose of 0.4 mg/kg (Harris and Newman, 1987). We concluded from these experiments that the $\partial 2$ adrenergic receptor is involved in separation-induced vocalization in the squirrel monkey.

Table 1   Clonidine Dose Response Results (Calls/15 minutes)

Dose of Clonidine mg/kg

	0.0	0.05	0.075	0.10	0.15
Subject 1	14	0	0	8	0
Subject 2	15	29	0	0	0
Subject 3	110	50	62	0	0
Subject 4	17	0	0	0	0

Table 2: Summary of Adrenergic Effects on Vocalization (Calls/15 min)

	Clonidine (0.15 mg/kg)	Yohimbine (0.2 mg/kg) +Clonidine	Prazosin (0.25 mg/k +Clonidine	Control
Subject 1	0	10	0	14
Subject 2	0	87	0	15
Subject 3	0	143	0	110
Subject 4	0	0	0	17

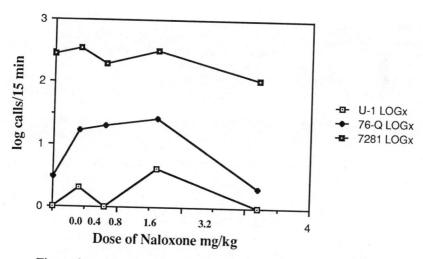

Figure 2 : Naloxone Dose Response Curve for Isolation Peeps

Second Experiment: Opiate Effects

Since Herman and Panksepp (1978) had reported that the opiate antagonist naloxone increased the rate of separation calls in chicks and guinea pigs, we tested whether the same results could be achieved in a primate, the squirrel monkey. Determination of the dose response relationship between naloxone and isolation call production demonstrated that a dose of 0.4 mg/kg and 1.6 mg/kg reliably increased calling over control levels, The other doses (0.8 and 3.2 mg/kg) either produced no increase or in fact a decrease in the rate of calling. (Figure 2)

Third Experiment: Test of Vocal Specificity of Drugs Activating Separation Calls

In the same experiments used to demonstrate enhancement of separation calls following effective doses of yohimbine or naloxone, the subjects were also tested for the effectiveness of these drugs in enhancing a vocal alarm response. Each subject was presented with a fur covered puppet shown to be effective in eliciting an alarm response in these same monkeys in the absence of drug. The puppet was presented five times to each animal; each trial consisted of 30 seconds of exposure to the puppet at 30 second intervals. In all subjects doses of yohimbine or naloxone that increased isolation calls were ineffective in the alarm call test. In other experiments the anticholinergic drug, benactyzine, which does not effect isolation calls reliably produced increases in alarm calls (Glowa and Newman, 1986).

CONCLUSIONS

This chapter reviews previous studies and our own data relevant to pharmacological control of separation distress in primates and other animals On the basis of behavior presentation and pharmacological responses we conclude that separation distress in animals and separation anxiety in children may be controlled by homologous mechanisms. This suggests that animal models might be usefully employed to elucidate the mechanisms underlying separation anxiety and lead then to improved clinical management. If we are to utilize primate models to greatest advantage in developing an improved understanding of the factors controlling separation anxiety, it is necessary to clarify the contexts in which these behaviors occur. Our experiments and the literature review raise also the possibility of a homology between the alarm reaction of monkeys and panic attacks in humans. In our studies using squirrel monkeys, subjects emit characteristic vocalizations in the context of social separation, but when challenged with an alarm inducing stimulus they emit entirely different vocalizations. It is important in this regard to note that the pharmacological manipulation of this vocal behavior is context and vocalization specific. Consequently vocalizations may provide useful and reliable behavioral measures for differentiating between the nonhuman primate equivalent of both separation anxiety and panic behavior. We believe that this evidence of ethopharmacological specificity in a primate model for separation distress may lead to a useful approach in pharmacologically managing separation anxiety disorder in children.

To recapitulate, our review of previous studies together with our own experiments suggests that separation distress may be behaviorally and pharmacologically different than panic. Since the behavioral reaction of primates to an alarming stimulus includes both specific vocalizations as well as persistent and vigorous efforts to escape from the proximity of the stimulus alarm behavior in animals may be a model for panic. Consideration of these behavioral differences supports the view that separation distress and alarm are components of different emotional systems culminating respectively in depression and panic.

REFERENCES

American Psychiatric Association. Diagnostic and Statistical Manual of Mental Disorders (revised ed.), 1987,. Washington, D. C.

Breese, G. R., Smith, R. D, Mueller, R. A., Howard, J. L., Prange, A. J. Jr., Lipton, M.A., Young, L. D., McKinney, W. T. and Lewis, J. K., 1973, Induction of Adrenal Catecholamine synthesising enzymes following mother-infant separation. Nature New Biology. 246: 94.

Coe, C. L., Wiener, S. G., Rosenberg, L.T., and Levine, S. ,1985, Endocrine and Immune Responses to Separation and Maternal Loss in M. Reite and T. Field (Eds). Academic Press, New York.

Gittelman-Klein, R. and Klein, D.F. ,1971,Controlled imipramine treatment of school phobia. Arch. Gen.Psychiat. 25: 204.

Glowa, J. and Newman, J. , 1986, Benactyzine increases alarm call rates in the squirrel monkey. Psychopharmacology 90: 457.

Harris, J. C. and Newman, J. ,1987, Mediation of separation distress by Alpha 2 adrenergic mechanisms in a nonhuman primate. Brain Research 410: 353

Herman, B. H. , and Panksepp, J. , 1978, Effects of morphine and naloxone on separation distress and approach attachment: evidence for opiate mediation of social affect. Pharmac. Biochem. Behav. 9: 213.

Klein, D. F.,1981, Anxiety reconceptualized, in Anxiety: New Research and Changing Concepts. Klein, D.F., and Rabkin, J. Eds. Raven Press, N. Y.

Klein, D. F.,1964, Delineation of two drug responsive anxiety syndromes. Psychopharmacologia , 5: 397.

Klein, D. F., and Fink, M. ,1962, Psychiatric reaction patterns to imipramine. American Journal of Psychiatry. 119: 432.

Mineka, S. ,1985, Animal models of anxiety-based disorders: their usefulness and limitations. In Anxiety and the Anxiety Disorders, A. H. Tuma and J. Maser (Eds.) Lawrence Erlbaum Associates, Hillsdale, N. J.

Mineka, S,.In press a, A primate model of phobic fears. In Theoretical Foundations of Behavior Therapy, H. Eysenck and I. Martin, Plenum Press, New York.

Mineka, S, 1985, The frightful complexity of the origins of fears. In Affect, Condition, and Cognition, Brush T. R.and J. D. Overmeier.(Eds.) Lawrence Erlbaum Associates, Hillsdale, N. J.

Newman, J. D.,1985, The infant cry of primates: an evolutionary perspective. In Infant Crying: Theoretical and Research Prospectives, B. M. Lester and C. F. Z. Boukydis,(Eds) Plenum, New York.

Newman, J.D. and MacLean, P.D., 1982, Effects of tegmental lesions on the isolation call of squirrel monkeys Brain Research 232: 317.

Panksepp, J., Meeker, R., and Bean, N.J.,1980, The neurochemical control of crying. Pharmac.Biochem.Behav. 12: 437.

Redmond, D. E. Jr., 1985, Neurochemical basis for anxiety and anxiety disorders: evidence from drugs which decrease human fear or anxiety. In Anxiety and the Anxiety Disorders, A. H. Tuma and J. Maser (Eds.) Lawrence Erlbaum Associates, Hillsdale, N. J.

Reite, M. and Capitanio, J. P.,1985, On the nature of social separation and social attachment. In The Psychobiology of Attachment and Separation, M. Reite and T. Field (Ed) Academic Press, New York.

Rheingold, H.L.,1969, The effects of environmental stimulation upon social and exploratory behavior in the human infant. In Determinants of Infant Behaviour, B.M.Foss, (Ed.) Methuen, London

Rossi, J. III, Sahley, T L. and Panksepp, J., 1983, The role of brain norepinephrine in clonidine suppression of isolation-induced distress in the domestic chick. Psychopharmacology, 79: 338

Scott, J. P., Stewart, J. M., DeGhett, V. J.,1973, Separation in infant dogs: emotional response and motivational consequences. In Separation and DepressionPublication #94 of the American Association for the Advancement of Science. Washington, D. C.

Scott, J. P.,1974, Effects of psychotrophic drugs in separation distress in dogs. Proc. IX Congress Neuropsychopharmacology, (Paris), Excerpta Medica International Congress . Series No. 359: 735.

Suomi, S.J., Seaman, S.F., Lewis, J.K., DeLizio, R. D., and McKinney, W.T., 1978, Effects of imipramine treatment on separation-induced social disorders in rhesus monkeys. Arch. Gen. Psychiat., 35: 321.

Suomi, S.J., Kraemer, G.W., Baysinger, C.M., and DeLizio, R.D.,1981, Inherited and experiential differences in anxious behavior displayed by rhesus monkeys.In Anxiety: New Research and Changing Concepts, D. F. Klein and J. Rabkin, (Eds.) Raven Press, New York.

Suomi, S.J.,1986, Anxiety-like disorders in young nonhuman primates. In Anxiety Disorders of Childhood. Gittelman, R. (ed). Guilford Press, N. Y.

Symmes, D., Newman, J.D., Talmage-Riggs, G., Lieblich, A.K.1979, Individuality and stability of isolation peeps in squirrel monkeys. Anim.Behav. 27: 1142.

Winter, P., Ploog, D., and Latta, J.,1966, Vocal repertoire of the squirrel monkey (Saimiri Sciureus), its analysis and significance. Exp. Brain. Res., 1: 359.

Wolff, P., 1969, The natural history of crying and other vocalizations in early infancy. In Determinants of Infant Behaviour, Vol.4, B. M. Foss, (Ed.) Methuen, London.

RAT PUP ULTRASONIC ISOLATION CALLS AND THE BENZODIAZEPINE RECEPTOR

T. Insel, L. Miller, R. Gelhard and J. Hill

Laboratory of Clinical Science, NIMH
P. O. Box 289
Poolesville, MD   20837

Since their first description by Anderson (1954), rodent ultrasonic vocalizations have been noted in three social contexts. Adult rats in aggressive encounters emit short (3-55 msec), high frequency (40-70 kHz) pulses when attacking and longer (300-500 msec), lower frequency (22-30 kHz) calls during submission (Sales, 1972). In addition, following ejaculation, male rats embark on a long (1-3 sec) 22 kHz "song" which is associated with the refractory period between ejaculations (Barfield and Geyer, 1972). Finally, in the young of a wide variety of myomorph rodents, ultrasonic calls have been described in association with social isolation (reviewed by Sales and Pye, 1974). These calls, variously denoted as "isolation calls" or "distress vocalizations," are the focus of this chapter. We will briefly review some of the factors influencing these calls before describing several pharmacologic studies designed to test the hypothesis that these calls are mediated by the brain benzodiazepine receptor.

The ultrasonic vocalizations of infant rats are monotonic, whistle-like sounds, with a frequency range between 35 and 45 kHz. These sounds appear to be laryngeal in origin (Roberts, 1975) and, like the audible isolation calls of other mammals, are extremely potent stimuli for maternal retrieval (Allin & Banks, 1972; Elwood, 1979; Smotherman et al., 1974).

The various stimuli that elicit ultrasonic calls from the pup are still under investigation. Calls are evident within the first day of postnatal life, increase in number and intensity in the second week and decrease abruptly around day 14, about the time of eye opening (Fig. 1a). Within these first fourteen days of postnatal life, the physiologic responses to environmental conditions change rapidly in the pup. For instance, pups are poikilothermic right after birth and do not begin to develop homeothermy until day 5 or 6. Possibly for this reason, a decrease in ambient temperature has been noted to stimulate ultrasonic calls most noticeably near the end of the first week (Okon,

1971; Allin and Banks, 1971). The power of this effect can be seen in Fig. 1b, where data from a group of 6-day-old pups recorded at various temperatures demonstrate a near absence of calls at 36° C, the temperature within a huddled litter. One interpretation of this finding is that "isolation" for a 6-day-old rat pup, with immature visual and auditory systems, may be perceived primarily by the change in temperature. Between 10 and 14 days of age, thermal regulation has matured and yet ultrasonic calls can still be predictably elicited by isolating pups. Hofer and Shair (1987) have demonstrated that the isolation calls from pups at this stage are reduced by exposure to littermates as well as by exposure to the mother. Analytic studies of the sensory inputs from social contact indicate that texture, contour, warmth, and odor have additive effects for reducing isolation calls; no single component appears to be prepotent (Hofer and Shair, 1980). Furthermore, previous social experience appears to be unnecessary, as isolated pups raised without littermates respond to the addition of pups with a robust decrease in calling rate (Hofer and Shair, 1987).

Although the importance of hunger as a stimulus for pup ultrasonic calls has never been documented, recent studies have investigated a role for gustatory input. Blass and co-workers (1987) have recently demonstrated that intraoral infusions of 7.5% sucrose induced a rapid suppression of calls. As this effect was not apparent with intragastric infusions of sucrose or with intraoral infusions of water, it appeared that the tasting of sucrose was essential. Moreover, the opiate antagonist naltrexone prevented this sucrose effect on vocalization, suggesting that an opiate mechanism might mediate the neural and behavioral response to this particular gustatory stimulus.

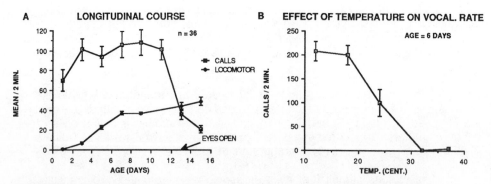

FIGURE 1 (A)Effects of age on number of ultrasonic isolation calls and locomotor activity. Isolation calls were recorded for two minutes at 24°C. Locomotor activity was recorded as crossovers into 2" x 2" squares on floor of recording chamber. (B) Effect of temperature on vocalization rate during two minute test of 6-day-old pups.

Investigators have consistently noted the high inter-litter variability in calling rates from pups of the same age. In our pups from 6 to 10 days of age, the mean rate of isolation calls varies between 10 and 80 calls/min at room temperature. To test whether genetic differences might contribute to this variability, we studied pups from an inbred rat strain selected for "fearfulness" or "emotionality." Maudsley Reactive (MR) rats were bred for high defecation (believed to reflect fearfulness) and low exploration in an open field. Maudsley Non-Reactive (MNR) congeners were selected for low defecation and high exploration (reviewed by Broadhurst, 1975). These adult measures of fearfulness are not useful in the first week of postnatal life before solid stool and locomotor exploration have developed. To determine if pups of these inbred strains might differ in their rate of ultrasonic isolation call production, 5-day-old rats from three litters of each strain were recorded during 2 minutes of isolation at room temperature. As shown in Fig. 2, MR pups called nearly five times as much as MNR pups (Student's t = 4.53, p < .001). These results not only suggest that genetic differences may contribute to inter-litter variance in the rate of isolation calls, they also imply a relationship between adult measures of emotionality or fearfulness and the rat pup isolation call.

ISOLATION CALLS AND ANXIETY

The high rate of isolation call production in the MR pups suggests that drugs with effects on anxiety and fear may affect this behavior. Among the anxiolytic drugs the benzodiazepines are of particular interest as recent studies

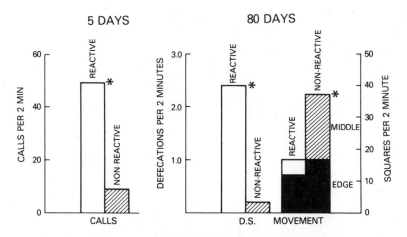

FIGURE 2. Differences in rate of isolation calls in MR and MNR 5-day-old pups. Note that adults (80-day-olds) differ in defecation score (D.S.) and movement (number of crossovers) in an open field test. MR pups have more isolation calls at 5 days, as well as more defecation and less exploration of the central portion of the open field arena in adulthood. * signifies p < .01.

have demonstrated that their behavioral properties are mediated through specific brain receptors which are linked to the GABA-A receptor and a chloride channel (Tallman et al., 1982). The current model is that diazepam binds to its receptor in the presence of GABA to affect a prolonged opening of the ion channel and hyperpolarization of the cell (i.e. inhibition of firing). Other agents, such as pentylenetetrazol, are known to increase anxiety clinically (Lal and Emmett-Oglesby, 1983), apparently via a direct action on the chloride channel, opposed to the benzodiazepine effect (Squires et al., l984). A third class of agents, represented by RO 15-1788, have neither anxiolytic nor anxiogenic effects yet bind to the benzodiazepine receptor and specifically block benzodiazepine effects. These three classes of compound, shown in Fig. 3, all affect the benzodiazepine-GABA receptor-chloride channel complex in different ways with strikingly different behavioral results.

To determine if a clinically anxiolytic drug would decrease rat pup isolation calls, we administered a range of doses of diazepam to pups between 6 and 10 days of age. Variance between pups and litters was reduced by testing each animal twice--once for a baseline measure and then 30 minutes after subcutaneous drug or saline administration. Baselines were matched across treatments to minimize differences in calling rate. The post-injection test was subtracted from the baseline to obtain a difference score for each pup. Each pup was injected only once and all doses were studied at 24° C. Tests were of 2-minute duration. Locomotor activity was scored simultaneously by equating the number of 2" x 2" squares entered during each 2-minute test. A more complete description of these methods has been published (Insel et al., 1986).

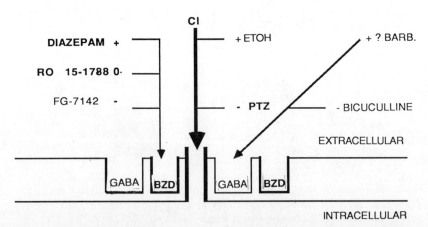

FIGURE 3. Model of the benzodiazepine receptor showing linkage to GABA receptor and chloride channel. According to this model, agents which increase ion channel opening, marked here with a +, decrease anxiety; whereas those that decrease channel opening, marked here with a -, increase anxiety.

In a parallel set of experiments, the clinically anxiogenic drug pentylenetetrazol was administered. The method was essentially unchanged, except that the temperature was increased to 34° C to avoid ceiling effects.

In a third set of experiments, RO 15-1788 was given either 5 minutes before diazepam (to determine if diazepam effects were mediated via the benzodiazepine receptor) or alone (to investigate if the receptor was physiologically activated by isolation).

Figure 4 demonstrates the dose-dependent decreases in calling rate following diazepam and corresponding increases following pentylenetetrazol. The diazepam effect was not due to sedation as locomotor scores did not significantly decrease at any of the doses given. Conversely, the pentylenetetrazol dose was well below the convulsant range (CD^{50} = 50 mg/kg for pups of this age). Most importantly, neither of the drugs significantly affected body temperature. RO 15-1788 (5.0 mg/kg) given 5 minutes before diazepam (0.5 mg/kg) entirely blocked the diazepam effect on calling rate (mean $\pm$ SEM decrease = 2.1 $\pm$ 13.3 calls/2 min., n = 10) demonstrating that the profound decrease following diazepam alone was mediated by the brain benzodiazepine receptor and not via a peripheral (e.g. laryngeal) or nonspecific (i.e. other neurotransmitter) site.

These results along with the MNR-MR differences are generally consistent with the hypothesis that factors that decreased anxiety or fear are associated with fewer isolation calls, whereas those that increase anxiety or fear are associated with more isolation calls. However, pharmacologic studies such as these, may have little relevance to the physiologic mediation of this species-typical behavior. Recent studies have isolated endogenous ligands for the benzodiazepine receptor which may activate this complex during stress (Guidotti et al., 1983; Ferrero et al.,1984; Ferrero et al., 1986). If an endogenous ligand activated the benzodiazepine receptor during the pup isolation test, then RO 15-1788 (an "inactive" compound in the resting state) might be expected to alter the rate of calling. This is precisely what we found as shown in Fig. 5.

Pharmacologic blockade of the receptor decreases the rate of calling without affecting locomotor activity. This weak diazepam-like effect of RO 15-1788 implies that an endogenous ligand might physiologically drive this system to produce isolation calls. To further test this hypothesis, we adopted a technique for in vivo receptor labeling (Goeders & Kuhar, 1985) to investigate receptor occupancy during states of low and high isolation calls.

IMAGING THE RECEPTOR

^{3}H-RO 15-1788 (3 μCi animal) was injected into 10-day pups either when unseparated or separated for 25 minutes. In a subset of pups, nonspecific binding was determined by preinjections of diazepam (5 mg/kg). Twenty minutes post-injection all pups were decapitated, then brains were immediately removed and either macrodissected for proteolytic digestion and counting or frozen on powdered dry ice for autoradiography. Autoradiograms were generated

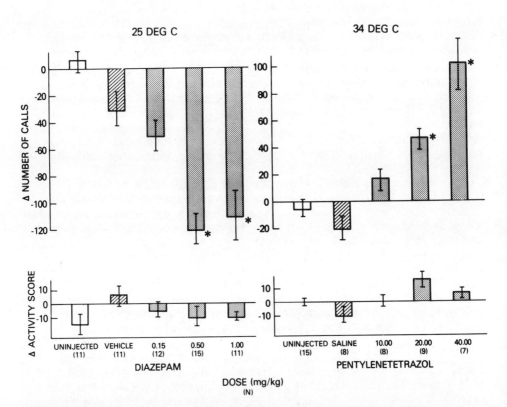

FIGURE 4. Dose dependent decrease in isolation calls following administration of diazepam and increase in calls following administration of pentylenetetrazol. Changes in locomotor activity were not significant with either drug. * p< .05.

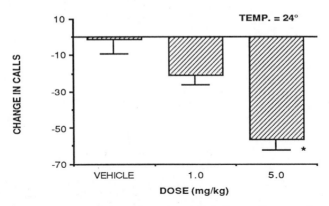

FIGURE 5. RO 15-1788 decreases rate of isolation calls at a dose generally lacking intrinsic behavioral effects. * signifies p< .05.

using frozen sections (24 μ thick) cut in a cryostat, thaw-mounted onto slides, and exposed to ^{3}H sensitive film for 8 weeks. The resulting autoradiograms were digitized with the Loats Image Analysis System and quantified using a set of ^{3}H standards to convert optical density to equivalents of fmole binding/mg protein.

Recordings of pups in the two conditions demonstrate highly significant differences in the number of vocalizations (Fig. 6A). Counts from macrodissected tissue indicate a decrease in cortical binding (Fig. 6B). A regional receptor analysis by autoradiography demonstrated decreases in ^{3}H-RO 15-1788 binding in cingulate and frontal-parietal-motor cortex in the separated group (Fig. 6C). Nonspecific binding was relatively uniform and equal across the two testing conditions.

These quantitative autoradiographic results extend the pharmacologic studies with unlabeled RO 15-1788 to demonstrate first that some benzodiazepine receptors are, in fact, less available during the period of isolation when ultrasounds are being produced and second, that certain receptor fields in limbic and neocortex are involved whereas other regions show little change.

SPECIFICITY OF THE BENZODIAZEPINE RESPONSE

Previous pharmacologic studies of distress vocalizations in several species have implicated the brain opiate system (Panksepp et al.,1978; Newman, 1988; Kehoe and Blass, 1986). To determine whether the benzodiazepine effect on rat pup ultrasonic calls was unique or simply one of several compounds that might alter this behavior, several other drugs with clinical effects on anxiety or analgesia were tested. The method was essentially as described for the benzodiazepine study above, using pups between 6 and 10 days of age.

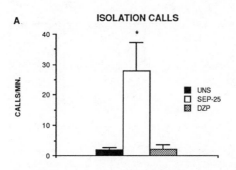

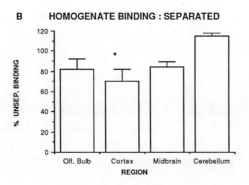

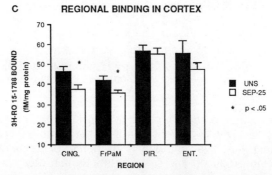

FIGURE 6 Results of in vivo receptor labelling of brain benzodiazepine receptor in isolated pups vs. socially caged littermates. (A) Isolation calls were significantly (p< .05) increased in 10-day-old pups at 25 minutes of separation. This increase was entirely prevented by pre-treatment with diazepam (0.50 mg/kg). (B) Counts of homogenized tissue in 3 independent studies showed a significant decrease in label bound to cortex in the separated pups. (C) Autoradiographic analysis of binding to cortex revealed decrease primarily in cingulate and convexity (frontal-parietal-motor) regions in separated pups.

Table 1 lists the results from trials with several different compounds. Morphine decreases vocalizations, but only at doses that also decreased locomotor activity. Naloxone does not increase vocalizations as might be expected if a brain opiate system were mediating this behavior. Pentobarbital, with effects mediated via the benzodiazepine-GABA receptor-chloride channel complex, appears similar to diazepam. Adrenergic compounds have paradoxical effects: clonidine, a clinically anxiolytic drug, increases rather than decreases the rate of isolation calls. Yohimbine, which may be associated with increased anxiety in man, blocks the clonidine effect and, when given alone, decreases the rate of calling. These paradoxical effects have been previously noted with adrenergic drugs in developmental studies of locomotor behavior (Pappas and Walsh, 1979) and may reflect the immaturity of either the alpha adrenergic receptor or its second messenger. Finally, compounds working via the adenosine receptor appear to have weak effects on isolation calls.

These results may be summarized as follows: several agents affect rat pup ultrasonic calls; however, some (e.g. morphine) appear to do so by altering the level of arousal and others (e.g. clonidine) have effects that are highly age dependent. Although diazepam is not unique in its effects, it is distinguished by its potency for isolation calls relative to sedative effects and these call-reducing effects are mediated by a receptor system that matures early in ontogeny (Braestrup et al., 1978).

SUMMARY

Rat pups emit ultrasonic isolation calls throughout the first 2 weeks of postnatal life. These calls which are modulated by several environmental stimuli, appear to elicit maternal retrieval. Pups from the MR "fearful" strain emit about 5 times as many calls as their "nonfearful" MNR congeners. Drugs working through the benzodiazepine-GABA receptor-chloride channel complex to decrease (diazepam) or increase (pentylenetetrazol) anxiety in man, induce a potent and selective decrease or increase respectively in rat pup isolation calls. Pharmacologic blockade of the benzodiazepine receptor with an "inactive" antagonist also decreases the number of calls. In vivo labeling of the receptor with ^{3}H-RO 15-1788 demonstrates decreased binding to brain benzodiazepine receptors in limbic and neocortex during social isolation.

Taken together, these results suggest that the benzodiazepine-GABA receptor-chloride channel complex is physiologically important in the mediation of rat pup isolation calls. Other socially relevant stressors, such as isolation of adult rats, have already been shown to alter the conformation of the chloride channel (Trullas et al., 1986). The benzodiazepine system develops early in ontogeny, reaching mature levels of receptor density in the first postnatal week, and relatively late in phylogeny (Nielsen et al., 1979), roughly in parallel with the evolution of mother-infant attachment (MacLean, 1986). From a comparative perspective, this receptor system appears to have evolved for a role early in development to modulate some aspect of social behavior. Indeed, one

Table 1. Effects of Various Psychotropic Drugs on USV and Locomotor Performance (mean changes from baseline 30 min post-treatment)

DRUG	DOSE	N	% Δ VOC	% Δ MOV
OPIATES				
Morphine (mg/kg)	0.05	7	-12.9	-55.5
	0.1	12	-39.3	-80.1
	0.5	8	-98.1	-100.1
Naloxone (mg/kg)	.5+5.0	15	12.3	-39.1
Morphine	0.1	11	-1.3	-18.8
+ NAL	0.5			
Saline	- -	30	-8.3	-22.9
Untreated	- -	8	-2.4	-13.2
ALPHA 2 ADRENERGIC LIGANDS				
Clonidine (μg/kg)	0.5	5	-11.1	-10.8
	5.1	13	110.6	-49.6
	100	9	192.9	-70.6
Yohimbine (mg/kg)	0.04	6	-38.1	-81.9
	0.2	6	-84.8	79.1
	1.1	8	-79.4	-61.3
Clonidine	5.0 μg/kg	8	-47.1	-79.4
+ Yohimb	1.0 mg/kg			
ADENOSINE				
PIA (mg/kg)	0.01	17	-32.8	-32.5
Caffeine (mg/kg)	10.1	4	-27.6	29.1
BARBITURATES				
Pentobarb (mg/kg)	1.1	5	-21.9	-47.3
	2.5	11	-58.5	-73.8
	10.1	4	-100.1	-74.4

might wonder if the receptor's better known role in the pharmacology of anxiety is only an adult residue of these developmental effects.

In ongoing studies we are administering endogenous ligands for the benzodiazepine receptor into the lateral ventricle to further test the hypothesis that this receptor complex is involved in the mediation of isolation calls. With the development of better probes for both these endogenous ligands and for different components of the receptor complex, the future promises to provide several interesting keys into the neural mechanisms for this species-typical vocalization.

REFERENCES

Allin, J. T. and Banks, E. M. (1972), Functional aspects of ultrasound production by infant albino rats (rattus norvegicus). Anim. Behav. 20:175.

Anderson, J. W. (1954), The production of ultrasonic sounds by laboratory rats and other mammals. Science 119:808.

Barfield, R.J. and Geyer, L.A. (1972), Sexual behaviour: Ultrasonic postejaculatory song of the male rat. Science 176:1349.

Blass, E.M.,Fitzgerald, E., Kehoe, P. (1987), Interactions between sucrose, pain and isolation distress. Dev. Psychobiol. 20: 483.

Braestrup, C. and Nielsen, M. (1978), Ontogenetic development of benzodiazepine receptors in the rat brain. Brain Res. 147:170.

Broadhurst, P. L. (1975), The Maudsley reactive and nonreactive strains of rats: A survey. Behav. Genet. 5:229.

Darragh, A., Lambe, R., O'Boyle, C., Kenny, M., and Brick, I. (1983), Absence of central effects in man of the benzodiazepine antagonist RO15 1788. Psychopharmacology (Berlin) 80:192.

de Carvalho, L. P., Greksch, G., Chapouthier, G., and Rossier, J. (1983), Anxiogenic and non-anxiogenic benzodiazepine antagonists. Nature 301:64.

Elwood, R. W. (1979), Ultrasounds and maternal behavior in the Mongolian gerbil. Devel.Psychobiol. 12:281.

Ferrero, P., Cost, E., Conti-Tronconi, B., and Guidotti, A. (1986), A diazepam binding inhibitor (DBI)-like neuropeptide is detected in human brain. Brain Res. 399:136.

Ferrero, P., Guidotti, A., Conti-Tronconi, B., and Costa E. (1984), A brain octadecaneuropeptide generated by tryptic digestion of DBI functions as a proconflict ligand of benzodiazepine recognition sites. Neuropharmacology 23:1359.

Goeders, N.E. and Kuhar, M.J. (1985), Benzodiazepine receptor binding in vivo with [^{3}H]-Ro 15-1788. Life Sciences 37:345.

Guidotti, A. (1983), Isolation, characterization, and purification to homogeneity of an endogenous polypeptide with agonistic action on benzodiazepine receptors. PNAS 80:3531.

Hofer,M.A. and Shair,H.N. (1980), Sensory processes in the control of isolation-induced ultrasonic vocalization by 2-week-old rats. J. Comp. Physiol. Psychol. 94: 274.

Hofer,M.A. and Shair,H.N. (1987), Isolation distress in two-week-old rats: Influence of home cage, social companions, and prior experience with littermates. Devel.Psychobiol. 20:465.

Insel, T.R., Hill, J., Mayor, R.B. (1986), Rat pup ultrasonic isolation calls: Possible mediation by the benzodiazepine receptor complex. Pharm. Biochem., Behav. 24:1263.

Kehoe, P. and Blass, E. (1986), Opioid mediation of separation distress in 10-day-old rats: reversal of stress with maternal stimuli. Devel. Psychobiol. 19:385.

Lal, H. and Emmett-Oglesby, M. W. (1983), Behavioral analogues of anxiety: Animal models. Neuropharmacology 22:1423.

Newman, J.D. (1988), Ethopharmacology of vocal behavior in primates, in: "Primate Vocal Communication," D. Todt, P. Goedeking, and D. Symmes, eds., Springer-Verlag (Berlin).

Nielsen, M., Braestrup, C., and Squires, R. F. (1978), Evidence for a late evolutionary appearance of brain-specific benzodiazepine receptors: An investigation of18 vertebrate and 5 invertebrate species. Brain Res. 141:342.

Okon, E.E. (1971), The temperature relations of vocalization in infant golden hamsters and Wistar rats. J. Zool. Lond., 164: 227.

Oswalt, G.L. and Meier,G.W. (1975), Olfactory, thermal, and tactual influences on infantile ultrasonic vocalization in rats. Devel. Psychobiol. 8:129.

Panksepp, J., Herman, B., Conner, R., Bishop, P., and Scott, J. P. (1978), The biology of social attachments: Opiates alleviate separation distress. Biol. Psychiatry13:607.

Pappas, B. A. and Walsh, P. (1983), Behavioral comparison of pentylenetetrazol, clonidine, chlordiazepoxide and diazepam in infant rats. Pharmacol. Biochem. Behav. 19:957.

Roberts, L. H. (1975), Evidence for the laryngeal source of ultrasonic and audible cries of rodents. J. Zool. (Lond) 175:243.

Sales, G.D. (1972), Ultrasound and aggressive behaviour in rats and other small mammals. An. Behav. 20:88.

Sales, G. D. and Pye, D. (1974), "Ultrasonic Communication by Animals." Chapman and Hall, London.

Smotherman, W. P., Bell, R. W., Starzec, I., Elias, J., and Zachman, T. A. (1974), Maternal responses to infant vocalizations and olfactory cues in rats and mice. Behav. Biol. 12:55.

Squires, R. F., Saederup, E., Crawley, J. N., Skolnick, P., and Paul, S. M. (1984), Convulsant potencies of tetrazoles are highly correlated with actions on GABA/picrotoxin receptor complexes in brain. Life Sci. 35:1439 (1984).

Tallman, J. F., Paul, S. M., Skolnick, and Gallagher, D. W. (1980), Receptors for the age of anxiety: Pharmacology of benzodiazepines. Science 207:274.

Trullas, R., Havoundjian, H., Zamir, N., Paul, S., and Skolnick P. (1987), Environmentally-induced modification of the benzodiazepine/GABA receptor coupled chloride ionophore. Psychopharmacology 91:384.

DRUG EFFECTS ON PRIMATE ALARM VOCALIZATIONS

John R.Glowa*, Jack Bergman**,Thomas Insel***
and John D. Newman****

Biological Psychiatry Branch*
  National Institute of Mental Health
  Bethesda, MD 20892

Division of Behavioral Biology**
  Harvard Medical School
  New England Regional Primate Research Center
  Southborough, MA 01772

Laboratory of Clinical Science***
  National Institute of Mental Health
  Poolesville, MD 20837

Laboratory of Comparative Ethology****
  National Institute of Child Health and Human
  Development
  Poolesville, MD 20837

INTRODUCTION

Mammalian vocalization traditionally has been an
area of intense ethological analysis. Vocal behavior
often promotes predictable responses in conspecifics,
providing a convenient basis for classifying social
interactions. The current volume extends the analysis of
vocalizations to evaluate potential physiological
mechanisms involved in their production. A primary means
for addressing physiologic mechanisms is by pharmacological manipulation. Although a large literature has
described ethological determinants of vocalization,

relatively little is known of the effects of drugs on
these behaviors. If specific neuronal mechanisms mediate
vocalization, then neurochemically selective agents
might be expected to have specific effects on these
behaviors. In turn, orderly pharmacological effects on
vocal behavior might lead to a better understanding of
the role of underlying physiologic mechanisms. Furthermore, as specific types of calls typically occur in particular situations, a pharmacological analysis of vocalizations might lead to a better understanding of the
interaction of neurochemistry with environmental determinants of vocal behavior. The studies reported within
this chapter were initiated following the observation
that drugs can increase rates of specific vocalizations
under some conditions. The unique nature of these drug-
behavior interactions has encouraged further characterization of conditions under which pharmacological
enhancement of vocalization occurs. Emphasis is placed
on the squirrel monkey alarm call, because it is well
characterized. Not surprisingly, drugs that affect
vocalizations also have other behavioral effects, and
some comparisons provide a basis for evaluating similarities and differences in the determinants of these
behaviors.

Primates exhibit a rich repertoire of different
types of calls, including isolation calls, alarm calls,
display vocalizations, infant vocalizations, distress
calls, and other calls associated with agonistic encount-
er or group cohesion. Calls produced in the laboratory
closely resemble those produced in the wild (Winter et
al., 1966; Winter, 1972). Identification of these calls
has typically been both structural and functional. Sonographic analysis characterizes the temporal structure of
the full range of frequencies emitted, providing an
objective way to categorize calls. Situational determinants detail the conditions under which calls occur,
providing a different level of analysis. Primates and
other social species often emit a characteristic alarm
call in the presence of a predator or other alarm stimulus (Klump and Shalter, 1984). In some species this call
has been differentiated into several sub-types based on
both sonographic and situational characteristics (Winter
et al., 1966; Winter, 1969; Schott, 1975; Newman, 1985).
For example, squirrel monkeys emit alarm peeps, high-
pitched calls of short duration, when rapidly moving
objects suddenly appear in view; yaps, barks, and
cackles, conspicuous, closely spaced calls with a low
fundamental frequency plus harmonics, when confronted
with a stationary or slowly moving object; noisy

shrieks, if recently captured or defeated; and keckers, repeated FM components interspersed with noisy elements, when more aggressive, dominant individuals are confronted. Although stereotyped calls can be easily recognized by the trained observer, inter-observer reliability scores for some types of calls can be quite low when, for example, drugs are given (Crowley, 1978). Thus, in addition to identification of the call type, sonograms may also be helpful in their quantification. We have also found, using sonograms, that while drugs may alter call rates, the structure of the call remains within normal species-typical limits over a wide range of doses. Thus, sonographic analysis provides an objective basis for assessing the reproducibility of vocalizations.

Situational analyses sometimes prompt speculation on the adaptive significance of alarm calls. The successful escape of the caller and its groupmates from a noxious situation is assumed to maintain the call in the species repertoire, and well-developed alarm calls in the newborn of some species supports this notion. In other species however, characteristics of the call develop with experience (Hinde, 1954), and differences in both the alarm call and response to it can depend upon the exact circumstances of the situation. A question arises as to how vocalizations in the presence of a predator might increase the likelihood of escape. In squirrel monkeys, different varients of the alarm call may occur when threat is from above or below (Newman, 1985). Marler (1959), in noting the structural properties of avian alarm calls, speculated that the acoustic properties of some may enhance the difficulty of their localization by a predator. Several authors have suggested the distraction provided by multiple calls (often called mobbing) may aid in group flight. As shown below, the alarm call need not require the presence of other individuals, raising the question of its "altruistic" foundations. Nevertheless, the potential adaptive significance of vocal behavior elicited by strongly arousing situations seems compelling.

The resemblance between situations leading to alarm calls in non-human primates and those which might produce analogous responses in man has maintained additional interest in primate vocalization as a metric of response to "stress" induced by a noxious situation. In this light, it would be of interest to link these types of behaviors to physiological responses subserving stress reactions in both species. To address such issues in the laboratory, it will be necessary to determine the

range of conditions under which vocalizations can be
produced. This chapter enumerates some of its determinants and compares the effects of drugs on vocal behavior with other behaviors under the control of noxious
stimuli.

EFFECTS OF DRUGS ON THE ALARM CALL

    Although there is a growing interest in the effects
of drugs on social interactions (Miczek, 1978; Suomi,
1983), relatively few studies have addressed drug
effects on vocalizations. Of these, the majority have
focussed on rodent (Herman and Panksepp, 1978), canine
(Panksepp et al., 1978), or avian (Panksepp et al.,
1980; Sahley et al., 1981) calls. Most studies report
that drugs decrease rates of vocalization, but fail to
determine whether this is a specific effect of the drug
on vocalizations. For example, sedative-hypnotic drugs
decrease many behavioral end points and a decrease in
vocalization might easily be replaced by a more convenient measure such as motor activity or food consumption
if there is no behavioral specificity. A few studies
have reported increases in vocalizations following certain drugs, raising similar questions of the ability of
drugs to increase a wide range of behaviors. For example, Sahley et al. (1981) demonstrated that the antimuscarinic agent scopolamine could increase the frequency
of separation-induced distress vocalizations in domestic
chicks. This study is of particular interest, not only
because of the agent studied, but also because situational variables (separation) apparently enhanced the
likelihood that the drug would specifically affect vocalizations. Thus, situational variables may be very
important in obtaining the desired effect of a particular drug.
    Several reports clearly indicate that drugs have
clear effects on vocalizations in primates. For example,
increased vocalization rates were reported following
administration of d-amphetamine (in Ceropithecus
aethiops; Kjellberg and Randrup, 1972), apomorphine (in
Macaca artoides, Schlemmer et al., 1980), and ß-
 carbolines (Ninan et al., 1983), although no indication
of the type of vocalization was given. In another study,
d-amphetamine only decreased infant distress calls in
Ceropithecus (Schiorring and Hecht, 1979). More recently, Harris and Newman (1987) have demonstrated
imipramine- and clonidine-induced decreases in isolation
calling in Saimiri sciureus. These findings, which differ from earlier reports that showed imipramine

increased calling in <u>Macaca</u> <u>mulatta</u> (Porsolt et al.,
1984), suggest that effects of drugs on primate vocalizations may depend upon the species studied.

Effects of benactyzine on squirrel monkey alarm calls

Recently, we reported that the anticholinergic drug,
benactyzine, increased alarm call rates in <u>Saimiri</u>
<u>sciureus</u> (Glowa and Newman, 1986). The report followed
the serendipitous observation that a squirrel monkey was
vocalizing at an unusually high rate after receiving a
dose of benactyzine. The effect was clearly unusual, as
individual squirrel monkeys rarely vocalize under normal
laboratory conditions. A second observation, that covering the monkey arrested the vocalizations, was also of
interest, as the subsequent covering and uncovering of
the monkey arrested and reinstated calling, respectively. Following sonographic analysis,   benactyzine was
found to specifically increase <u>alarm call</u> rates. Interestingly, the effect depended upon the environmental
context. Threat stimuli, such as monkey puppets, brooms,
nets, and other large objects (including the experimenter) apparently served well as alarm stimuli, but high
rates of vocalization only occurred when the animal had
been given benactyzine. In contrast, drug alone had little effect on alarm calling in the absence of such stimuli. Several additional experiments were designed to
better characterize these effects.
Initially, four good responders were studied inten-
sively. A monkey puppet was chosen as the alarm stimulus. Dose-effect functions for benactyzine HCl were
obtained for each monkey in a systematic fashion, replicating the effects of a wide range of doses twice. Monkeys were dosed and handled by methods commonly used in
behavioral pharmacology (i.e. the monkeys were tethered
on a leash in their home cages, and transported to the
cage on a pole). This allowed gentle restraint for
injections and a minimum of direct handling or undue
arousal. Injections were given i.m. in the calf muscle,
using sterile saline as a vehicle. The monkey was then
placed in a wire cage, and the cage was placed within a
sound-attenuating chamber equipped with a microphone.
After a 10 min post-injection period the vocalization
test began by simply presenting the puppet at eye-level
to the squirrel monkey, at a distance of approximately 1
m. The puppet was presented for a 30-s period, and then
withdrawn for 30 s. Ten such cycles constituted a short
and effective testing period.Sessions were taped using a
full-spectrum recorder for sonographic analysis. Figure

1 shows the relationship between dose of benactyzine and
alarm call rate. Normally, alarm calls were virtually
non-existent or, at most, occurred once or twice a
minute, typically only in the presence of the alarm
stimulus. With increasing dose of benactyzine alarm call
rate increased dramatically, reaching asymptotic levels
at doses of 0.3-3.0 mg/kg. Generally, at doses of 3
mg/kg, no untoward effects were observed. In one monkey

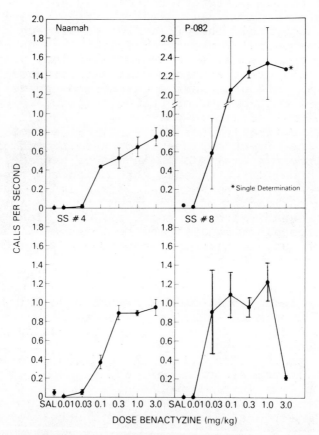

Fig 1. Effects of benactyzine on alarm call rate in
       four squirrel monkeys. For each monkey, the
       effects of benactyzine were assessed in
       random order over the range of doses, and then
       the effects of each dose were replicated. The
       data represent the mean effect of two
       sessions, and the bars indicate the S.D. of
       the effect. Ordinate, alarm call rate in calls
       per sec. Abscissa, dose in mg/kg. (Glowa and
       Newman, 1986).

(SS#8) 3 mg/kg, and in all other monkeys tested, 10
mg/kg decreased call rates, produced profuse salivation,
and resulted in pronounced agitation.

The pharmacological specificity of benactyzine-
induced calling was then assessed by attempting blockade
with cholinesterase inhibition, using physostigmine and
neostigmine. Figure 2 shows that neither of these drugs
alone increased alarm call rates. However, in combination with benactyzine, physostigmine was able to block
the rate-increasing effects of the anticholinergic on
calling in a dose-dependent manner. In contrast, similar
doses of neostigmine did not block the effects of benactyzine. These results suggested that the pharmacological induction of the alarm call was mediated by central
mechanisms, as neostigmine penetrates the blood brain
barrier poorly.

Cholinergic mechanisms have been implicated in
other vocalizations as well. In addition to the earlier
mentioned studies in which scopolamine induced distress
vocalizations in chicks (Sahley et al., 1981), cholinergic participation in song has also been suggested by the
presence of cholinergic binding in brain regions associated with vocalization (Ryan and Arnold, 1981). Earlier
studies with cats have also implicated the involvement
of central cholinergic systems by documenting vocalizations associated with attack and aggressive behavior
after i.c.v. administration of carbachol or muscarine
(Beleslin and Samardic, 1977, 1979; Beleslin et al.,
1986). Although these results suggest that cholinergic
mechanisms are related to mechanisms of both avian and
mammalian vocalization, they do little to narrow the
range of conditions under which vocalizations are most
likely to occur.

The combined effect of drug and alarm stimulus to
increase alarm calling demonstrates a unique drug-
behavior interaction, as alarm call rates during the
stimulus-off periods were much lower than rates during
stimulus presentations. While such results reiterate the
importance of situational variables in *in vivo* pharmacology, cause and effect relationships remain obscure.
For example, situational variables may have effectively
increased the "noxiousness" of the alarm stimulus by
increasing the sensitivity of the monkey to its presence
or acted on some property of the behavior itself, such
as its rate of occurrence.

Benzodiazepine withdrawal-induced alarm calling

In order to obtain a more complete profile of drug
effects on the alarm call, the effects of several other

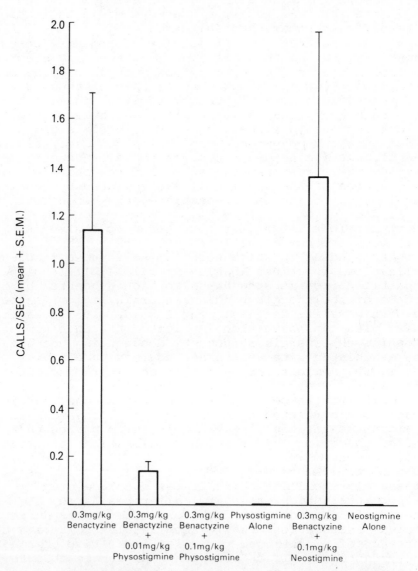

Fig.2. Effects of 0.3 mg/kg benactyzine, 0.01-
0.1 mg/kg physostigmine, and 0.1 mg/kg
neostigmine alone, and in combination on mean
alarm call rates in four squirrel monkeys.
Data are one determination per point, bars
indicate S.E.M.(Based on data in Table 1 of
Glowa and Newman, 1986).

drugs were also assessed. Cook and Davidson (1973) have
shown that benactyzine increased suppressed responding,
an effect that is usually associated with anxiolytic
properties of benzodiazepine agonists such as chlordiazepoxide or diazepam. These results, together with a
potential link between alarm calls and anxiety-producing
situations, suggested that other agents which affect
anxiety should be assessed on the alarm call. More
recently inverse benzodiazepine agonists, agents with
neuropharmacological effects opposite to those of the
benzodiazepine agonists, also have been described. One
of these, ß-CCE, has been reported to produce
"experimental anxiety," including increased vocalization
rates, in rhesus monkeys (Ninan et al., 1983). Finally,
two agents reported to produce anxiety in humans, caffeine and the inverse agonist FG 7142, also were
assessed for their ability to increase alarm calls. None
of these agents appeared to increase alarm call rates
under the current conditions.

One of the more relevant aspects of the clinical
pharmacology of benzodiazepines is that withdrawal from
repeated administration of anxiolytic drugs may be associated with an increase in anxiety. Recent reports have
shown that withdrawal from chronic benzodiazepine treatment, induced by challenge with the benzodiazepine
receptor antagonist Ro 15-1788, resulted in a abstinence
syndrome in the baboon (Lukas and Griffiths, 1982). In
additional studies, Ro 15-1788-induced withdrawal also
was observed to increase the frequency of squirrel monkey vocalizations (Bergman, 1987). The observation
prompted another series of studies in which diazepam was
given daily to four monkeys. After 5-6 days of chronic
administration, a 1 mg/kg dose of Ro 15-1788 was substi-
tuted for diazepam on the next day. All other conditions
were similar to those during the benactyzine experiments, except 5-min testing sessions were used. Figure 3
shows when the daily dose of diazepam was increased from
0.1 to 3 mg/kg, the challenge dose of Ro 15-1788
increased alarm call rates to levels near those previously seen with suitable doses of benactyzine.

Further comparisons of the ability of benactyzine and
Ro 15-1788 to increase alarm call rates were made by
studying the effects of a 0.3 mg/kg benactyzine challenge following sub-acute (6-day) treatment with diazepam (1 mg/kg) or saline. Figure 4 shows that the
benactyzine response was significantly greater following
sub-acute diazepam than sub-acute saline, suggested a
potential interaction of chronic diazepam and benactyzine in potentiating alarm calling. Figure 4 also shows
the effects of several putative benzodiazepine antago-

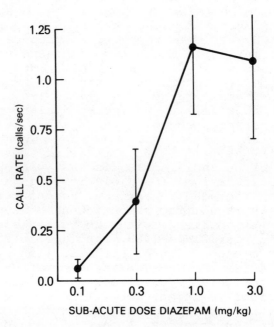

Fig.3. Effects of 1 mg/kg Ro 15-1788 on alarm call
        rates in four squirrel monkeys, when given
        before sessions preceded by 5-6 daily doses
        (indicated) of diazepam. The data represent
        the mean effect of one session per monkey; the
        bars indicate the S.E.M. Ordinate, alarm
        call rate in calls per sec. Abscissa, daily
        dose of diazepam in mg/kg.

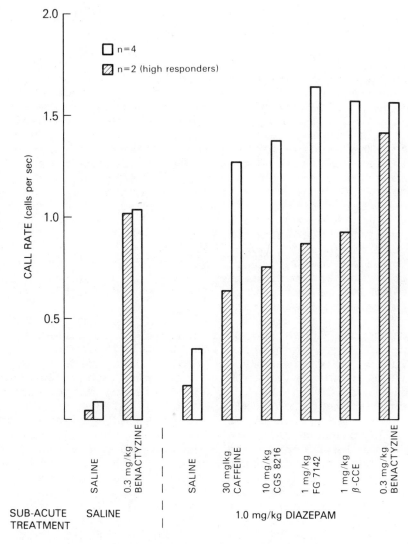

Fig 4. Effects of several drugs on alarm call rates in squirrel monkeys when given 10 min before daily sessions preceded by 5-6 daily injections of saline (left) or 1 mg/kg diazepam (right). The data represent mean effects in one session in four monkeys (stippled bars) or in two particularly focussed high-responding monkeys. Ordinate, alarm call rate in calls per sec. Abscissa, drug, dose, and treatment.

nists on alarm call rates following sub-acute
diazepam. In contrast to the effect of each agent when
given alone, following sub-acute diazepam each was quite
effective in increasing alarm call rates.

Few studies have directly linked benzodiazepine-
mediated effects and cholinergic mechanisms of action,
although physostigmine has been shown to antagonize
benzodiazepine-induced myoclonus in the baboon (Rektor
et al., 1984). Benzodiazepine and cholinergic receptors
are both heavily represented in the septum and medial
forebrain bundle, further suggesting potential interactions. The studies with squirrel monkey vocalizations
presented here also suggest some common features,
although vocalizations are only increased either in the
presence of benactyzine or during benzodiazepine withdrawal. Other benzodiazepine-cholinergic interactions
have been reported. The significant difference in the
effects of benactyzine following chronic saline versus
chronic diazepam support additive, but separate
mechanisms. However, it remains entirely possible that
benactyzine and benzodiazepine withdrawal produce the
same behavioral effect through completely unrelated
pharmacological substrates.

In other studies involving chronic administration
of diazepam, Lucas and Griffiths (1982) reported that
baboons (Papio anubis), given 10 mg/kg twice daily,
exhibited mild signs of withdrawal after 7 days, and
intense withdrawal including tremor and convulsion after
35 days, following Ro 15-1788 challenge. No vocalizations were reported. Gallager et al. (1986) reported
similar findings in the rhesus monkey (Macaca mulatta).
From these results it might seem that the squirrel monkey alarm call represents a useful model for the study
of the pharmacological induction of vocalization in primates, as increases in this behavior have not been
reported in other primate species. However, more
recently investigations have reported opiate-withdrawal
induced vocalizations in the rhesus monkey. Katz (1985)
and Katz and Valentino (1986) have reported increased
vocalization ("screams") provoked by handling during
naloxone-precipitated withdrawal, whereas physostigmine
and UM1046 (a cholinergic agent) produced a quasi-
withdrawal syndrome that failed to elevate vocalization
levels. These observations raise the question of whether
vocalizations may represent a sensitive end point for
"symptoms" of withdrawal. However, it is noteworthy that
narcotic antagonist administration alone has been
reported to increase rodent distress calls in non-
dependent subjects (Herman and Panksepp, 1978).

These results indicate that a spectrum of different pharmacological treatments are effective in inducing alarm calls. As these agents probably operate through different neurochemical and neuroanatomical substrates, the question arises as to whether each may be separately involved in different components of the neuronal substrates of vocalization, or whether their effects collectively represent a more global response of the organism to "stress."

Individual differences in effects

An important clue to differences in the effects of different agents on alarm calling may reside in differences in individual responses to drug. Throughout these studies individual differences in the effects of drugs on vocalization were noted. For example, differences in the efficacy of benactyzine were apparent in P-082, as maximal call rate was about twice that of the other monkeys. Differences in sensitivity also was seen in the minimal dose required to elevate call rates. Lower doses increased calling in SS#8 and P-082, than in Naamah or SS#4. Additionally, SS#8 appeared slightly more sensitive to the toxicity associated with higher doses. In these studies Bolivian and Columbian sub-species, both sexes, and a wide range of ages, were represented. The individual differences in response to benactyzine and the other drugs did not appear to be related to any of these variables. Failure to produce the expected effects with benactyzine has occurred in a few monkeys. When a fuller picture of variables related to drug-induced increases in alarm calling is obtained, such individuals may be tremendously important in developing treatment strategies for coping with noxious environments.

Further differences in effect were noted during the benzodiazepine withdrawal experiments, as shown in figure 2. Although benactyzine had effects similar to those seen in the monkeys tested previously, two monkeys consistently exhibited higher rates of vocalization than two other monkeys when tested with the inverse agonist challenges.

Although the form of a vocal response may be very similar within a species, the rate at which it occurs obviously can differ across individuals. Individual differences often provide an empirical basis of investigation. For example, Suomi has found large differences in individual reactivity to early separation in macaques (Suomi, 1983), and has maintained these differences in subsequent generations by selective breeding. Hinde (1954) has noted individual differences in the onset of

stimulus-induced alarm calls in the chaffinch. Factors
such as social status, prior history, and differences in
individual sensitivity probably play a role in
determining the effect of drugs on alarm calls. In addition, the role of the current environment and prior
experience should also not be underestimated. Because of
the complex nature of drug-behavior interactions, it is
quite possible that many earlier studies failed to
observe drug effects on vocal behavior because the
appropriate combination of conditions was not present.

The pharmacological production of vocalization in
individuals has several implications. Obviously, the
observation of vocalizations occurring in the absence of
conspecifics promotes a question regarding the functional relevance of the call. Such results may also
raise questions regarding the likelihood of physiological substrates specifically involved in communication.
By studying vocal behavior in the individual, the complexity of its ethological determinants may be reduced
by the elimination of potential interaction with calls
from other individuals. Thus, regardless of the final
disposition of the nature of the alarm call, methods to
study its modification by drugs seem to be well developed.

COMPARISONS OF DRUG EFFECTS ON OTHER TYPES OF BEHAVIORS

The ability to compare the behavioral effects of
drugs under different conditions allows determination of
the behavioral specificity of a drug effect. All drugs
will decrease all behavior if given in high enough
doses. However, an effect that occurs at doses that have
little or no effect on other behaviors is perhaps more
revealing of selective pharmacological activity. For
example, drugs with anxiolytic properties selectively
increase responding suppressed by noxious consequences,
at doses that have less of an effect on non-suppressed
responding (Kelleher and Morse, 1968). The effects of
drugs that increase certain types of vocalization can be
compared to their effects on different behaviors. However, these types of comparisons encompass additional
difficulties. The behavioral effects of drugs often have
multiple determinants, and can depend on such factors as
the ongoing rate of behavior, the context in which it
occurs, and even the influence of prior events (Barrett,
1985). Comparisons of drug effects should be obtained
across a range of conditions in order to arrive at meaningful conclusions.

The study of drug effects on operant behavior has
provided a useful vantage point for behavioral analysis

of drug effects on learned performances, in particular
because it allows an analysis of situational determinants of drug effects across a wide range of conditions.
Similar techniques may be of advantage in the study of
drug effects on vocalizations. Vocalization behavior is
clearly affected by situational factors as several
studies have used these factors to directly control
vocalization. For example, operant control of vocal
behavior has been demonstrated in the budgerigar
(Ginsberg, 1960), chicken (Lane, 1960), guinea pig
(Burnstein and Wolff, 1967), rat (Lal, 1967), cat
(Molliver, 1963), dog (Salzinger and Waller, 1962), sea
lion (Schusterman and Feinstein, 1965), dolphin (Lilly,
1965), and the cebus monkey, (Myers et al., 1965;
Leander et al., 1972) by arranging vocalization
-dependent delivery of species-appropriate reinforcers.
In one study (Leander et al., 1972), the vocal behavior
of three jungle-born Cebus monkeys was maintained under
various schedules of food-pellet presentation; under
each condition the rates and patterns of responding
appropriate to the schedule in effect were well maintained. Furthermore, stimuli known to elicit species-
characteristic behavior, such as the presentation of an
alarm call in the chaffinch, also have been used to control behavior (Thompson, 1969). These results suggest
that vocalization, like other performances, can be
modified by their consequences. Clearly, these behaviors
also are under stimulus control, as well-defined classes
of stimuli set the occasion for vocalizations. Unfortunately, no studies have assessed the effects of drugs on
operantly maintained vocal behaviors. However, several
reports have described the effects of drugs on other
types of performances. The following descriptions outline some of these effects and the conditions under
which they occur.

Anticholinergics

Several reports have described the effects of benactyzine and other anticholinergic drugs on complex learning and memory performances (McDonough, 1982; Penetar
and McDonough, 1983; Penetar, 1985). In rhesus monkeys
these drugs disrupt performances designed to assess memory, but only at relatively high doses. Earlier reports
indicated that benactyzine could increase the occurrence
of several different operant behaviors (Boren and Navarro, 1959; Boren, 1961). Subsequent reports have shown
that similar doses of benactyzine also can increase
responding that is suppressed by response-dependent
delivery of noxious stimuli (Cook and Davidson, 1973).

As discussed previously, this type of effect is often produced by drugs with anxiolytic action, such as the barbiturates and benzodiazepines (McMillan, 1975). Responding that postpones the delivery of noxious stimuli (continuous avoidance) also is increased by benactyzine (Stone, 1964). Such results clearly indicate that benactyzine can increase behaviors other than vocalization, including some that are controlled by noxious events.

Some effects of benactyzine appear similar to those of other antimuscarinic agents, such as scopolamine and atropine. These agents also increase operant responding (Boren, 1961; Carlton, 1963; Stone, 1964; Vaillant, 1967; Willis and Windland, 1968), although these increases may occur less reliably than those produced by other types of drugs. Continuous avoidance responding is also inconsistently increased by scopolamine (Herrnstein, 1958; Stone, 1964) and atropine (Carlton, 1962; Heise and Boff, 1962; Scheckel and Boff, 1964), supplementing the point. Although Herrnstein (1958) suggested that these rate-increasing effects of anticholinergic drugs are independent of increases in shock frequency, subsequent studies have demonstrated a relationship between the rate-increasing effects of these drugs and changes in shock frequency (Pradham and Roth, 1968; Stone, 1965). McKim (1973) has demonstrated that the rate-increasing effects of scopolamine are related to baseline rates of responding, with lower rates being increased proportionally more by these drugs. Other data corroborate this notion, as higher response rates are typically only decreased by scopolamine (Hanson et al., 1967; Miczek, 1973). These findings are consistent with a large body of data supporting the notion that drug effects on behavior can depend both upon the manner in which behavior is maintained and the normally occurring baseline frequencies of the response (Kelleher and Morse, 1968).

Unfortunately, there are few other reports of the effects of benactyzine on operant behaviors. To the extent that comparisons can be made, the effects of benactyzine seem similar to those of other anticholinergic drugs. It would appear that antimuscarinics can increase responding maintained by escape from noxious stimuli, as well as responding that is maintained by conventional means and suppressed by noxious stimuli. However, when comparable rates and patterns of responding are maintained under appetitive conditions, similar rate-increasing effects are produced.

Benzodiazepine withdrawal. As discussed earlier, the
benzodiazepine antagonist, Ro 15-1788, is a relatively
silent drug at low doses in untreated monkeys, but can
induce vocalization in subjects treated with repeated
administration of diazepam. In experiments with squirrel
monkeys, changes in the behavioral effects of diazepam
and Ro 15-1788 were evaluated after three months of
daily injections of 10 mg/kg diazepam (Bergman and
Dorsey, 1986). Initially, diazepam (0.03-3.0 mg/kg) produced dose-related decreases in suppressed responding
maintained by termination of a noxious stimulus, whereas
the antagonist had little effect until high doses (17
mg/kg or more) were administered. After three months of
chronic administration of diazepam, the dose-effect
curve for diazepam was shifted more than 10-fold to the
right. In contrast, the dose-effect curve for Ro 15-1788
shifted leftward and responding was disrupted by doses
as low as 0.03 mg/kg in all monkeys. Gross observation
of the subjects revealed that vocalization (and sometimes, tremor) occurred after rate-decreasing doses of
the antagonist were administered. Interestingly, both
the rate-decreasing and vocalization-producing effects
of the antagonist in these monkeys could be prevented by
administration of 30-100 mg/kg diazepam prior to the
antagonist. Furthermore, the dose-effect curve for Ro
15-1788 regained its initial position following discon-
tinuation of chronic administration of diazepam. Taken
together, these results suggest that disruptions in
behavior produced by low doses of Ro 15-1788 in
chronically-treated monkeys can effectively serve as a
marker for antagonist-produced withdrawal.

CONCLUSIONS

From the studies reported here it is clear that the
squirrel monkey alarm call can be altered by both pharmacological and behavioral factors. Studies of the pharmacological induction of the alarm call may lead to a
better understanding of physiological mechanisms underlying vocalization. In addition, the functional significance of drug-induced increases in calling may also be
clarified. The pharmacological induction of the alarm
call in the absence of conspecifics questions the likelihood that the alarm call may serve as a metric of nat-
uralistic response to noxious environments. Further
studies are needed to address the functional significance of changes in vocal response and relate the occurrence of these behaviors to underlying physiological
substrates.

One measure of the responsiveness of organisms to noxious stimuli is the assessment of change in neuro-endocrine functioning. During acute stress corticotropin-releasing hormone (CRH) can be released into the hypophyseal portal system, stimulating the anterior pituitary to release adrenocorticotropin (ACTH) and ß-endorphin. ACTH, in turn, stimulates the release of glucocorticoids, in particular, cortisol. Both ACTH and cortisol are considered good peripheral indices of a stress response in the organism. Conditions eliciting some primate vocalizations have been clearly related to neuroendocrine release. For example, Hennessy (1986) has shown that brief maternal separation results in marked elevations of cortisol levels in the squirrel monkey. CRH and other stress-related peptides (including ACTH and ß-endorphin) also exist in extrahypothalamic CNS. Their role, either in initiating or coordinating responses to stress, has been suggested by a variety of behavioral and pharmacological studies. For example, central administration of CRH can decrease appetitive, sexual, and exploratory behaviors while increasing loco-motor activity and aggression (Koob and Bloom, 1983; Weiss et al, 1986). These types of agents are of particular interest in terms of their potential permissive role in behavioral response. Cholinergic mechanisms also may be involved in the response to stress. Chronic atropine treatment has been shown to increase the number of central CRH receptors (DeSouza and Battaglia, 1986). The central blockade of benactyzine's effects in the present studies further suggests that some form of stress may be mediated by central components.

The nature of the pharmacological induction of alarm vocalization in the primate encourages speculation that this model can provide a unique method to study human response to stress-provoking stimuli. It is well established that drugs like caffeine and ß-carbolines can precipitate panic-like attacks in man, although the situational variables controlling these effects are unknown. The availability of a primate model of stress reaction would be of obvious value for mental health research, in as much as somatic and psychiatric disorders including anxiety, depression and post-traumatic stress disorder (Post et al., 1981), have long been thought to result from or be exacerbated by exposure to uniquely stressful situations. Both benzodiazepine-mediated and cholinergic mechanisms have been implicated in these types of illnesses (Janowsky, 1985; Dilsaver, 1986). Physiologic and behavioral profiles of stress-related illnesses include hypercortisolism, decreased

appetitive and sexual behavior, increased arousal and
sleep disturbances, and suppressed immune response (Gold
et al., 1987). The pharmacological induction of an analogous response to stressful situations in the non-human
primate will allow a more direct assessment of stress-
related disorders and potential strategies for treatment.

Vocalization is a pharmacologically sensitive behavior that may serve as a unique indication of the physiological state of the organism. Unfortunately, very little is known of the underlying physiology of this
response, or the state it is purported to reflect.
Although the functional significance of the pharmacological potential of vocalization is not presently clear,
the effects of drugs may aid our understanding of
mechanisms involved in vocalizations. In the current
chapter we have focussed attention on the alarm call of
the squirrel monkey, which seems to occur more frequently under conditions in which the organism is confronted
by noxious events. Further studies in this area should
directly address the issue of eliciting variables, by
attempting to manipulate the "noxiousness" of the environmental event and directly relating behavioral
response to physiological parameters.

ACKNOWLEDGEMENTS: Portions of this manuscript were
supported by research grants #DA03774, and DRR 00168.

REFERENCES

Barrett, J.E., 1985, The effects of drugs on squirrel
     monkey behavior, in " Handbook of Squirrel Monkey
     Research", L.A. Rosenblum and C.L. Coe eds.,
     Plenum Publishing Co., New York.
Beleslin, D.B., Stefanovic-Denic, K. and Samardic, R.,
     1986, Comparative behavioral effects of anticholin-
     ergic agents in cats: psychomotor stimulation and
     aggression. Pharmacol.Biochem. Behav.,24:581.
Beleslin, D.B., Samardic, R., 1977, Muscarine- and
     carbachol- induced aggression: fear and irritable
     kinds of aggression.Psychopharmacology, 55: 233.
Beleslin, D.B., Samardic, R., 1979, Effects of para-
     chlorophenylalanine and 5,6-dihydroxytrptamine on
     aggressive behavior evoked by cholinomimetics and
     anticholinesterases injected into the cerebral
     ventricle of conscious cats.Neuropharm.,18:251.

Bergman, J. and Dorsey, L. 1986. Behavioral effects of
    Ro 15-1788 and pentobarbital in diazepam-tolerant
    squirrel monkeys. Fed. Proc.,45: 663.
Boren, J.J., 1961, Effects of adiphenine, benactyzine,
    and chlorpromazine upon several operant behaviors.
    Psychopharmacologia,2:416.
Boren, J.J. and Navarro, A.P., 1959 The action of
    atropine, benactyzine,and scopolamine upon fixed-
    interval and fixed-ratio behavior.J. Exper. Anal.
    Behav., 2:107.
Burnstein, D.D. and Wolff, P.C., 1967, Vocal responding
    in the guinea pig. Psychonom. Sci., 8:39.
Carlton, P.L., 1962, Some behavioral effects of
    atropine and methylatropine. Psychol. Rep. 10:579.
Carlton, P.L., 1963, Cholinergic mechanisms in the
    control of behavior by the brain. Psychol. Rev.,
    70:19.
Cook, L. and Davidson, A.D., 1973, Effects of
    behaviorally active drugs in a conflict-punishment
    procedure in rats, in_ "The Benzodiazepines," S.
    Garattini, E. Mussini, and L.O. Randall, eds. Raven
    Press, New York.
Crowley, T.J., 1978, Substance abuse research in monkey
    social groups,in_ "Ethopharmacology: Primate Models
    of Neuropsychiatric Disorders," K.A. Miczek, ed.,
    Alan R. Liss, Inc. New York.
DeSouza, E. and Battaglia, G., 1986, Increased
    corticotropin-releasing factor receptors in rat
    cerebral cortex following chronic atropine
    treatment. Brain Res., 397:401.
Dilsaver, S.C., 1986, Cholinergic mechanisms in
    depression. Brain Res.Rev., 11:285.
Gallager, D.W., Heninger, K. and Heninger, G., 1986,
    Periodic benzodiazepine antagonist administration
    prevents benzodiazepine withdrawal symptoms in
    primates. Eur. J. Pharmacol., 132:31.
Ginsberg, N.,1960, Conditioned vocalization in the
    budgerigar. J. Comp.Physiol. Psych., 53:183.
Glowa, J.R. and Newman, J.D., 1986, Benactyzine
    increases alarm call rates in the squirrel monkey.
    Psychopharmacology, 90:457.
Gold, P.W., Goodwin, F.K. and Chrousos, G.P., 1987,
    Clinical and biochemical manifestations of
    depression: relationship to the neurobiology of
    stress. New Eng. J. Med. (in press).
Hanson, H.M., Witoslawski, J.J., and Campbell, E.H.,
    1967, Drug effects in squirrel monkeys trained on a
    multiple schedule with a punishment contingency. J.

Exp. Anal. Behav., 10:565.

Harris, J.C. and Newman, J.D., 1987, Mediation of separation distress by a2- adrenergic mechanisms in a non-human primate. Brain Res., 410:353.

Heise, G.A. and Boff, E., 1962, Continuous avoidance as a baseline for measuring behavioral effects of drugs. Psychopharmacologia, 3:264.

Herrnstein, R.J., 1958, Effects of scopolamine on a multiple schedule. J. Exp. Anal. Behav., 1:351.

Hennessy, M.B., 1986, Multiple, brief maternal separations in the squirrel monkey: changes in hormonal and behavioral responsiveness. Physiol. Behav., 36: 245.

Herman, B.H. and Panksepp, J., 1978, Effects of morphine and naloxone on separation distress and approach attachment: evidence for opiate mediation of social affect. Pharmacol. Biochem. Behav., 9:213.

Hinde, R., 1954, Factors governing the changes in strength of a partially inborn response, as shown by the mobbing behavior of the chaffinch (Fringilla coelebs). I. The nature of the response, and an examination of its course. Proc. R. Soc. B., 142:306.

Janowsky, D.S., and Risch, S.C., 1985, An acetylcholine hypothesis of stress modulation. Integr. Psychiatry, 3:3.

Katz, J.L., 1985, Effects of clonidine and morphine on opioid withdrawal in rhesus monkeys. Psychopharmacology, 251:17.

Katz, J.L. and Valentino, R.J., 1978, Pharmacological and behavioral factors in opioid dependence in animals, in, "Behavioral Analysis of Drug Dependence," S.R. Goldberg and I.P. Stolerman, eds., Academic Press, New York.

Kelleher, R.T. and Morse, W.H., 1968, Determinants of the specificity of the behavioral effects of drugs. Ergb. Physiol. Pharmakol. Chemie., 60:1.

Kjellberg, B. and Randrup, A., 1972, Changes in social behavior in pairs of vervet monkeys (Cercopithecus) produced by single, low doses of amphetamine. Psychopharmacolia, 26:127.

Klump, G.M. and Shalter, M.D., 1984, Acoustic behavior of birds and mammals in the predator context. Z. Tierpsychol., 66:189.

Koob, G. and Bloom, F., 1983, Memory, learning and adaptive behaviors, in, "Brain Peptides," D. Krieger, M.J. Brownstein, and J.B. Martin, eds., John Wiley & Sons, New York.

Lal, H., 1967, Operant control of vocal responding in

rats. Psychonom. Sci., 8:35.

Lane, H.L., 1960, Control of vocal responding in
    chickens.Science, 132: 37.

Leander, J.D., Milan, M.A., Jasper, K.B. and Heaton,
    K.B., 1972, Schedule control of the vocal behavior
    of Cebus monkeys. J. Exp. Anal. Behav., 17:229.

Lilly, J.C., 1965, Vocal mimicry in Turiops: ability to
    match numbers and durations of human vocal bursts.
    Science, 147:300.

Lukas, S.E. and Griffiths, R.R., 1982, Precipitated
    withdrawal by a benzodiazepine receptor antagonist
    (Ro 15-1788) after 7 days of diazepam. Science,
    217:1161.

MacLean, P. D., 1957, Chemical and electrical
    stimulation of the hippocampus in unrestrained
    animals. II. Behavioral findings. AMA Arch.
    Neurol., 78:128.

Marler, P. Developments in the study of animal
    communication, in "Darwin's Biological Work," P.R.
    Bell, ed. Cambridge Univ. Press.

McDonough, J.H. Jr., 1982, Effects of anticholinergic
    drugs on DRL performance of rhesus monkeys. Pharm.
    Biochem. Behav., 17:85.

McMillan, D.E., 1975, Determinants of the effects of
    drugs on punished responding. Fed. Proc. 34:1870.

McKim, W.A., 1973, The effects of scopolamine on fixed-
    interval behavior in the rat: a rate dependency
    effect. Psychopharmacology, 32:255.

Miczek, K.A, 1973, Effects of scopolamine, amphetamine,
    and benzodiazepines on conditioned suppression.
    Pharm. Biochem. Behav., 1:401.

Miczek, K.A. 1978 "Ethopharmacology: Primate Models of
    Neuropsychiatric Disorders," Alan R. Liss, Inc.
    New York.

Molliver, M.E., 1963, Operant control of vocal behavior
    in the cat. J. Exper. Anal. Behav., 6:197.

Myers, R.D., Horel, J.A. and Pennypacker, H.S., 1965,
    Operant control of vocal behavior in the monkey
    Cebus alifrons. Psychonom. Sci., 3: 389.

Newman, J.D., 1985, Squirrel monkey communication, in
    "Handbook of Squirrel Monkey Research," L.A.
    Rosenblum and C.L. Coe, eds. Plenum Publishing Co.,
    New York.

Ninan, P.T., Insel, T.R., Cohen, R.M., Cook, J.M.,
    Skolnick, P. and Paul, S.M. Benzodiazepine-receptor-
    mediated experimental anxiety in primates. Science,
    218:1332.

Panksepp, J. Meeker, R. and Bean, N.J., 1980, The
    neurochemical control of crying. Pharmacol.

Biochem. Behav., 12:437.
Panksepp, J., Herman, B., Conner, R., Bishop, P. and
    Scott, J.P., 1978, The biology of social
    attachments; opiates alleviate separation distress.
    Biol. Psychi., 13:607.
Penetar, D.M., 1985, The effects of atropine,
    benactyzine, and physostigmine on a repeated
    acquisition baseline in monkeys.
    Psychopharmacology, 87:69.
Penetar, D.M. and McDonough, J.H. Jr., 1983, Effects of
    cholinergic drugs on delayed match-to-sample
    performance of rhesus monkeys. Pharm. Biochem.
    Behav., 9:963.
Porsolt, R.D., Roux, S. and Jalfre, M., 1984, Effects of
    imipramine on separation- induced vocalizations in
    young rhesus monkeys. Pharm. Biochem. Behav.,
    20:979.
Post, R.M., Ballenger,J.C., Uhde, T.W., and Putman,
    F.W., Jr., 1981, Kindling and drug sensitization:
    implications for the progressive development of
    psychopathology and treatment with carbamazepine,
    in, "The Psychopharmacology of Anticonvulsants,"
    M. Sandler, ed., Oxford Univ. Press, Oxford.
Pradham, S.N. and Roth, T., 1968, Comparative behavioral
    effects of several anticholinergic agents in rats.
    Psychopharmacologia, 17:49.
Rektor, I., Bryere, P., Valin, A., Silva-barrat, C.,
    Naquet, R., and Menini, Ch., 1984, Physostigmine
    antagonizes benzodiazepine-induced myoclonus in the
    baboon, Papio papio. Neurosci. Let., 52: 91.
Ryan, S.M. and Arnold, A.P., 1981, Evidence for
    cholinergic participation in the control of bird
    song: acetylcholinesterase distribution and
    muscarinic receptor autoradiography in the zebra
    finch brain. J. Comp. Neurol., 202:211.
Sahley, T.L., Panksepp, J., and Zolovick, A.J., 1981,
    Cholinergic modulation of separation distress in
    the domestic chick. Eur. J. Pharmacol., 72:261.
Salzinger, K. and Waller, M.B., 1962, The operant
    control of vocalization in the dog. J. Exp. Anal.
    Behav., 5:383.
Scheckel, C. and Boff, E., 1964, Behavioral effects of
    interacting imipramine and other drugs with d-
    amphetamine, cocaine and tetrabenazine.
    Psychopharmacologia, 5:198.
Schiorring, E. and Hecht, A., 1979, Behavioral effects
    of low, acute doses of d- amphetamine on the didac-
    tic interaction between mother and infant vervet
    monkeys (Cercopithecus aethiops) during the first

six postnatal months. Psychopharmacology,64:219.

Schott, D.,1975, Quantitative analysis of the vocal repe-
toire of squirrel monkeys. Z. Tierpsychol.38:225.

Schlemmer, R.F., Jr., Narasimhachari, N. and Davis,
J.M., 1980, Dose-dependent behavioral changes
induced by apomorphine in selected members of a
primate social colony. J. Pharm. Pharmacol.,32:285.

Schusterman, R.J. and Feinstein,1965, Shaping and
discriminative control of underwater click
vocalizations in a California sea lion.Science,
150:1743.

Stone, G.C., 1964, Effects of drugs on non-discriminated
avoidance behavior I. Individual differences in
dose-response relationships.Psychopharmacologia,
6:245.

Stone, G.C., 1965, Effects of drugs on avoidance
behavior II. Individual differences in
susceptibilities. Psychopharmacologia, 7:283.

Suomi, S.J., 1983, Social development in rhesus
monkeys: consideration of individual differences,
in "The Behavior of Human Infants," A. Oliverio
and M. Zappella, eds. Plenum Press, New York.

Thompson, T.I., 1969, Conditioned avoidance of the
mobbing call by chaffinches. Anim. Behav., 17:517.

Vaillant, G.E., 1967, A comparison of antagonists of
physostigmine-induced suppression of behavior. J.
Pharmacol. Exper. Ther., 157:636.

Weiss, S.R.B., Post, R.M., Gold, P.W., Chrousos, G.,
Sullivan, T.L., Walker, D. and Pert, A., 1986, CRF-
induced seizures and behavior: interaction with
amygdala kindling. Brain Res., 372:345.

Willis, R.D. and Windland, L.M., 1968, Effects of
repeated administrations of atropine on two
multiple schedules. Psychonom. Sci., 13:139.

Winter, P., Ploog, D. and Latta, J., 1966, Vocal
repertoire of the squirrel monkey (Saimiri
sciureus): its analysis and significance. Exp.
Brain. Res., 1:359.

Winter, P., 1972, Observations on the vocal behavior of
free-ranging squirrel monkeys (Saimiri sciureus).
Z. Tierpsychol., 31:1.

Winter, P., 1969, Dialects in squirrel monkeys:
vocalizations of the roman arch type. Folia
Primatol., 10:216.

ENDOCRINE AND NEUROCHEMICAL SEQUELAE OF PRIMATE VOCALIZATIONS

Sandra G. Wiener, Christopher L. Coe*,
and Seymour Levine

Department of Psychiatry & Behavioral Sciences
Stanford University School of Medicine
Stanford, C.A.

*Department of Psychology
University of Wisconsin
Madison, W.I.

INTRODUCTION

There is now an extensive literature on the behavioral effects of separation of non-human primate infants from their mothers (see review by Mineka and Suomi, 1978). These studies have been conducted in a variety of species, both New and Old World monkeys. Early research focused primarily on behavioral variables, in particular the infant's activity and vocalization during the separation. More recently, measures of physiological function have been included in the examination of the infant's response to removal from its mother (Reite et al., 1982; Coe et al., 1985a,b). By assessing behavior and physiology simultaneously, our laboratory has taken a psychobiological approach to this field of study. In this chapter, we will review a series of studies conducted during the past 10 years in the Laboratory of Developmental Psychobiology at Stanford University on the physiological and behavioral responses to separation in the infant squirrel monkey (<u>Saimiri</u> <u>sciureus</u>) and the infant rhesus monkey (<u>Macaca</u> <u>mulatta</u>). By using two species of monkeys, we have been able to generalize some of our findings across non-human primate species.

The infant's behavioral response following separation has been characterized as biphasic. The first phase observed immediately following separation has been termed "protest."

This phase is characterized by high rates of vocalization and an increase in general activity. The second phase has been called either "depression" or "despair". This phase is characterized by a decrease in activity, a cessation of calling, a hunched-over posture and an increase in self-directed behaviors (e.g., huddling, rocking, self-orality, etc.) The intensity and duration of each phase varies with the separation environment, the infant's prior experience with separation, the species studied, and genetic factors (Suomi et al., 1981; Mineka and Suomi, 1978). Although the "protest" phase is almost always observed, the "depression" or "despair" phase does not always occur. During the brief separations we have used in the squirrel monkey and rhesus macaque, we have not observed a "despair" reaction. Thus, we will focus on the initial "protest" behaviors, especially vocalizations, and their relationship to physiological indices of arousal.

The physiological measures we have examined are the activity of the pituitary-adrenal system and that of the monoamines of the central nervous system. The former is assessed by plasma cortisol levels and the latter by the monoamine metabolites in the cerebrospinal fluid (CSF). Our laboratory has found that the pituitary-adrenal system is a sensitive and reliable indication of an organism's response to changes in its environment (Hennessy and Levine, 1978, Hennessy et al., 1979; Hennessy and Levine, 1979). More recently, the monoamine metabolite of norepinephrine, MHPG, has also proven to be sensitive to changes in the separation environment (Levine, 1987).

Based on behavioral data, the vocalizations emitted by the separated infant have been interpreted to reflect "distress." Thus, infants that vocalize the most are viewed as the most stressed and those that call less are viewed as less stressed. However, the physiological indices examined often do not indicate that this is the case. As we will demonstrate in the studies to be described, we have observed that in many cases high vocalization rates are associated with lower elevations in plasma cortisol and CSF MHPG. This lack of concordance between the behavioral and physiological responses has led us to reevaluate the function of vocalizations during separation.

Instead of viewing infant vocalizations emitted during separation as a measure of "distress", we have hypothesized that these vocalizations are a coping response. From our

perspective, any response made during a stressful situation
which results in a diminution in the physiological indices of
arousal is a coping response. Infants which stray from their
mothers during their attempts to explore the environment will
vocalize when there is a threatening occurrence in their
environment. This ususally results in retrieval of the infant
by its mother. Thus, the infant has learned that
vocalizations elicits contact with the mother. Contact with
the mother following separation has been shown to
significantly reduce the physiological measures of arousal
(Mendoza et al., 1978; Levine and Coe, in press; Coe et al.,
1985b). Thus, vocalization becomes associated with reduced
arousal. When we have imposed a separation, under certain
conditions (i.e., in the presence of the mother), the infant
produces a high rate of vocalization in an active attempt to
elicit reunion. Although reunion is not successful because we
have imposed a physical barrier, none the less, vocalizations
appear to act as a coping response which reduces arousal.

We have examined the infant monkey under numerous
conditions of separation. First, we have examined the time
course of the separation response from 30 min to 24 hr in the
squirrel monkey and up to 96 hr in the rhesus. Second, we
have examined the response to multiple separations under
identical conditions at 10 day intervals in the squirrel
monkey. Third, we have examined the importance of other
social partners by allowing the separated infant squirrel
monkey to remain in its home social group following removal of
the mother. Fourth, we have examined the effects of maternal
cues present during separation in both species. This involved
placing the infant in an adjacent cage to its mother, allowing
visual, olfactory and auditory communication while preventing
tactile contact. Fifth and finally, we have manipulated the
endogenous opiate system of the separated infant squirrel
monkey and observed the potential changes in behavioral and
physiological measures. This last set of studies on the
endogenous opiate involvement in separation are based on the
work of Panksepp and co-workers (see review by Panksepp et
al., 1985) which proposed an endogenous opiate theory of
social attachment.

In order to simplify our description of the specific
studies, we have briefly described some methods general to the
experiments conducted in our laboratory. Unless otherwise
noted, all the studies on infant squirrel monkeys were
conducted between 3.5-7 months of age. Only monkeys derived

from adults imported from Guyana in the early 70's were
tested. The animals were bred in small social groups with 5-6
adult females (feral or lab-born) and 1-2 males in large mesh
pens. Once pregnancy was confirmed, the males were removed.
Infants reared in social groups remained in these breeding
groups until weaned at 6-7 months of age. Infants reared only
with their mothers were transferred out of their social group
at 1.5-3 months of age into individual primate cages.

The rhesus monkeys were bred in large outdoor cages
containing 8-10 adult females and one adult male. Since it
was difficult to rapidly capture the mother and infant
directly out of these large cages, it was necessary to house
the dyad in a smaller primate cage for the studies. The dyads
were allowed to acclimate to this new housing situation for at
least a week prior to the start of the study. The experiments
were conducted when the infants were 4-9 months old.

All behavioral observations were conducted from behind
one-way glass. Using standardized checksheets, the posture of
the infant was noted every 30 sec (e.g., moving, active,
inactive but alert, inactive curled with head down,
stereotypic movements) and the total frequency of
vocalization, eating, drinking, and object exploration was
noted. In addition, in a number of studies the vocalizations
produced by the infant were recorded on tape. These were
subsequently analyzed, in collaboration with Dr. Francoise
Bayart of our laboratory and with Dr. Charles Snowden of the
University of Wisconsin, by spectrographic procedures.

The CSF and blood samples were taken following rapid
anesthetization with ethyl ether in squirrel monkeys and
ketamine in the rhesus macaques. CSF was collected first at
the cervical level between C1 and C2. Subsequently a blood
sample was taken. Both the CSF and blood samples were
collected within 3 min of capture in order to minimize the
effects of disruption due to capture. Both samples were
centrifuged and then frozen until assay. The CSF samples were
analyzed for the monoamine metabolites of norepinephrine
(MHPG), dopamine (HVA); and serotonin (5HIAA) by a gas
chromatography/mass spectrography method in collaboration with
Drs. Kym Fall and Jack Barchas of the Nancy Pritzker
Laboratory for Behavioral Neurochemistry (Faull et al.,
1979). The plasma cortisol levels were determined by a
radioimmunoassay procedure (see Coe et al., 1978a for
details). Both the blood and CSF sampling procedures are

routinely used in our laboratory without any detrimental
consequences for the infant since we have microtized the
assays so that less than 0.5 ml of blood or 0.2 ml of CSF are
required.

Temporal Factors

When we first began our squirrel monkey mother-infant
experiments, we chose to examine very brief separations of 30
min (Coe et al., 1978b; Mendoza et al., 1978; Levine et al.,
1978). The blood samples taken at the end of this brief
separation demonstrated a marked elevation in plasma cortisol
levels. By combining the results of several different studies
using the total isolation condition (i.e., no contact with the
mother or other conspecifics), we have generated a time
course of the response of infants separated for 1 hr, 4 hr, 6
hr and 24 hr. As illustrated in Figure 1, plasma cortisol
levels increased as length of the separation increased. In
contrast, the number of species-specific infant isolation
vocalizations (Winter et al., 1966) decreased over time (Fig.
2). This negative relationship between cortisol and
vocalization levels indicates that high levels of vocalization
do not necessarily reflect heightened physiological arousal
levels. This result was one of our first examples where
vocalization levels was not a good indication of distress.
However, if vocalization is viewed as a communicative process,
then the decrease with time observed in total isolation would
be predicted because the infant has no cues to reinforce its
calling. The negative relationship between the behavior and
physiological data also fits well with a coping theory which
states that when an animal fails in its coping response, in
this case having its call not result in reunion with the
mother, then it will be highly aroused.

Repeated Separations

The effects of repeated, identical separations were
analyzed in a paper by Coe et al. (1983). Infant squirrel
monkeys were separated from their mothers under conditions of
total isolation for 1 hr six times at 10 day intervals. As
illustrated in Figure 3, these infants displayed a marked
decrease in calling over the first 3 separations and then
plateaued at lower levels for the last 3 separations. In
contrast, agitated activity levels did not change with
repeated separations. Similarly, the plasma cortisol levels
of the separated infants were consistently elevated above

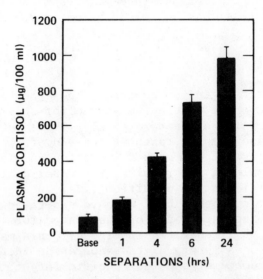

Fig. 1.   Time course of the infant plasma cortisol
(μg/100 ml) response ($\overline{x}$±SEM) to total isolation
from the mother. (Coe et al., 1985a)

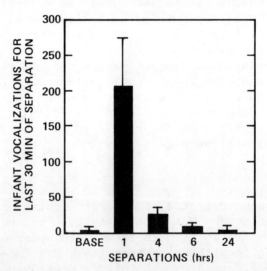

Fig. 2.   Time course of the infant vocalizations
($\overline{x}$±SEM) emitted to total isolation during the last 30
min of separation. (Levine et al., 1987)

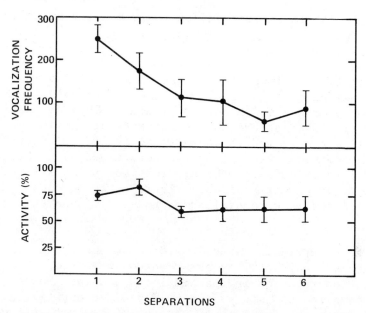

Fig. 3.   Vocalization frequency and activity levels
(x̄±SEM) of infant squirrel monkeys separated in total
isolation for 1 hr six times at 10 day intervals. (Coe et
al., 1983)

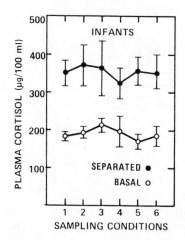

Fig. 4.   The plasma cortisol (μg/100ml) levels
(x̄±SEM) of infant squirrel monkeys separated in total
isolation for 1 hr six times at 10 day intervals. (Coe et
al., 1983)

those infants not separated from their mothers but blood
sampled immediately upon removal from the home cage at 10 day
intervals (see Figure 4).

As in the previous time course data, vocalizations appear
to decrease under total isolation when repeatedly separating
an infant over a 2 month period of time. This decrease in
vocalization was not due to the maturity of the infant at 6
months of age compared to when it had its first separation at
3.5 to 4 months of age. This was determined by separating the
previously non-separated "basal" cortisol animals for the
first time at 6 months of age. Their rates of vocalization
during separation were similar to the first separation at 3.5
months.

In this particular study, we did not observe an increased
pituitary-adrenal activity as a consequence of decreased
vocalization rates as in the time course data. However, since
separations in this study were only 1 hr in duration, it is
possible that the duration of separation was not sufficiently
long to detect an inverse relationship between cortisol levels
and vocalization. However, this data does indicate that even
during separations that produce low levels of vocalization
(i.e., the last 3 separations), the separated infant is still
highly aroused as demonstrated by the elevated cortisol
levels.

Social Interactions During Separation

In one of our earliest studies, we noted that infant
squirrel monkeys allowed to remain in their home social group
during separation appeared behaviorally quiescent compared to
when they were separated under conditions of total isolation
(Coe et al., 1978b). During the home separation, a late
pregnant female in the group was observed to permit the
separated infant to ride on her back. This phenomenon is
termed "aunting." Although the infant was quiescent during
the home separation condition, it was not possible to
differentiate its cortisol response from that of the total
isolation because the separation lasted only 30 min. However,
a subsequent study which increased the duration of separation
to 4 hr, indicated that those infants allowed to remain in the
social group during separation showed lower cortisol levels
than when placed in total isolation (Coe et al., 1985a).

Another study (Wiener et al., 1987) addressed the issue of

whether the aunting behavior was the reason for this decreased
behavioral and physiological arousal. Aunting of the infant
was prevented by composing the social group of only other
mother-infant dyads. This study also tested whether
familiarity with the separation environment was an important
factor. This was accomplished by comparing group-reared
infants to infants which were reared only with their mothers
in a small primate cage. Each group of infants were separated
from their mothers in either their home cage (HOME CAGE) or in
total isolation (NOVEL CAGE).

As illustrated in Figure 5, the group-reared subjects
vocalized less in their familiar home environment than in the
total isolation novel cage condition. However, at 1 hr the
individually-reared infants actually vocalized more in the
home environment than in total isolation. By 6 hr these
individually-reared infants displayed a lower rate of
vocalization in the home environment than in total isolation.
Although all infants displayed marked elevation of plasma
cortisol levels that increased with time, the group-reared

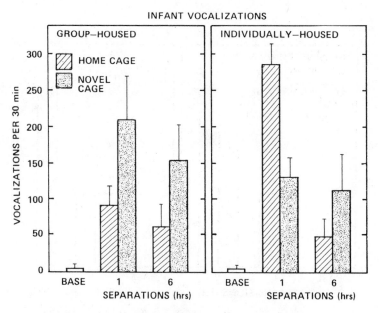

Fig. 5.   The vocalizations (x±SEM) emitted by
    group-housed and individually-housed infant squirrel
    monkeys following separation from their mothers in either
    total isolation (NOVEL CAGE) or when allowed to remain in
    the HOME CAGE. (Wiener et al., 1987)

infants allowed to interact with its home social group during
separation showed lower elevations than when totally isolated
(see Figure 6). In contrast, the individually-reared infants
displayed equal elevations in the two separation conditions.
Thus, the familiar home cage without social interaction did
not serve to buffer the physiological response to separation.

These social interaction studies are the first clear
indication of a positive relationship between the rate of
vocalization and plasma cortisol levels. When the infant is
allowed social interactions during separation then the
cortisol elevations and vocalizations are lower than in the
total isolation condition. We believe these non-vocal social
interactions are an important factor which permits both
behavioral and physiological responses to be attenuated
following loss of mother. The predictability of the social
interactions with familiar conspecifics may serve to reduce
arousal for the infant in the home separation condition.
These studies also rule out a possible role of familiarity
with the separation environment and point out the importance
of social interactions. However, placement of an infant into

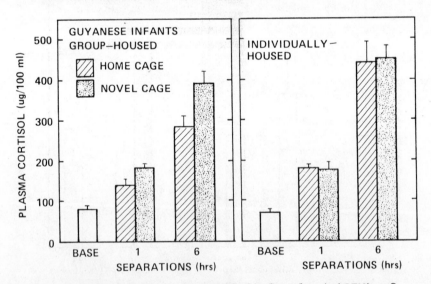

Fig. 6.   Plasma cortisol (μg/100ml) levels (x±SEM) of
    group-housed and individually-housed infant squirrel
    monkeys following separation from their mothers in either
    total isolation (NOVEL CAGE) or when allowed to remain in
    the HOME CAGE. (Wiener et al., 1987)

a strange social group during separation does not attenuate
the physiological response. In fact, these infants display the
most elevated cortisol levels found during separation observed
to date (Levine and Wiener, in press).

Presence of Maternal Cues

As stated in our introduction, we have examined the
importance of maternal visual, olfactory and auditory cues on
the separation response of infants placed in an adjacent cage
to their mothers which did not permit tactile contact. We
have conducted similar studies with both rhesus and squirrel
monkeys comparing total isolation to separation with the
mother present in an adjacent cage.

Levine et al. (1985) reported a study that examined rhesus
infants separated from their mothers at 4 months of age for 24
hr under four conditions: mother present without tactile
contact (ADJ), mother present with tactile contact (TAC), peer
present (PEER) or total isolation (ISO). Infants were
observed to rarely vocalize in the total isolation condition,
but were highly vocal when the mother was present with or
without tactile contact (see Figure 7). In the rhesus, the
species typical vocalization is known as a whoo or coo call
(Rowell and Hinde, 1962). In the mother present conditions,
the infants displayed lower cortisol elevations above baseline
compared to infants totally isolated or in the presence of a
peer that showed higher cortisol elevations (see Figure 8).

The rhesus infants were again tested at 9 months of age,
and the length of separation was extended to 3 days. The
total isolation and mother adjacent without tactile contact
conditions were used in this second phase of the experiment.
Infants were blood sampled at the following times following
separation: 1 hr, 3 hr, 20 hr (Day 2 AM), 27 hr (Day 2 PM), 44
hr (Day 3 AM) and 51 hr (Day 3 PM). The results indicated
again that infants vocalized more frequently when the mother
was present than when she was absent (see Figure 9). The
plasma cortisol levels were elevated above base on the first
day (1 hr & 3 hr) for both separation conditions. However,
the totally isolated animals displayed higher elevations than
when tested with the mother present (see Figure 10). By Day 2
the mother present condition had returned to baseline cortisol
values, similar to the results at 4 months of age. In
contrast, the isolated infants continued to show cortisol
elevations in the mornings of Day 2 and 3.

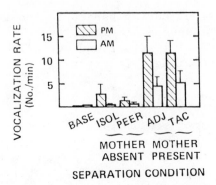

Fig. 7.   Vocalization rate (x̄±SEM) of rhesus infants
    separated from their mother, in the presence of their
    mothers (ADJacent or TACtile), or in the absence of their
    mothers (ISOlation or PEER). (Levine et al., 1985)

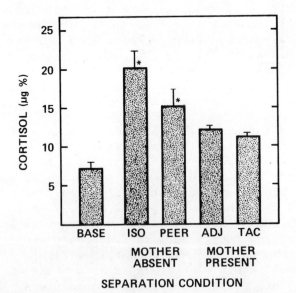

Fig. 8.   Plasma cortisol (μg %) levels (x̄±SEM) of
    rhesus infants separated from their mothers, in the
    presence of their mothers (ADJacent or TACtile), or in the
    absence of their mothers (ISOlation or PEER) compared to
    nondisturbed BASE levels. Asterisks indicate significant
    differences from base. (Levine et al., 1985)

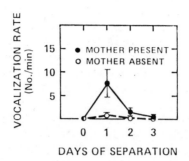

Fig. 9.   Vocalization rate (x̄±SEM) of rhesus infants
separated from their mothers either in presence or absence
of the mother in the adjacent cage. (Levine et al., 1985)

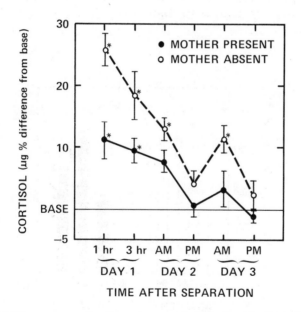

Fig. 10.   Difference of plasma cortisol (μg%) levels from
base of rhesus infants separated from their mothers either
in presence or absence of the mother in the adjacent
cage.   Asterisks indicate a significant difference from
base. (Levine et al., 1985)

A subsequent rhesus experiment (Levine et al., 1987)
extended the length of separation to 96 hr and included
analysis of the CSF monoamine metabolites: HVA for dopamine,
MHPG for norepinephrine, and 5HIAA for serotonin (Levine,
1987). These monoamine metabolites were analyzed in order to
determine whether or not there was a central nervous system
representation of the response to separation that was
concordant with either the vocalization behavior or the
pituitary-adrenal response we have observed.

Blood and CSF samples were obtained 24 and 96 hr following
separation under conditions of total isolation or mother
present in an adjacent cage. Both the behavioral and
endocrine responses were consistent with previous results.

The rate of vocalization was greater when the infants were
separated in the presence of the mother than in total
isolation. Likewise, the plasma cortisol was significantly
greater and persisted for a longer period of time when the
infant was totally isolated (see Figure 11).

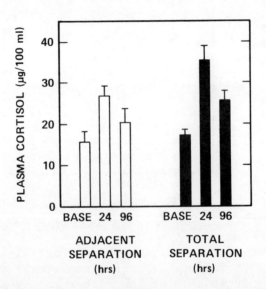

Fig. 11. Plasma cortisol (μg/100ml) levels of infant
     rhesus monkeys prior to (BASE) and following separation
     (24 hr and 96 hr) when the mother was in the adjacent cage
     or when the infant was totally isolated from the mother.
     (Levine, 1987)

The CSF monoamine metabolite analysis indicated that the norepinephrine metabolite MHPG clearly discriminated between the two separation conditions. While the CSF metabolites of dopamine (HVA) and serotonin (5HIAA) displayed a transient elevation and return to baseline in both conditions, MHPG was significantly elevated in total isolation and only showed a transient elevation under the adjacent separation.

Although we initially proposed that the monoamine metabolites would discriminate between the behavioral and pituitary-adrenal response to these two conditions of separation, it is not possible to make such a discrimination at this time on the basis of the limited amount of data. However, it appears in this study that the MHPG elevation and the cortisol elevations are responding similarly, with greater elevations observed in the total isolation condition.

A parallel series of experiments were conducted in the infant squirrel monkey. In the first study (Wiener et al., in press), infant squirrel monkeys were separated either adjacent to their mothers or in total isolation for 6 and 24 hrs. As observed in the rhesus, the rate of vocalization was greater in the presence of the mother. In contrast, the totally isolated infant had higher cortisol elevations than the infant adjacent to its mother. However, unlike the rhesus infants, separated squirrel monkey infants adjacent to their mothers did show a cortisol elevation above base at the two time points examined.

In a second experiment, we examined infant squirrel monkeys separated for 24 hr under the two conditions discussed above and an additional condition of allowing the infant to remain in its home social group following removal of the mother (Wiener et al., submitted). This social group consisted only of other mother-infant dyads and no potential aunts. This last condition, known as "home separation" was not possible with the rhesus since it was impossible to capture the monkeys from the large outdoor cage without a major disruption of the social group which would influence the physiological measures. As discussed in the previous section, separation with the possiblity of social interaction with familiar conspecifics appears to be a more benign form of separation. As a result, vocalizations were the least in the home separation, with higher levels in the total isolation condition and the highest observed in the presence of the mother (see Figure 12).

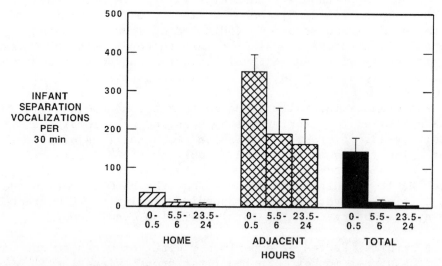

Fig. 12.   Infant squirrel monkey vocalizations ($\overline{x}\pm$SEM)
emitted during the first half-hour, 5-1/2-6 hr and last
half hour of 24 hr separations when the infant is left in
the HOME social group, ADJACENT to the mother, or TOTALly
isolated from the mother and conspecifics.

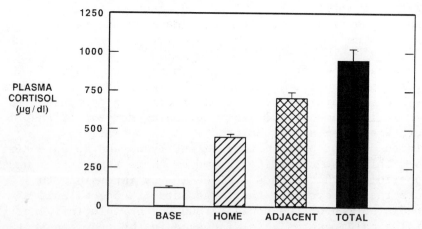

Fig. 13.   Plasma cortisol (μg/dl, $\overline{X}\pm$SEM) of separated
infant squirrel monkeys prior to (BASE) and following 24
hr separation when the infant is left in the HOME social
group, ADJACENT to the mother, or TOTALly isolated from
the mother and conspecifics.

The plasma cortisol levels indicated that the home separation resulted in the lowest elevation, and that similar to previous results the adjacent separation was lower than the total isolation condition (see Figure 13). Again, the CSF norepinephrine metabolite, MHPG, differentiated the conditions similar to the cortisol results. The total isolation condition resulted in a higher elevation than the adjacent condition. One difference between MHPG and cortisol response occurred in the home separation condition in which MHPG levels were not elevated above baseline.

Both species of monkey infants demonstrate a higher number of vocalizations when the mother is present. This is accompanied by a lower elevation of cortisol levels in the squirrel monkey and rhesus monkey and sometimes no change from basal levels in the rhesus. The total isolation condition results in lower levels of calling and marked cortisol elevations. Again, we appear to have an inverse relationship between vocalization rate and plasma cortisol elevations much like observed with the time course data. As the infant continues to vocalize in the presence of the mother, it appears to benefit from this calling by reducing its physiologic arousal level by having lower elevations of both plasma cortisol and CSF MHPG. This reaction would fit nicely with the hypothesis that the infant's vocalization is an active coping response to separation.

However, spectrographic analysis of the infant rhesus and squirrel monkey vocalizations revealed that the rate of vocalization, per se, does not truly characterize the behavior of the infant under the two separation conditions. The type of vocalization of the infant rhesus was strikingly different, with two types of whoo or coo calls only occuring while the infant is adjacent to the mother and a third totally different call only occuring when the infant is totally isolated (see Figure 14). Lillehei and Snowdon (1978) also noted distinctive coo calls made by stumptail macaques during separations from the mother, one when alone and another as they approached their mothers in a free-ranging group. Thus, there appears to be calls which may be related to communication with the mother, possibly to elicit retrieval,and another distinct call emitted during total isolation which might be better characterized as a distress vocalization.

Preliminary spectrographic analysis of the infant squirrel monkey vocalizations produced in the total isolation and

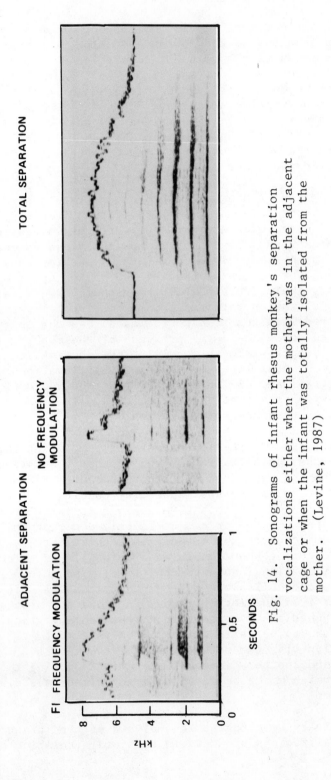

Fig. 14. Sonograms of infant rhesus monkey's separation vocalizations either when the mother was in the adjacent cage or when the infant was totally isolated from the mother. (Levine, 1987)

adjacent to the mother conditions (it was not possible to have clear recordings in the home separation condition due to background colony noises) indicated that the differences in the calls made under the two conditions were much more subtle than those observed in the rhesus studies. Only the peak frequency was significantly different, with the calls made during total isolation 60 hz higher than in the adjacent condition. However, it was noted that the number of doublets observed in the presence of the mother was significantly lower than in the total isolation condition. Since the squirrel monkey infant vocalizes at a rapid rate, in the past we have counted doublets, triplets, etc., as a single call if there was less than a 3 sec interval between calls. Most researchers have only analyzed each call individually and have ignored the apparent grouping nature of the calls.

In addition to the number of calls, the infants appear to make distinctive calls in response to the two different separation conditions. Although the rhesus infant's calls are audibly different to the human observer, the squirrel monkey calls require detailed spectrographic analysis to differentiate the calls. However, if one analyzes the number of multiple calls in the squirrel monkey, there appears to be a shift in the multiple calls which does not require spectrographic analysis. Thus, there may be some communicative value for the different calls the infant monkeys make during different conditions of separation. This is currently being investigated by playing back the various infant calls to the mother and then observing her behavior and her pituitary-adrenal response.

Endogenous Opiate Manipulation

Based on the hypothesis of Panksepp and co-workers (1985) that the endogenous opiate system is involved in social attachment and the distress response to separation, we have manipulated this system with opiate agonists (e.g., morphine) and antagonists (e.g., naloxone) (Wiener et al., in preparation). In doing so, we hoped to manipulate the rate of vocalization independent of environmental conditions, and then assess whether our physiological measures (i.e., plasma cortisol and CSF monoamine metabolites) would track the behavioral changes. Just prior to a 4 hr separation, the infant was injected with one of 4 substances: (-)naloxone (an active opiate antagonist), (+)naloxone (an inactive form of the drug), morphine (opiate agonist), and saline (vehicle).

The two forms of naloxone were used to control for a potential
non-opiate action of naloxone. All drugs were injected
intravenously in a volume of 0.1 ml with a dose of 1.7 mg/kg
for naloxone and 0.9 mg/kg for morphine. The infants were
treated with the same drug prior to each of the 6 separations
at 10 day intervals, with the exception of the
morphine-treated infants which received morphine on the first
3 separations and then received saline on the subsequent
separations.

The vocalization results indicated that the opiate
antagonist naloxone increased the rate of vocalizations and
the opiate agonist morphine decreased calling (see Figure 15),
as predicted by prior work with chicks (Panksepp et al.,
1980), and guinea pigs (Herman and Panksepp, 1978). The
inactive form of naloxone did not differ from the saline
treated infants. However, both the plasma cortisol values and
those of the monoamine metabolites failed to differentiate the
drug conditions. All separated infants, regardless of their
drug treatment, displayed equivalent cortisol elevations above
the levels of non-separated infants (see Figure 16). Levels

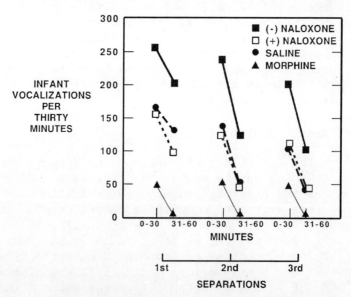

Fig. 15. Infant squirrel monkey vocalizations during the
first and second half hr of separation following
separations 1 to 3 of drug-treated [(-)naloxone and
morphine] and controls [saline and (+)naloxone].

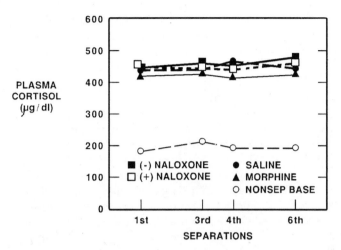

Fig. 16.   Plasma cortisol (μg/dl, $\bar{x}\pm$SEM) levels
    following 4 hr of separation during the 1st, 3rd, 4th, and
    6th separation of drug-treated [(-)naloxone and morphine]
    and controls [saline and (+)naloxone].

of MHPG and HVA in the CSF were also elevated above
non-separated basal levels, but again these additional
physiological indices of arousal did not differ between the
drug conditions. Thus, it appears that the opiate agonists
and antagonists are acting at some site in the brain mediating
vocalization which apparently does not influence the
physiological indices of arousal examined in this study.

   The physiological results of this opiate agonist and
antagonist study raise questions about the theory proposed by
Panksepp and coworkers (1985) of an endogenous opiate
modulation of social attachment. This theory hypothesizes
that the separation response is similar to opiate withdrawal
since it shares many of its behavioral characteristics,
including increased behavioral arousal. The results supporting
his theory are based primarily on the infant's increased
behavioral activity and vocalization responses observed
following maternal separation or separation from juvenile
peers. However, when we assess the physiological response of
the infants following the drug-treated separations, we did not
find either an inverse relationship between vocalization rates
and the physiological indices of arousal, as predicted by our
coping model, or a positive relationship that would fit the
Panksepp hypothesis. The failure in this study to find any
relationship between the vocalization rates and the

physiological responses measured raises further questions
about whether vocalization rates accurately reflect the degree
of distress of separated infants.

DISCUSSION AND CONCLUSIONS

     This final section will attempt to reconcile the observed
relationships between the behavior of the infant as
characterized by its vocalizations and the physiological
measures of plasma cortisol and CSF monoamine metabolites. In
order to summarize these findings we have provided a 2 x 2
table of all the squirrel monkey studies discussed (see Table
1). The axes are high/low vocalization and high/low cortisol.
By far, most of our studies are located in the high
vocalization/low cortisol and low vocalization/high cortisol
cells. This inverse relationship was derived from both the
time course data and the adjacent/total isolation studies.
These studies support our hypothesis that vocalizations on the
part of the infant are an active coping response which serve
to reduce the physiological arousal of the organism. In the
nonseparated condition, infant squirrel monkeys often use
calling to elicit retrieval by the mother. When there are no
cues from the mother, this response diminishes within a test
session and across repeated identical separations. The
physiological data on these totally isolated infants indicates
an increasing cortisol response over time or a constant
response over repeated separations. In contrast, infants
exposed to maternal cues continue to vocalize at high rates
even during long separations and display an attenuated
cortisol elevation in the squirrel monkey or in the rhesus no
elevation by 24 hr. It thus appears that by calling, an
infant can reduce the indices of physiological arousal.

     Although most of the data presented concurs with the
theory that the infant's vocalizations during maternal
separation serve as a coping response which reduces the
physiological indices of arousal, there are two exceptions to
this inverse relationship between behavioral and physiological
responses. First, the apparent reduction of <u>both</u> the behavior
(vocalizations) and physiology (plasma cortisol and CSF MHPG)
when the infant is permitted to remain in their home social
group following removal of its mother. However, the familiar
social home environment is unique compared to our other
environmental manipulations. Since familiarity <u>per</u> <u>se</u> with
the separation environment is not important because

TABLE 1

INFANT SQUIRREL MONKEY VOCALIZATIONS AND PLASMA CORTISOL LEVELS
DURING SEPARATION FROM THE MOTHER

PLASMA CORTISOL LEVELS	RATE OF VOCALIZATION	
	High	Low
High	1. Infant during first 30 min of separation in a novel environment (Levine et al., 1978; Mendoza et al., 1978)	1. Infant isolated in a novel cage for 4-24 hours (Wiener et al., in press) 2. Infant after three repeated separations (Coe et al., 1983) 3. Infant aunted during 1/2-hour separation (Coe et al., 1978) 4. Infant placed in an unfamiliar social group (Levine & Wiener, in press)
Low	1. Infant adjacent to mother during separation (Wiener et al., in press) 2. Surrogate-reared infant following removal of surrogate (Hennessy et al., 1979)	1. Infant aunted during 1-4-hour separation (Coe et al., 1985a) 2. Infant allowed familiar social partners during 1-6-hour separation (Wiener et al., 1987)

individually-reared infants did not display reduced behavioral
or physiological measures when left at home during separation,
then the social interactions with other members of the group
appears to be the important variable. In addition, the home
social group is a highly predictable environment based on the
past experience of the infant during its development. Both
predictability (Hennessy and Levine, 1979) and social
interactions can produce reduction in the physiological
measures of arousal (Coe et al., 1982; Stanton et al., 1985).
Thus, we have proposed that a non-vocal coping response, the
interaction with familiar conspecifics, and the predictability
of the environment accounts for the reduction in both the
infant's behavioral and physiological reaction to separation
from its mother when the infant is left at home.

The second inconsistency in our data involves the results
of the drug treatment with opiate agonists and antagonists.
Although we were able to either increase vocalization rate
with naloxone or decrease vocalization with morphine, the
physiological responses were unchanged despite the differences
in calling. If our hypothesis that vocal expression serves to
reduce arousal, then naloxone treatments should have reduced
plasma cortisol and CSF MHPG levels and that morphine
treatment should have resulted in an increase in these
physiological measures. The only way we can reconcile the
failure of the physiological response to be altered following
drug exposure, is to hypothesize that these drugs are acting
at some central nervous system site which regulates
vocalizations. As demonstrated by electrical stimulation
studies, the midline limbic cortex and midline thalamus are
involved in the production of isolation vocalizations (Jurgens
and Ploog, 1970). On the other hand, lesions of certain parts
of the thalamic tegmentum and adjacent core gray have been
demonstrated to disrupt the production of isolation
vocalizations (Newman and MacLean, 1982). If opiate agonists
and antagonists act on these CNS sites directly, it may be
more akin to the electrical stimulation or lesion of these
neural circuits. Vocalizations produced under these
conditions may not be a voluntary response and one which the
infant has no control over. Since a coping response involves
an active participation on the part of the subject, these
drug-induced calls may not serve the same function as
vocalizations produced under nondrug situations. Since we
have not analyzed the calls made during these drug treatments,
an alternative explanation is that there is some alteration in
their sonic characteristics and may not serve the same coping

function as non-drugged calls. However, until we conduct the appropriate studies, this drug experiment is not consistent with our theory that vocalizations serve as a coping response based on environmentally-induced changes in vocalization.

The challenge of future psychobiological research will be to reconcile the behavioral and physiological findings. Since we cannot ask our animals how they feel, we are forced to use their behavioral response to ascertain how they react to our experimental manipulations. In this case, many researchers have interpreted the vocalizations emitted in response to maternal separation as "distress" vocalizations. The term distress has the connotation of an affective state of high arousal. As we have demonstrated with our physiological data, an increase in vocalization rate is not necessarily associated with increased levels of either plasma cortisol or CSF monoamine metabolites. When a separated infant vocalizes more in the presence of the mother it is probably trying to elicit reunion. When it stops vocalizing in total isolation it is probably conserving resources. In addition, the type of calling in these different situations appears to be different. Thus, just quantifying the number of vocalizations may be misleading. Our laboratory no longer assumes that because the human observer may not be able to hear the differences in the call, that just counting the number of calls is not sufficient. At least in the rhesus, there appears to be a distinctive coo or whoo call made in isolation that may be a true distress vocalization. Further research will be necessary to determine whether there is a similar distress call in the squirrel monkey. Until such time, we would urge, as has Newman (1985), the use of the term "infant isolation call" instead.

ACKNOWLEDGMENT

This research is supported by grants HD-02881 from NICH&HD, MH-23645 from NIMH, and USPHS Research Scientist Award MH-19936 from NIMH to S. Levine, MH-23861 to J. D. Barchas, and MH-41659 from NIMH and RR-00167 from NIH to C. Coe. We wish to thank Ms. Edna Lowe for her assistance in the blood and CSF sampling. Ms. Helen Hu for her assay of plasma cortisol and Ms. Nina Pascoe for her analysis of the CSF monoamine metabolites. Additionally, we express our appreciation for the assistance in collecting the behavioral data to numerous undergraduate research assistants.

REFERENCES

Coe, C. L., Mendoza, S. P., Davidson, J. M., Smith, E. R.,
    Dallman, M.F., and Levine, S., 1978a, Hormonal response to
    stress in the squirrel monkey (<u>Saimiri</u> <u>sciureus</u>),
    <u>Neuroendocrinology</u>, 26:367.
Coe, C. L., Mendoza, S. P., Smotherman, W. P., and Levine, S.,
    1978b, Mother-infant attachment in the squirrel monkey:
    adrenal response to separation, <u>Behav. Biol.</u>, 22:256.
Coe, C. L., Franklin, D., Smith, E. R., and Levine, S., 1982,
    Hormonal responses accompanying fear and agitation in the
    squirrel monkey, <u>Physiol. Behav.</u>, 29:1051.
Coe, C. L., Glass, J. C., Wiener, S. G., and Levine, S.,
    1983, Behavioral, but not physiological, adaptation to
    repeated separation in mother and infant primates,
    <u>Psychoneuroendocrinology</u>, 8:401.
Coe, C. L., Wiener, S. G., Rosenberg, L. T., and Levine, S.,
    1985a, Physiological consequences of maternal separation
    and loss in the squirrel monkey, <u>in</u>: The handbook of
    squirrel monkey research, C. L. Coe and L. A. Rosenblum,
    eds., Plenum Press, New York.
Coe, C. L., Wiener, S. G., Rosenberg, L. T., and Levine, S.,
    1985b, Endocrine and immune responses to separation and
    maternal loss in nonhuman primates, <u>in</u>: The psychobiology
    of attachment and separation, M. Reite and T. Field, eds.,
    Academic Press, New York.
Faull, K. F., Anderson, P. J., Barchas, J. D., and Berger, P.
    A., 1979, Selected ion monitoring assay for biogenic amine
    metabolites and probenecid in human lumbar cerebospinal
    fluid, <u>J. Chromatography</u>, 163:337.
Hennessy, M. B., and Levine, S., 1978, Sensitive
    pituitary-adrenal responsiveness to varying intensities of
    psychological stimulation, <u>Physiol. Behav.</u>, 21:295.
Hennessy, M. B., Heybach, J. P., Vernikos, J., & Levine, S.,
    1979, Plasma corticosterone concentrations sensitively
    reflect levels of stimulus intensity in the rat, <u>Physiol.
    Behav.</u>, 22:821.
Hennessy, J. W., and Levine, S., 1979, Stress, arousal, and
    the pituitary-adrenal system: a psychoendocrine
    hypothesis, <u>in</u>: Progress in psychobiology and
    physiological psychology, Vol. 8, J. M. Sprague, and A. N.
    Epstein, eds., Academic Press, New York.
Hennessy, M. B., Kaplan, J. N., Mendoza, S. P., Lowe, E. L.,
    and Levine, S., 1979, Separation distress and attachment
    in surrogate-reared squirrel monkeys, <u>Physiol. Behav.</u>,
    23:1017.

Herman, B. H., and Panksepp, J., 1978, Effects of morphine and naloxone on separation distress and approach attachment: evidence of opiate mediation of social affect, Pharmac. Biochem. Behav., 9:213.

Jürgens, U., and Ploog, D., 1970, Cerebral representation of vocalization in the squirrel monkey, Exp. Brain Res., 10:532.

Levine, S., 1987, Psychobiologic consequences of disruption in mother-infant relationships, in: Perinatal development: A psychobiological perspective, N. Krasnegor, E. Blass, M. Hofer, and W. Smotherman, eds., Academic Press, New York

Levine, S., Coe, C. L., Smotherman, W. P., and Kaplan, J. N., 1978, Prolonged cortisol elevation in the infant squirrel monkey after reunion with mother, Physiol. Behav., 20:7.

Levine, S., Johnson, D. F., and Gonzales, C. A., 1985, Behavioral and hormonal responses to separation in infant rhesus monkeys and mothers, Behav. Neurosci., 99:399.

Levine, S., Wiener, S. G., Coe, C. L., Bayart, F. E. S., and Hayashi, K.T., 1987, Primate vocalization: a psychobiological approach, Child Development, 58:148.

Levine, S., and Coe, C. L., in press, Psychosocial modulation of neuroendocrine activity, in: Biorhythms and stress in the physiopathology of reproduction, P. Pancheri, ed., Hemisphere Publ., New York.

Levine, S., and Wiener, S. G., in press, Psychoendocrine aspects of mother-infant relationships in nonhuman primates, Psychoneuroendocrinology.

Lillehei, R. A., and Snowdon, C. T., 1978, Individual and situational differences in the vocalizations of young stumptail macaques (Macaca arctoides), Behaviour, 65:270.

Mendoza, S. P., Smotherman, W. P., Miner, M. T., Kaplan, J., and Levine, S., 1978, Pituitary-adrenal response to separation in mother and infant squirrel monkeys, Dev. Psychobiol., 11:169.

Mineka, S., and Suomi, S. J., 1978, Social separation in monkeys, Psychol. Bull., 85:1376.

Newman, J. D., 1985, Squirrel monkey communication, in: The handbook of squirrel monkey research, C. L. Coe and L. A. Rosenblum, eds., Plenum Press, New York.

Newman, J. D., and MacLean, P. D., 1982, Effects of tegmental lesions on the isolation call of squirrel monkeys, Brain Res., 232:317.

Panksepp, J., Bean, N.J., Bischof, P., Villberg, T., Schley, T.L., 1980, Opioid blockade and social comfort in chicks, Pharmac. Biochem. Behav., 13:673.

Panksepp, J., Siviy, S. M., and Normansell, L. A., 1985,

Brain opioids and social emotions, in: The psychobiology
of attachment and separation, M. Reite and T. Field,
eds.,   Academic Press, New York.

Reite, M., Short, R., Kaufman, I. C., Stynes, A. J., and
Pauley, J. D., 1982, Heart rate and body temperature in
separated monkey infants, Biol. Psychiat., 13:91.

Rowell, T. E., and Hinde, R. A., 1962, Vocal communications
of the rhesus monkey (Macaca mulatta), Proc. of the Zool.
Soc. of London, 138:279.

Stanton, M. E., Patterson, J. M., and Levine, S., 1985,
Social influences on conditioned cortisol secretion in the
squirrel monkey, Psychoneuroendocrinology, 10:125.

Suomi, S. J., Kraemer, G. W., Baysinger, C. M., and DeLizio,
R. D., 1981, Inherited and experiential factors associated
with individual differences in anxious behavior displayed
by rhesus monkeys, in: Anxiety, new research and changing
concepts, D.F. Klein, and J. G. Rabkin, eds., Raven Press,
New York.

Wiener, S. G., Johnson, D. F., and Levine, S., 1987,
Influence of postnatal rearing conditions on the response
of squirrel monkey infants to brief perturbations in
mother-infant relationships, Physiol Behav., 39:21.

Wiener, S.G., Coe, C.L., and Levine, S., in press, Temporal
and social factors influencing the behavioral and hormonal
responses to separation in infant squirrel monkeys, Amer.
J. Primatol.

Wiener, S. G., Bayart, F. E. S., Faull, K. F., and Levine,
S., submitted, Behavioral and physiological responses to
maternal separation in the squirrel monkey, Behav.
Neurosci.

Winter, P., Ploog, D., and Latta, J., 1966, Vocal repertoire
of the squirrel monkey (Saimiri sciureus), its analysis
and significance, Exp. Brain Res., 1:359.

EARLY DETECTION OF THE INFANT AT RISK THROUGH CRY ANALYSIS

Barry M. Lester, Ph.D.
Michael Corwin, M.D.
Howard Golub, M.D., Ph.D.

Brown University Program in Medicine
Bradley Hospital and
Women & Infants' Hospital, Providence RI

Boston University Medical School
Boston City Hospital, Boston, MA

Pediatric Diagnostic Services, Inc.
Cambridge, MA

INTRODUCTION

The study of the infant cry has been approached from two general perspectives. The first is as an indicator of the biological integrity of the infant, and the second, as an influence on the caregiving environment. Figure 1 shows a theoretical model for the study of the biological and caregiving or social aspects of the cry. This model allows us to postulate direct and indirect relationships between the cry and later developmental outcome. Direct relationships are shown by the path from medical status to cry acoustics to outcome and suggest the use of the cry as a measure of the biological integrity of the infant. Indirect effects refer to the cry as a determinant of parenting behavior which in turn affects developmental outcome. For example, the acoustic characteristics of the cry as well as the amount of crying affect parenting behavior which in turn relate to later outcome.

The biological and social aspects of the cry may also have diagnostic implications. As a measure of the biological integrity of the infant, these include the early detection of the infant at risk for adverse developmental outcome. Prematurity is as prototype of the infant at risk and we will discuss a follow-up study with premature infants later. Some preliminary work with term infants who suffered birth asphyxia suggests that changes in the cry over the first few weeks indicate which infants recover from the effects of birth asphyxia (C. Jackson, C. Garcia-Coll and B. Lester, unpubl.). The toxic effects of bilirubin in term infants has been related to changes in the cry and it has been suggested that the cry may indicate CNS involvement in infants with presumably safe levels of serum bilirubin (Golub and Corwin 1982; Rapisardi, et al 1987; Wasz-Hockert, et al 1971). Abnormalities in the cry have also been reported in a few cases of victims of the sudden infant death syndrome (Corwin, et al 1983; Colton and Steinschneider 1981; Stark and Nathanson 1972; Corwin, Golub, Kelly, et al 1986). These findings will also be discussed in this chapter.

Examples in which the cry may have implications related to the development of social interaction include parental cry perception and its effects on parenting behavior, colic, temperament, and failures in parenting such as abuse and neglect. This aspect of the cry as a social signal will not be discussed here but can be found elsewhere (Lester 1984; Lester and Boukydis 1985).

BACKGROUND

The scientific study of the cry started with the use of the sound spectrograph (Figure 2). Figure 2

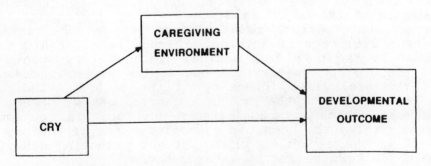

Figure 1   BIOSOCIAL MODEL OF INFANT CRY

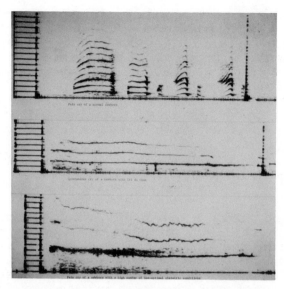

Figure 2

shows spectrograms from three infants. On the
spectrogram, energy is plotted on the vertical axis.
The dark markings on the spectrogram represent areas in
the frequency spectrum where energy is present. The
frequency bands are in 500 Hz or cycle per second
increments as shown by the horizontal bars on the
vertical axis. Time is plotted on the horizontal axis
and each spectrogram represents about 2 seconds of
time. The spectrogram on the top is from a normal
healthy term infant. The spectrogram in the middle is
from an infant with the genetic syndrome of cri du
chat ("Cat Cry Syndrome"), and shows a cry that is
clearly abnormal. It was this kind of finding, that
the acoustic characteristics of the cry were altered by
brain damage, that lead to the initial hypothesis that
the cry might have diagnostic utility.

Research since the 1960's using the sound
spectrograph has identified acoustic characteristics of
the cry that are correlated with medical abnormalities
(cf. Wasz-Hockert, et al 1968). In addition to cri
du chat there are other well known examples such as
asphyxia, hyperbilirubinemia and various forms of brain
damage. Since this pioneering work, most of which was
done by Scandinavian researchers, first in Stockholm
and later in Helsinki (Wasz-Hockert, 1985), there have
been a number of advances in the field which have

broadened the potential application of cry analysis. One advance is represented by the lower graph in Figure 2 and is the extension of the study of cry features beyond infants with known abnormalities to infants at risk for adverse outcome.   This lower spectrogram is from a healthy term infant who was part of a group of infants with poor obstetric histories and also showed abnormal cry characteristics (Zeskind and Lester 1978). Changes in the cry have also been associated with prematurity, illness, low birthweight, small for gestational age, malnutrition, and low ponderal index (see Lester and Boukydis 1985).

A second advance has been in our understanding of the mechanisms of cry production.   Conceptual models that describe the anatomical and physiological basis for the production and neurological control of the cry have been developed which lead to hypotheses about the relationship between the cry and the outcome of the infant (Bosma, et al 1965; Golub and Corwin 1985; Lester 1984).   For conceptual purposes the cry measures that we study are divided into three categories as shown in Figure 3.   The first is the subglottal system and relates to the respiratory influences on the cry. Crying occurs during the expiratory phase of respiration.   Respiration directly effects the duration of each cry unit and the amplitude or intensity of the cry.

Respiration influences the fundamental frequency characteristics of the cry which is the second category

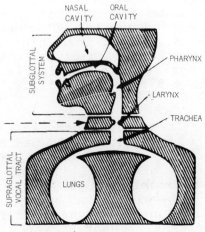

Figure 3

of measures.   The fundamental frequency is the number of glottal openings per second or the frequency of vocal fold vibration and is what we hear as voice pitch.   When we say that a cry is high pitched that is our perception of the physical phenomenon that the vocal cords are oscillating at a higher frequency.   The fundamental frequency is determined in part by subglottal pressure but primarily by vocal fold tension from the intrinsic muscles of the larynx.

The third category of cry measures are the formant frequencies which are determined by the contour and cross sectional area of the supraglottal airway.   The formants are the sound resonances that occur as a result of the filtering by the vocal tract and reflect motor innervation of the supraglottal airway.   The acoustically important muscles of the larynx, pharynx neck and chest are controlled throughout the cry by the 9th, 10th, 11th, and 12th cranial nerves and by the phrenic and thoracic nerves.   Damage to any of these nerves or their nuclei especially the nuclei of the cranial nerves located in the medulla, will directly affect the sound of the cry.   For example, if the nucleus of the vagus, the 10th cranial nerve is damaged, this would alter neural input to the vocalis, cricothyroid and cricoarytenoid muscles of the larynx. These muscles determine tension of the vocal folds which affect measures of the fundamental frequency.

A third advance in the field has been technological.   While the spectrogram provides a good visual image of the cry it has a number of disadvantages such as poor dynamic range, inadequate frequency resolution and difficulty in the measurement of acoustic information.   The application of high speed computer technology has improved the measurement as well as the efficiency of cry analysis (Golub and Corwin 1985).

GENERAL METHOD

The infant is placed in supine position with a microphone held 15 cm from the infants mouth.   The first 30 seconds of crying following the stimulus is recorded on audio cassette.   This cry signal is filtered above 5 Hz and digitized at 10 kHz using a cry analysis system developed in collaboration with Pediatric Diagnostic Service (P.D.S.,Cambridge, MA). For each cry unit defined as the cry that occurred during the expiratory phase of the respiration, the

Fast Fourier Transform is used to compute the log
magnitude spectrum for each 25 msec block of the cry
unit.   Figure 4 is a schematic of the computer analysis
for a single 25 msec block.

   Summary   variables   that   measure   acoustic
characteristics are computed across the 25 msec blocks.
For the fundamental frequency we measure both the
average and the percent change in the fundamental
during the cry.   These measures are thought to reflect
neural control of the cry.   The first formant also
includes measures of the average and percent change.
The first formant is determined by the airways that
form the vocal tract and by neural input that controls
the degree of vocal tract mobility.   Amplitude and
duration are also measured.   Amplitude is the intensity
of the cry and duration is the length of each cry unit.
Both amplitude and intensity are related to the
respiration influences on the cry.

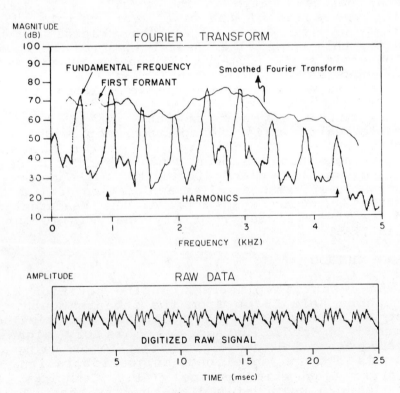

Figure 4

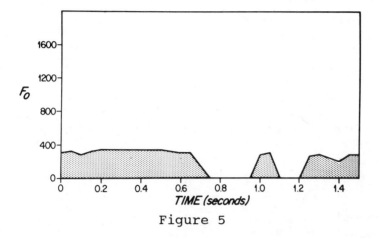

Figure 5

Figure 5 shows a fundamental frequency by time plot of the cry of a preterm infant recorded at 40 weeks gestational age. Frequency is on the vertical axis and about 2 seconds of time is shown on the horizontal axis. The fundamental frequency average is about 375 hz which is well within the normal range. This infant was born at 32 weeks gestational age, had been sick but by term the cry appeared normal. This infant was part of the follow-up study discussed below and was normal at follow-up. The infant in Figure 6 from the same study, had a similar medical course but showed an abnormally elevated and variable fundamental frequency at the same age and showed abnormal developmental outcome.

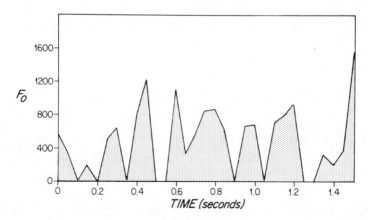

Figure 6

TABLE 1. Medical Problems in Preterm Infants*

Subject No.	Gestational Age (wk)	Birth Wt (g)	Apgar Score		Respiratory Problems	Time Intubated (d)	Neurologic Problems
			1 min	5 min			
1	32	1,650	9	10	−	0	−
2	30	1,350	7	8	+	11	+
3	28	950	7	8	+	18	+
4	33	1,190	7	8	−	0	−
5	34	2,080	9	10	−	0	−
6	34	2,090	9	10	+	3	−
7	28	825	2	6	+	4	−
8	34	1,970	9	10	−	0	−
9	34	2,440	7	8	−	0	−
10	28	1,080	7	8	−	0	−
11	32	1,820	7	8	+	4	−
12	33	1,930	9	10	−	0	−
13	30	1,350	9	10	+	0	−
14	31	1,300	9	10	−	0	−
15	30	1,310	2	6	+	15	+
16	32	1,900	7	8	−	0	−
17	30	1,480	2	6	+	9	−
18	32	2,340	2	6	+	3	−

* Symbols: +, present; −, none.

In a series of studies cry analysis has been applied to the study of the infant at biological risk for poor developmental outcome (see Lester and Boukydis 1985). In contrast to most previous work, where cry features were associated with known CNS impairment and the prognosis was more obvious, this work has shown that cry features are also associated with factors that place the infant at risk such as prematurity, but where the prognosis is less certain. We have conducted a longitudinal follow-up study in which cry analysis in the neonatal period was related to developmental outcome at 18 months and 5 years of age (Lester 1987).

LONGITUDINAL STUDY

The sample included 13 normal healthy term infants and 18 appropriate for gestational age preterm infants. The term infants averaged 40 weeks gestational age with an average birthweight of 3.3 kilograms. The gestational age of the preterm infants averaged 31.5 weeks with an average birthweight of 1.6 kilograms. The medical problems of the preterm are shown in Table 1. Nine of the 18 preterm infants had respiratory problems including 6 with hyaline membrane disease and 3 with bronchopulmonary dysplasia. The number of days

TABLE 2. Classification of 18-Month Bayley Scores by Neonatal Cry Measures*

Measure	High Bayley Score	Low Bayley Score
High av fundamental frequency	2	14
Low av fundamental frequency	14	1
High change fundamental frequency	5	10
Low change fundamental frequency	11	5
High change first formant	12	4
Low change first formant	4	11
High av amplitude	11	5
Low av amplitude	5	10

* Results are numbers of infants.

intubated ranged from 3 - 18. Three of the nine infants also had neurological problems including 2 with intraventricular hemorrhage and one with hydrocephalus. The cries were recorded at term conceptional age and were elicited by the administration of standard neurological reflexes.

RESULTS

Table 2 shows the results of the 18 month follow-up. At 18 months corrected age the Bayley scales were administered to the infants. To test the hypothesis that infants could be correctly classified into those scoring high or low on the Bayley, the term and preterm groups were combined into a single group of 31 infants. This group was then divided at the median on each cry measure and on the Bayley to form a high Bayley group and a low Bayley group.

The results of Chi Square analysis showed that a significant number of infants were correctly classified as scoring high or low on the Bayley on the basis of the acoustic characteristics of the cry. As shown in Table 2, infants with a high average fundamental frequency were more likely to score low on the Bayley ($p<.0001$). More changes in the fundamental frequency was related to low Bayley scores ($p<.05$). Infants with less change in the first formant were more likely to score low on the Bayley ($p<.05$). Infants with a low amplitude cry were also more likely to score low on the Bayley ($p<.05$).

TABLE 3. Classification of 5-Year McCarthy General
Cognitive Index by Neonatal Cry Measures*

Measure	High Cognitive Index	Low Cognitive Index
High change fundamental frequency	3	8
Low change fundamental frequency	8	2
High av first formant	3	8
Low av first formant	8	2
High av amplitude	9	1
Low av amplitude	2	9

* Results are numbers of infants.

At five years of age the McCarthy scales of
children's abilities were administered to 9 term and 12
preterm infants. The 21 infants were divided at the
median on each cry measure and on the McCarthy scales
which includes the general cognitive index or IQ, as
well as subscales for verbal, perceptual, and
quantitative performance. Tables 2 - 5 show the number
of infants correctly classified on the McCarthy scales
on the basis of the cry measures. Because of the
smaller sample size the Fishers Test was used.

Table 3 shows that infants with more change in the
fundamental frequency were more likely to score low on
the general cognitive index ($p<.007$). Infants with a
higher average first formant cry were more likely to
score low on the general cognitive index ($p<.02$).
Infants with a lower amplitude cry were also more
likely to score low on the general cognitive index
($p<.007$).

Table 4 shows the results on the verbal scale of
the McCarthy. More change in the fundamental frequency

TABLE 4. Classification of 5-Year McCarthy Verbal
Scores by Neonatal Cry Measures*

Measure	High Verbal Score	Low Verbal Score
High change fundamental frequency	3	8
Low change fundamental frequency	7	3
High change first formant	7	3
Low change first formant	3	8

* Results are numbers of infants.

TABLE 5. Classification of 5-Year McCarthy Perceptual Scores by Neonatal Cry Measures*

Measure	High Perceptual Score	Low Perceptual Score
High change fundamental frequency	3	7
Low change fundamental frequency	8	3
High av first formant	3	8
Low av first formant	8	2
High av amplitude	8	2
Low av amplitude	3	8

* Results are numbers of infants.

of the cry was found in infants who scored low on the verbal scale ($p<.05$). Infants with less change in the first formant were also more likely to score lower scores on the verbal scale ($p<.05$).

Table 5 shows the results for the perceptual performance scale of the McCarthy. More change in the fundamental frequency of the neonatal cry predicted infants with lower scores on the perceptual performance scale ($p<.05$). A higher average first formant in the cry was related to lower perceptual performance scores ($p<.02$). Infants with a low amplitude cry were also more likely to score low on the perceptual performance scale at age 5 ($p<.05$).

Table 6 shows the results of the quantitative scale. Infants whose cries during the neonatal period

TABLE 6. Classification of 5-Year Quantitative Scores by Neonatal Cry Measures*

Measure	High Quantitative Score	Low Quantitative Score
High av first formant	2	9
Low av first formant	8	2
High av amplitude	8	3
Low av amplitude	2	8
High av duration	8	2
Low av duration	2	9

* Results are numbers of infants.

showed a higher average first formant were more likely to score low on the quantitative scale at 5 years (p<.007). A lower amplitude cry was related to lower quantitative scores (p<.02). Infants with a short duration cry duration were also more likely to receive low quantitative scores (p<.02).

Additional analyses were conducted to determine if prematurity alone was related to the developmental outcome scores at 18 months or 5 years. There were no significant relationship between prematurity and any of the developmental outcome scores. Newborn neurological scores, medical risk factors and socioeconomic status also failed to significantly predict developmental outcome in this sample.

DISCUSSION

This study suggests a relationship between the acoustic characteristics of the cry measured at 40 weeks conceptional age in term and preterm infants and developmental outcome at 18 months and five years of age. Measures of the frequency characteristics of the cry, the fundamental frequency and the first formant, which are thought to be mediated, in part by neural mechanisms, and measures of the amplitude and duration of the cry which reflect respiratory control, were significant predictors of developmental outcome in a prospective longitudinal design. The speculation is that certain acoustic characteristics of the cry may reflect the neurophysiological status of the infant and could be useful in the early detection of the infant at risk for adverse developmental outcome.

The finding that variability in the frequency characteristics of the cry (F0 and F1) were related to developmental outcome is interesting because it has been suggested that the neurologic maturity of the infant is revealed by the stability of laryngeal coordination and vocal tract maturity (Bosma, et al 1965). Elevations in F1 are thought to indicate constriction in the upper airways. This leads to hypotheses about the potential relationship between acoustic cry characteristics and the sudden infant death syndrome (SIDS).

Cry Analysis and SIDS

In contrast to the preterm infant who has already been identified as at risk there is no warning for the

tragic death of victims of SIDS.   SIDS, the sudden,
unexpected and unexplained death of apparently healthy
babies is the leading cause of death for infants
between one month and one year of age.   In the United
States, SIDS, sometimes referred to as crib death or
cot death, is responsible for the death of
approximately 7,000 infants each year.   It has been
estimated that the incidence of SIDS in the United
States is approximately 1.3 deaths per 1000 live births
(Wegman 1986).

          The notion that infants at risk for SIDS may have
a distinctive cry is based on a few case studies and on
our understanding of the mechanisms of cry production.
Colton and Steinschneider (1981) and Stark and
Nathanson (1972) each reported a single case study of
an infant who had shifts in the formant frequencies and
later died of SIDS.   Infants who have anatomical or
functional alterations in their vocal tract will have a
shift in the sound resonances or formants that are
determined by the cross sectional area of the vocal
tract (Golub and Corwin 1985).   An upward shift in the
F1 could result either from a constriction in the lower
pharynx or from a dilatation in the mouth.

          In the present study (Corwin, et al 1983), we
analyzed the cries of 6 SIDS victims.   Cases 1 and 2
were normal term infants whose cries were recorded
during the first week of life and who died of SIDS at 4
and 6 months.   Cases 3, 4, and 5 were also normal
infants born at term.   These infants suffered a severe
apneic event between 2 - 4 weeks of age after which the
cry was recorded.   All 3 infants died of SIDS within 1
month of the cry recording.   Case 3 was atypical of
SIDS.   The infant had gastroesophageal reflex and had
two prior siblings who died of SIDS in the first month
of life.   Though it was not proven, child abuse was
suspected in this case.   Case 6 was the larger and
healthier of a set of twins born at 34 weeks
gestational age.   The cry was recorded by the infants
father at 69 days of age.   The infant died of SIDS one
week later.

Results

          We compared the mean first formant (F1) of the 6
SIDS victims with 1238 age matched controls.   The
results are shown in Figure 7.   The mean F1 for the
SIDS victims was 1815 (SD=218).   The mean F1 for the
controls was 1395 (SD=253).   The difference was
statistically different (p<.0001 by t test).

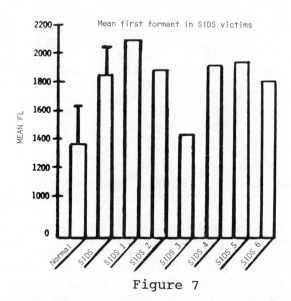

Figure 7

The values for each SIDS victim are also shown in the Figure 6. The only SIDS victim who did not have an elevated F1 was case 3 who was not typical for SIDS.

Discussion

The elevated first formant in the SIDS victims could be due to abnormal airway constriction perhaps as a consequence of impaired airway expansion due to a deficit in respiratory inspiration. The areas of the brain stem that are responsible for the control of the cry are in close proximity to those responsible for the control of heart rate and breathing rate (e.g. nucleus ambiguous). Other studies have documented abnormal regulation of heart rate and breathing rate in infants at risk for SIDS (Shannon and Kelly 1977; Gordon, et al 1982). Gliosis has been described in this region of the brain stem in SIDS victims (Kinney, et al 1983). It is possible that some infants at risk for SIDS have an abnormality in the brain stem which may lead to defective control of heart rate and respiration and abnormal regulation of the structures that control the production of the cry.

Conclusions

The cry is clearly a complex motor performance that involves respiratory, anatomical, and peripheral as well as central nervous system mechanisms. The work reviewed in this chapter supports the hypothesis that acoustic features of the infant cry may be a benchmark of the biological integrity of the infant. In the first study, analysis of the cry recorded at term gestational age was related to developmental outcome at five years of age in term and preterm infants. The second study showed that the cry in SIDS victims was different from controls.

Although other pathways are undoubtedly involved, it is likely that abnormalities in the brain stem may be responsible for some of the effects shown in both of these studies. Brain stem activity as mediated by the cranial nerves is thought to determine sound qualities of the cry including the fundamental frequency and the formant frequencies. Cranial nerves IX (glossopharyngeal), X (vagal), XI (accessory) and XII (hypoglossal) control the laryngeal muscles and are part of the vagal complex in the medulla.

We recently studied the relationship between the brainstem auditory evoked response (BAER) and acoustic cry characteristics (Vohr, et al 1988). Because of the anatomical proximity in the brainstem of cranial nerves 8 (auditory) and 9-12 (vagal complex) it was hypothesized that changes in BAER would reflect changes in the cry. The study showed significant correlations between BAER latencies, brainstem conduction time and the percent of dysphonation in the cry, providing evidence that the cry is mediated by brain stem activity.

While the exact mechanisms that relate cry analysis to developmental outcome are clearly different than those that cry analysis relate to SIDS, it is interesting to speculate that both conditions may reflect brain stem involvement. It is possible that the cry as a measure of brain stem involvement is the final common pathway through which a variety of clinical conditions are expressed.

Cry analysis may be useful as an early detection device in two different situations, as represented by the preterm and SIDS studies. In the case of the preterm infant, the infant has already been identified as at risk by virtue of being born prematurely and, in many cases, the added risk associated with medical illness that often accompanies prematurity. Since not all high risk preterm infants have abnormal outcomes,

the task is to identify, among those already determined
to be at risk, <u>which</u> individual infants will go on to
develop normally and <u>which</u> will have abnormal outcomes.
The preterm infant is a prototype of the infant at risk
and there are many other conditions (e.g. asphyxia,
hyperbilirubinemia, etc.) in which the infant is
thought to be at risk where the cry may be useful in
detecting those infants who are truly headed for
handicap.

The situation represented by SIDS is wholly
different, there is no prior warning. Most SIDS
victims come from the population of apparently normal,
healthy infants; the infant is not thought to be at
risk for SIDS. In this situation cry analysis may be
useful in determining which infants are at risk for
SIDS so that preventive measures can be taken.

Research on infant cry is revealing important
information about the biological status of the infant,
information often not provided by other medical data.
Cry analysis is showing promise as a non-invasive
measure of the neurophysiological integrity of the
infant that may be useful in the early detection of the
infant at biological risk.

References

Bosma, J. F., Truby, H. M., and Lind, J., 1965, Cry
motions of the newborn infant. <u>Acta</u> <u>Paediatrica</u>
<u>Scandinavia</u> <u>Supplement</u>, 163: 61.

Colton, R. H. and Steinschneider, A., 1981, The cry
characteristics of an infant who died of the sudden
infant death syndrome. <u>Journal</u> <u>of</u> <u>Speech</u> <u>and</u>
<u>Hearing</u> <u>Disorders,</u> 46: 359.

Corwin, M. J., Golub, H. L., Kelly, D. and Shannon, D.
C., 1983, Spectral analysis of a cry is abnormal
in infants at risk for SIDS. <u>Pediatric</u> <u>Research,</u>
17: 373.

Golub, H. L. and Corwin, M. J., 1982 Infant Cry: A
clue to diagnosis. <u>Pediatrics</u>, 69: 197.

Gordon, D., Kelly, D. H., Akselrod, S., Ubel, A.,
Kenet, R., Cohen, R. J. and Shannon, D. C., 1982,
Abnormalities in the HR and respiratory power
spectrum in SIDS. <u>Pediatric</u> <u>Research</u>, 16:350A.

Kinney, H. C., Burger, P. C., Harrell, F. E., and Hudson, R. P., 1983, Reactive gliosis in the medulla oblongata of victims of the sudden infant death syndrome. Pediatrics, 72:181.

Lester, B. M., 1984, A biosocial model of infant crying. Advances in infancy research In L. Lipsitt, ed., Ablex, NJ.

Lester, B.M., 1985, There's more to crying than meets the ear. "Infant Crying: Theoretical and Research Perspectives" In B. M. Lester and C. F. Boukydis, eds., Plenum Publishing Corp., New York.

Lester, B. M., 1987, Developmental outcome prediction from acoustic cry analysis in term and preterm infants. Pediatrics, 80: 529.

Shannon, D. C.and Kelly, D., 1977, Impaired regulations of alveolar ventilation and the sudden infant death syndrome. Science, 197:367.

Stark, R. E. and Nathanson, S. N., 1972, Unusual features of cry in an infant dying suddenly and unexpectedly. "Development of Upper Respiratory Anatomy and Function: Implications for SIDS. "In J.F. Bosma and T. Showacre, eds., US Department of HEW, Washington.

Wasz-Hockert, O., Lind, J., Vuorenkoski, V., Partanen, T. and Valanne, E., 1968, "The Infant Cry," (Clinics in Developmental Medicine, 1968, 29,) Spastics International Medical Publications, London.

Wegman, M. E., 1986, Annual summary of vital statistics - 1985. Pediatrics, 78:983.

Zeskind, P. S. and Lester, B. M., 1978, Acoustic features and auditory perceptions of the cries of newborns with prenatal complications. Child Development, 49: 580.

INFLUENCE OF INFANT CRY STRUCTURE ON THE HEART RATE OF THE LISTENER

Yvonne E. Bryan and John D. Newman

Laboratory of Comparative Ethology
National Institutes of Child Health and Human Development
NIH
Bethesda, MD 20892

INTRODUCTION

The cry of the human neonate is of great survival value, since
this signal is the primary means by which the young infant communi-
cates its wants, needs, and demands to its caregiver. How the
caregiver responds to the cries has profound implications for
the infant's well being, for development of the infant-caregiver
interaction process, and ultimately, for setting the infant on
an optimal developmental trajectory. In essence, infant crying
initiates what becomes a complex reciprocal feedback process
through which infant and caregiver build their relationship; it is
this complex reciprocal process which underscores the infant's
developmental outcome.

Previous work suggests that although infant cries, in general,
are perceived as aversive or unpleasant sounding, it appears that
caregivers have certain "expectations" with respect to the
normalcy of cries. If cries fall outside the expected boundaries,
these are clearly differentiated, and conceivably could result
in inappropriate responding on the part of caregivers.

Efforts to determine the properties of the cries that elicit
appropriate caregiver responses have adopted a strategy where
recordings of infant cries are presented to adult listeners who
are asked to evaluate cries on a set of perceptual scales. In
several previous studies, the cries of fullterm newborns who
were clinically healthy, but who on the basis of their pre- and
perinatal experiences were categorized as high or low-risk,
have been shown to be differentiated by acoustic parameters and

by adult listeners who perceived the cries of infants at risk as
more urgent, sick, arousing, and distressing (Zeskind, 1983),
and in addition, as more aversive, grating, piercing, and discom-
forting (Zeskind and Lester, 1978). Yet, data from the few studies
comparing the cries of term and preterm infants suggest that
these groups are less well differentiated.

Although Frodi et al. (1978b) reported that the cry of a preterm infant recorded just prior to discharge from the hospital
nursery was perceived as relatively more aversive than the cry
of a fullterm newborn, this finding was not replicated in a
later study (Frodi et al., 1981). These conflicting results
may reflect unreliability of responses associated with presenting
cries of only one preterm and one fullterm infant in each study;
moreover, cries of different infants were used.

Using four examples of each cry type, Friedman et al. (1982)
found that moderate-risk preterm cries were consistently rated
more negatively than either fullterm or low-risk preterm cries,
but that some low-risk preterm cries were consistently rated
more favorably (specifically more mature, and less urgent,
sick, arousing, and grating) than fullterm cries.

The fact that moderate-risk preterm cries were rated most negatively in the Friedman et al. study is consistent with Zeskind
and Lester's (1978) previous finding that greater aversiveness of
the fullterm infant's cry is associated with a higher level of
prenatal and perinatal medical risk. However, data from another
study conflict with that of Friedman et al. Bryan, Taylor, and
Seraganian (1984;Unpublished Ms.) investigated a sample of six
moderate-risk preterm cries and found no evidence that cries
recorded at either 38 or 44 weeks postconceptional age were
perceived as more aversive than the cries of newborn fullterm
infants. One possible explanation of these conflicting results
is that different complications were represented in the moderate-
risk samples of each study. In addition, the two studies used
different global criteria of risk in the preterm samples, and
neither of these studies controlled for level of medical risk
in the fullterm sample except for selecting healthy fullterm
infants. It should be noted that a further possible explanation
for the conflicting results across studies may be the diverse
adult populations that were used as subjects (parents of
either mixed or undefined parities versus college nonparent
students, groups of mothers whose parities were undefined, and
primiparous mothers versus nonmothers).

Recently, in a search for more objective and sensitive indices
of caregiver responsivity, self reports have been combined with
physiologic measures. This strategy has been pursued in the
hope of providing an understanding of the roles of physiologic

and subjective processes in adult responsivity to cries of
infants that differ in their stimulus characteristics. In
particular, researchers have monitored heart rate reactivity on
the assumption that this may constitute a sensitive measure of
maternal autonomic and behavioral state. The rationale for focus-
ing on heart rate stems from reports in the psychophysiological
literature which indicate that the direction of cardiac change
elicited by sensory stimulation can serve as an index of attentional processes (Graham and Clifton, 1966), or alternatively,
as an index of motivational dispositions (Obrist, 1976). However,
on the basis of a relatively small number of studies the heart
rate data are far from clearcut. First, it appears that response
to infant cries is influenced by diverse factors which are not
well understood. For example, relatedness of the listener to the
infant (Wiesenfeld et al., 1981), infant gestational status (pre-
term/fullterm; Frodi et al., 1978b), and infant risk status
(low- vs high-risk; Zeskind, 1987), have all been separately
implicated as factors which influence heart rate response to
cries. It is not clear, however, how these factors interact
with, or are differentiated by heart rate reactivity patterns,
since there have been contradictory reports of each of these elict-
ng cardiac acceleration, cardiac deceleration or both. Second,
the pattern of maternal cardiac response has not been readily
interpretable according to current psychophysiological models;
the most poignant example of this being evidence that cardiac
acceleration the response typically elicited by crying, which
on the basis of Graham and Clifton's (1966) model is thought to
reflect a defensive response or evidence of aversion, is also
elicited in response to supposedly pleasant infant signals ——— coos
(Bryan et al., 1984) and infant smiles (Wiesenfeld and Klorman,
1978). Perhaps one reason for the difficulty in interpreting
cardiac responses to infant signals is that models based on
autonomic response to steady state stimuli such as noise and
tones may be inadequate for analyzing responses to the temporal
and acoustic complexities of infant signals.

On the basis of the preceding review of the literature it
is apparent that more systematic empirical analyses of
cardiac responses to infant cries are warranted. The study
detailed in the next section was an attempt to explore in a
systematic way the relationship between medical risk, cry acoustics
and maternal cardiac response patterns.

PRESENT INVESTIGATION

The findings being presented here are based on audiospectro-
graphic analyses of the taped-recorded cries of 16 3-day-old
preterm and fullterm infants, and reanalyses of data generated
from a comprehensive study of mothers' and nonmothers' heart
rate responses to these cries (Bryan, 1986).

Table 1   Characteristics of Infants Providing Cry Samples

| | Fullterms | | Preterms | |
| | Complications | | Complications | |
	Low	High	Low	High
Number of Nonoptimal Obst. Conditions				
Mean	0.50	5.75	1.00	5.50
Gestational Age (Weeks)				
Mean	39.3	39.6	35.6	35.0
Range	39-40	39-40	34.5-36.4	33.5-36.5
Birthweight (Grams)				
Mean	3444	3715	2572	2481
Range	3061-3940	3260-4480	2154-2948	1980-3420
1-Min Apgar Score				
Mean	9	7.5	8.5	6.2
Range	9-9	7-8	8-9	4-8
5-Min Apgar Score				
Mean	9.8	9.2	9.8	8.5
N per Group	4	4	4	4

All infants were recorded while being weighed at a postnatal age of 3 days

Method, Stimulus Material, and Design

Subjects were twenty-four primiparous mothers (mean age 27.9 years; age range = 20 - 36 years) each with a fullterm infant, thirteen months of age or under (mean age of infant = 7.3 mos; age range = 2.5 - 13 mos), and 24 nonmothers with prior caretaking experience of an infant limited to a maximum of two weeks.

The experimental room was a temperature and humidity-controlled, electrically shielded enclosure. A 4-channel Beckman 511A Dynograph recorder (polygraph) was employed to monitor heart rate. A Sony TC-630 tape recorder equipped with a Sony stereo speaker was used for experimental presentation of the stimuli. The analog output from the Beckman and Sony (sound processed through an EMG coupler; Type 9852A) recorders were fed into a Transduction (Model No. PCB-00819) board, mounted in an IBM PC chassis. This configuration provided digitalized readings of heart rate, as well as the auditory stimuli. A Uher Report Monitor (Model No. 4400) and a Uher Unidrectional microphone (Model No. 534) placed 6 inches from the infant's mouth were used for the master recordings of the infant cries.

Characteristics of the infants from whom the cries were recorded are presented in Table 1. Infants categorized as high-risk had experienced 5 or more nonoptimal prenatal or

Table 2   Obstetric Complications Found for Sample of Infants

Providing Cries

Maternal Factors	
Age (>30)	(5)[a]
Single Marital Status	(3)
Parity (>6)	(1)
Infection in Pregnancy	(1)
Maternal Disease	(1)
Edema	(1)
Previous C-section	(1)
Cephalo-Pelvic Disproportion	(2)
Low Socio-Economic Status	(2)

Parturitional Factors	
Multiple Birth	(2)
Induced Delivery	(4)
Prolonged Labour	(1)
Rapid Labour and Delivery	(1)
Abnormal Presentation	(1)
Drugs (Other Than Local Ones)	(10)
Forceps	(2)
Artificial Membrane Rupture	(5)
Premature Membrane Rupture	(2)
Wrapped Cord	(2)
C-Section	(4)

[a] Number of Infants

perinatal risk factors, while low-risk infants had experienced 2 or fewer nonoptimal risk conditions (Zeskind and Lester, 1978). Table 2 shows the specific complications found for the sample. Cries were recorded from infants in the preterm and fullterm newborn nurseries approximately one hour after feeding, while the infant was undressed and placed on a scale for weighing. This procedure was chosen rather than the traditional procedures for eliciting a pain cry since it was felt that the cry so elicited would be more similar to those normally heard by the caregiver. Cry stimuli consisted of 30-s bouts taken after the infant had begun crying.

Four experimental tapes were used, each consisting of four
different 30-s cries: one high- and one low-risk preterm cry
and one high- and one low-risk fullterm cry. Order of the tapes
was systematically varied to meet the requirements of a balanced
randomized Latin square (each order consisting of the cries of
four different infants). In addition, there was the constraint
that no two preterm or no two fullterm cries were played in
succession.

Each tape began with a series of instructions followed by a
practice trial cosisting of two infant cries. These two cries
(1 30-s segment of fullterm infant cry and another segment of a
preterm cry) were not included in the experimental stimuli.
Each cry was separated by a 5-min interstimulus interval, and a
5-min interval also separated practice trials from the first
segment of experimental stimuli.

Measures

Although a multidimensional approach that employed a variety of
subjective measures and heart rate was used in the original study,
for purposes of this discussion what ensues is a detailed description of cry acoustics and heart rate responses to these stimuli.

Heart Rate

Cardiac response was determined online by the computer which
measured interbeat intervals in milliseconds and subsequently
converted them to heart rate in beats per minute. The last 10
s preceding each experimental stimulus constituted baselines
for comparison to each of the 10 s of the corresponding stimulation
period. The data were subsequently converted to change scores
which were computed by subtracting each of the 10 s baseline
scores from each of the first 10 s of the corresponding cry-
elicited heart rate samples.

Acoustic Analysis

Structural analysis of the cry stimuli was performed by printing out the full 30-s sample using a UNISCAN II Real-time audio
spectrograph and Epson RX-80 printer. More detailed analysis
was performed by making measurements directly off the screen of
the analyzer using the cursor controls.

RESULTS

General Description of the Stimuli

Structural analysis of the 16 infant cries obtained during
weighing revealed that these cries are generally distinguishable
from those reported on from infants experiencing a painful

stimulus. These nonpain cries show an almost complete absence
of "shifts" (an abrupt upward or downward shift in frequency
during some part of a voiced cry unit). Similarly, the frequency
range of most voiced cry units in the stimulus sample lead to the units
being classifiable as "phonation" or "dysphonation" rather than
"hyperphonation" (Truby and Lind, 1965).

Description of Cries in Each of the Four Subgroups

Cries from Low-risk Fullterm (LF) Infants:

Figure 1 shows the structure of the first 10 s of each of the four
lowrisk fullterm cries.

Low-risk Fullterm 1 : The predominant character of the cry
elements is "dysphonation", with turbulence-related noise obscuring
varying parts of each unit. The melody form is characterized
as "rising" and "falling". The duration and rhythm of each unit
are stable. The first and second units evidence what is typically
referred to as a "double harmonic break" (Lester and Zeskind, 1982).

Low-risk Fullterm 2: These units evidence only weak turbulence
and thus the predominant character of the cry is "phonation".
The melody form is predominantly "falling". The frequency,
duration and interval between units all appear relatively stable.

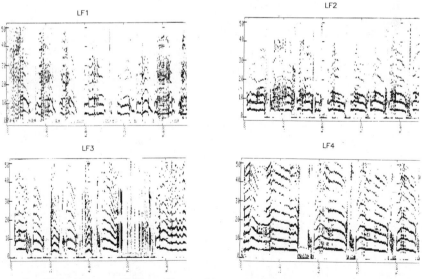

Figure 1. Structure of the first 10 seconds of each of the four
           low-risk fullterm cries (LF1-4 respectively). Seconds are
           displayed on the horizontal axis with frequency ranging
           from 0-5000 Hz on the vertical axis.

Low-risk Fullterm 3:   The cry units are more variable in duration,
fundamental and melody pattern, although all are phonations.   There
is a break in the rhythm filled with brief cough-like sounds
several seconds into the cry.

Low-risk Fullterm 4:   The duration of each unit is longer than in
LF1-3, with the first unit being the longest.   All 4 units
during the first 10 s of the cry are voiced.   The first unit
has an early "glide" feature; otherwise, the melody pattern of
the first unit is predominantly falling.   Both the interval between units and the fundamental frequency are stable across units.

Cries from High-risk Fullterm (HF) Infants:

The structures of the first 10 s of the four high-risk fullterm
cries are displayed in Figure 2.   As a group, HF1-4 are distinguished from LF1-4 by less stable fundamental, duration and
interunit intervals.   All units are predominantly voiced ("phonations").

High-risk Fullterm 1:   The units are weaker, with the fundamental
barely discernible and frequently interrupted by even greater
decreases or complete absence of a voiced component.

High-risk Fullterm 2:   This is the only Fullterm cry containing
"shifts."   Duration varies between units.   The melody pattern is
unclear.

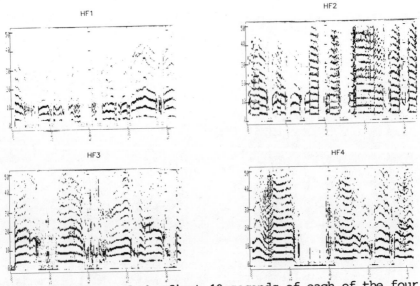

Figure 2. Structure of the first 10 seconds of each of the four
high-risk fullterm infant cries -- HF1-4 respectively.

High-risk Fullterm 3: This cry is more like those from low-risk
fullterm infants, although the fundamental is less distinct.
There is also greater emphasis on the higher harmonics.

High-risk Fullterm 4: This cry is similar to LF4, with the first
and second units showing brief "glides". After the first unit
there is a long interval before the next unit. Intervals between
subsequent units are shorter.

Cries of Low-Risk (LP) and High-Risk (HP) Preterm Infants:

Figure 3 displays the structure of the first 10 s of all 8 preterm
(low- and high-risk) cries. These cries have little in the way
of obvious shared features. Indeed, cries from infants of this
gestational age group are a variable assortment, irrespective
of risk category. With the exception of High-risk Preterm Cry
3, none of the preterm cries were characterized by units with
smoothly changing, tonal or voiced fundamental, a characteristic
of many of the fullterm cries. In the "low-risk" group, cries
ranged from dysphonic, short, repeated units (LP1 and 2) to cries
with variably long, predominantly voiced units lacking a clear melody pattern due to pitch instability. The "high-risk" set of
cry stimuli were likewise a mixed group, ranging from very
short, rhythmically repeated units (HP1) through cry units with
noticeable "shifts" (HP2) to cries with variable units, separated
periods with voiceless units, or "glottal roll" (fricative
subcomponents).

Heart Rate Changes During Presentation of Cry Stimuli

The first 10 s of heart rate responses elicited by each of the four
lowrisk fullterm cries are displayed in Figure 4. Although
cardiac deceleration appears to be the predominant overall
pattern of response elicited by these cries, there are also
definite unsustained periods of acceleration which makes for
interesting fine grain analysis of the relation between
cry structures, cardiac patterns and listener experience.

        The response to LF3 represents the clearest example of the
predominantly decelerative pattern. Not only is the response
decelerative, but both mothers and nonmothers exhibit an almost
identical pattern. Similarly, LF2 elicits an almost identical
response pattern in mothers and nonmothers; however, unlike
LF3, there are unsustained periods of attenuated acceleration.
Interestingly, LF3 is marked by relatively uncomplicated phonated
elements, while LF2, although the elements are marked by phonation,
has some weak turbulence present. LF4, on the other hand,
despite its characteristic phonated structure, elicited different
patterns in the two listener groups; mothers exhibited primarily
cardiac deceleration, while nonmothers exhibited definite periods
of both deceleration and acceleration. It may be worth noting

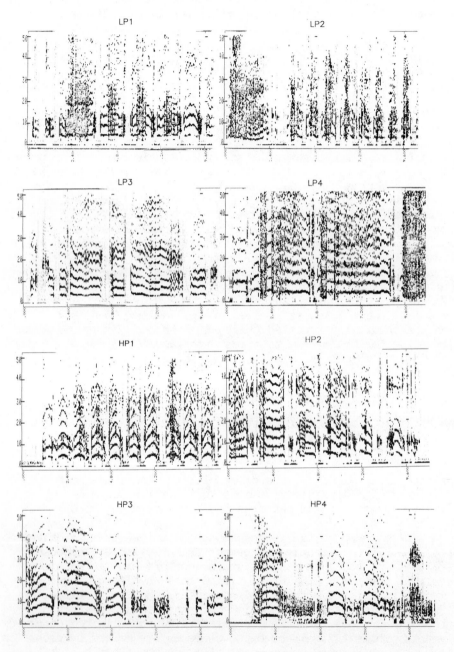

Figure 3. Structure of the first 10 seconds of each of the eight
preterm infant cries (LP1-4 and HP1-4 respectively).

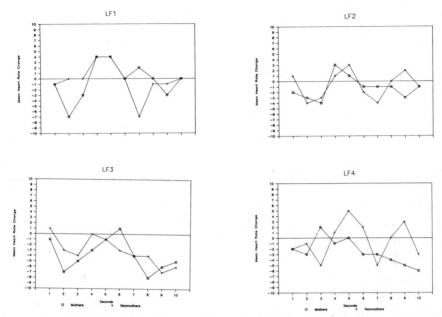

Figure 4. Mean heart rate change exhibited by mothers and non-
          mothers (subgroups of six women each) to each of the four
          low-risk fullterm cries.

that of the four low-risk cries, LF4 has the longest cry units,
and perhaps this difference in combination with an inexperienced
listener resulted in the nonmothers' bipolar cardiac response
pattern. Finally, LF1 which was marked by dysphonation, turbulence, and some obscured elements also elicited different patterns
of responses in the two listener groups. Although both mothers
and nonmothers evidenced similar unsustained cardiac acceleration
at seconds 4 and 5, the mothers' initial deceleratory response
was quite marked, while nonmothers heart rate hovered around baseline, with the reverse situation occuring at seconds 7 and 8.

     Figure 5 displays the response patterns elicited by the
four high-risk fullterm cries. In contrast to the deceleratory
cardiac pattern which essentially characterized the response to
the low-risk fullterm cries, acceleration appears to be the
predominant cardiac pattern elicited by the high-risk fullterm
cries. Again, it should be noted that there are definite deviations to this pattern, as is immediately evident in the
response pattern elicited by HF3, and to some extent HF4.

     Although the initial response to HF1 by both mothers and non-
mothers is deceleration, this is unsustained in both cases.
The nonmothers' heart rate level rose on second 3 to a level

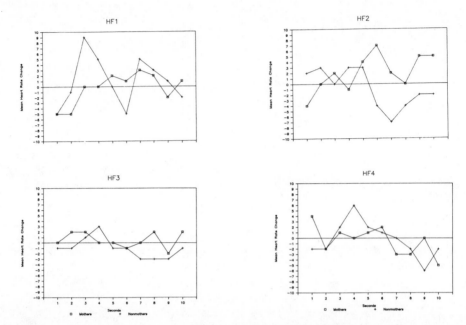

Figure 5. Mean heart rate change exhibited by mothers and non-
          mothers to each of the four high-risk fullterm cries.

well above baseline, falling below baseline at second 6, then
rising again to a level well above baseline; mothers' heart
rate, on the other hand, rose more gradually and showed a more
attenuated but sustained acceleration. The preceding patterns
emerged in response to a cry marked by weak elements and, at
times, the complete absence of voiced elements. Similarly, HF2
(marked by shifts and unclear melody patterns) elicited an
acceleratory response in nonmothers (although this was much
less marked than to HF1) over seconds 1-2 and 4-5, but which fell
below baseline for the remaining seconds; mothers' responses
again showed an initial unsustained deceleration, but rose to a
level well above baseline, and was essentially maintained. In
contrast, HF3, a cry which appears strikingly similar to the
low-risk fullterm cries, elicited in both mothers and nonmothers
only small fluctuations that hovered around the baseline.
Finally, HF4 (also similar in character to the low-risk cries,
but with brief "glides" evident in the first and second units)
elicited quite a marked but unsustained initial cardiac acceleration in mothers, and ended, after periods where levels hovered
around baseline, below baseline; the nonmothers' response was an
initial deceleration, followed by a marked but unsustained
acceleration at second 4, and ended with a gradual and sustained
decline to levels well below baseline.
     The top panel of Figure 6 displays the heart rate responses
elicited by the four low-risk preterm cries, while responses

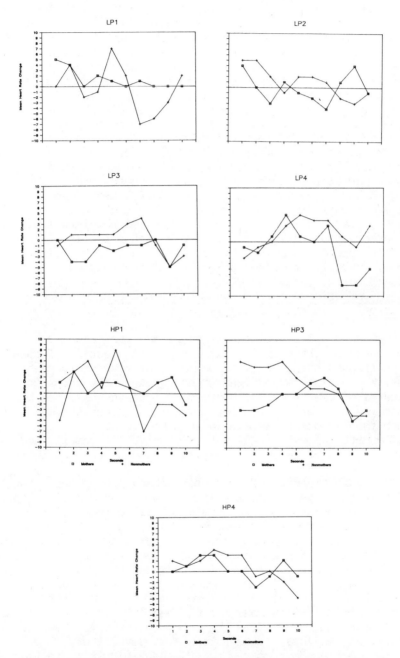

Figure 6. Mean heart rate change elicited in mothers and nonmothers by each of the four low-risk preterm cries (LP1-4
respectively) and three of the high-risk preterm
cries (HP1,3, and 4 respectively).

elicited by the high-risk preterm cries are displayed in the lower
panel. (Note that the heart rate response pattern elicited by
HP2 was unavailable). In contrast to the low- and high-risk
fullterm infant cries, but consistent with the variable assortment
independent of risk category which best characterize the structural
properties of the preterm group, no obvious differentiation is
apparent in the patterns of cardiac responses elicited by the
groups. Indeed, cardiac acceleration appears to be the predominant
response pattern evidenced by both mothers and nonmothers to
the two subgroups of infant cries, except in the case of LP3
and HP3. In the case of LP3 (which resembles low-risk fullterm
cries), it elicited in both mothers and nonmothers cardiac
response patterns that hovered below and above baseline, both
ending at levels below baseline. Similarly, HP3 the only high-risk
preterm cry marked mainly by smoothly changing tonal voiced
elements, elicited in mothers mainly cardiac deceleration, with some
attenuated, unsustained acceleration at seconds 6 and 7; nonmothers
initial response was marked by acceleration over the first 5
seconds, gradually falling to levels below baseline.

Detailed Comparisons of the Dynamics of Heart Rate and Cry
Structures

        Figures 7 and 8 depict a regrouping of the eight fullterm cries
on the basis of structural similarities. Inspection of these
configurations reveal that, independent of risk and gestation
status, there is a marked consistency between the acoustic
structures of the cries and heart rate patterns elicited by the
two subgroups. The clearest example of this consistency is
evident in the mothers' predominantly decelerative cardiac
response patterns exhibited to the relatively uncomplicated
voiced elements of HF3, HF4, LF3, and LF4 depicted in Figure 8.

        The dynamic nature of heart rate changes over the first 10
seconds suggest a temporal matching between the dynamic changes
in the cry structure and the physiological response of the
listener. For example, as demonstrated by Figure 9, the heart
rate changes of both subject groups to HP3 show a plateau between
6 and 8 seconds and a subsequent sudden deceleration that correlate
well with a transient absence of sound, and the sudden onset of
a new cry unit respectively. Because the cry patterns of most
of the fullterm and some of the preterm infants consist of
repeated, similar units, one might expect to see little in the way
of heart rate changes beyond the onset of the cry. However, it
is clear that the heart rate patterns to several cry stimuli
(for example see the response to LF1 and 2 displayed in Figure
10) are cyclic in their acceleration/deceleration patterns.
This suggests a kind of entrainment between the rhythm of crying
and the rhythm of associated heart rate changes in the listener.

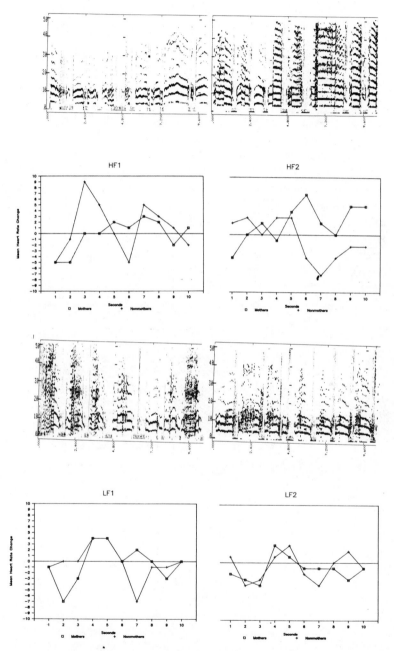

Figure 7. Mean heart rate change elicited by cries regrouped on the basis of structural similarities (HF1-2 and LF1-2 respectively).

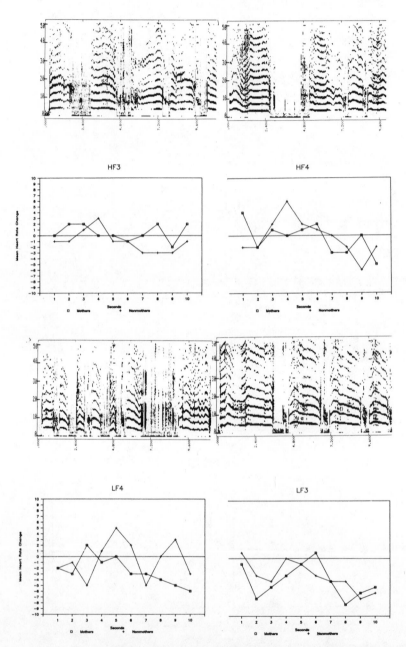

Figure 8. Mean heart rate change elicited by cries regrouped on
the basis of structural similarities (HF3-4 and LF3-4
respectively).

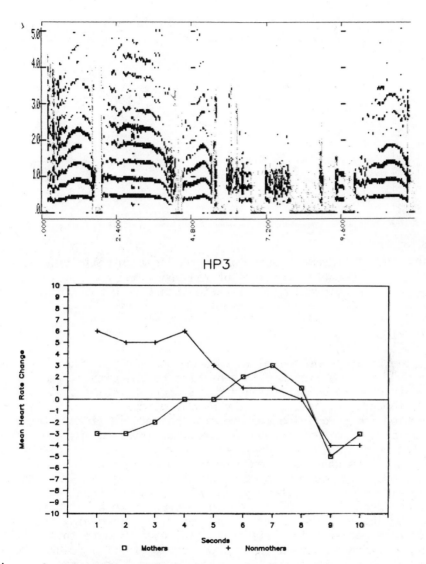

Figure 9. Temporal matching of the structure of HP3 and elicited mean heart rate change.

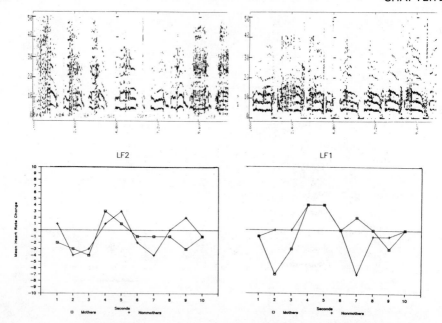

Figure 10.   Entrainment between the temporal rhythmicity of the
              acoustic structure of LF1 and 2 and the cyclic
              acceleration/deceleration heart rate patterns elicited.

DISCUSSION

       The findings presented in this chapter suggest that the heart
rate pattern of a listener is sensitive to the time-varying
acoustic pattern comprising a typical bout of infant crying.
This, in turn, suggests that the neural circuitry involved in
detecting and perceiving the acoustic pattern is linked over a
fairly direct pathway to neural circuitry involved in regulating
cardiac output. The temporal relationship between cry pattern
and heart rate changes appears to be independent of any differences
in the acoustic properties of cries from infants of differing gestational age or risk category, as well as the maternal experience
of the listener. It remains to be determined whether other
time-varying acoustic stimuli also can evoke temporally entrained
heart rate patterns in a listener. The exception to this fluctu-
ating heart rate pattern (the responses to cry HF3) occured to
a cry which matches most closely the "typical" cry pattern
reported in the literature-- a repeated series of nearly identical,
voiced cry units with little variability in duration or interval
between units. Perhaps this cry represents the closest match
of any stimulus used in this study to the expectancy in the
listener for a normal-sounding cry, and consequently failed to
elicit any significant deviation in heart rate from baseline
levels. It should be mentioned that the present study is, to

our knowledge, the first time that heart rate responses to cry stimuli have been presented so as to permit detailed comparison of the cry acoustic pattern and the corresponding time-synchronized heart rate responses. Previously published analyses (e.g., Zeskind 1987) have pooled heart rate responses over time as well as across stimuli of a given category, thereby masking the kind of stimulus-response relationships we have described here.

REFERENCES

Bryan, Y. E., 1986, The impact of cries of high-complications and low-complications preterm and fullterm infants on mothers and nonmothers: Perceived characteristics and psychophysiological reactivity, Doctoral Dissertation, Concordia University, Montreal.

Friedman, S. L., Zahn-Waxler, C., and Radke-Yarrow, H., 1982, Perceptions of cries of fullterm and preterm infants, Infant Behavior and Development, 5: 161.

Frodi, A. M., Lamb, M. E., Leavitt, L. A., Donovan, W. L.,

Neff, C., and Sherry, D. ,1978b, Fathers' and mothers' responses to the faces and cries of normal and premature infants, Developmental Psychology, 14:490.

Frodi, A. M., Lamb, M. E., and Wille, D., 1981, Mothers' responses to cries of normal and premature infants as a function of birth status of their own child, Journal of Research in Personality, 15:122.

Graham, F. K., and Clifton, R. K., 1966, Heart rate change as a component of the orienting response, Psychological Bulletin, 65:305.

Lester, B. M. and Zeskind, P. S., 1982, A biobehavioral perspective on crying in early infancy, in: "Theory and research on crying in early infancy", H. E. Fitzgerald, B. M. Lester and M. Yogman, Eds., Plenum Press: New York.

Obrist, P. A., 1976, The cardiovascular-behavioral interactions -- as it appears today, Psychophysiology, 3:95.

Truby, H. M., and Lind, J., 1965, Cry sounds of the newborn infant, in: "Newborn infant cry", J. Lind Ed., Aeta Poediatrica Scandinavica, Supplement 163.

Wiesenfeld, A. R., and Klorman, R., 1978, The mothers' reactions to contrasting affective expressions by her own and unfamiliar infant. Developmental Psychology, 14:294.

Wiesenfeld, A. R., Malatesta, C. Z., and DeLoach, L. L., 1981, Differential parental response to familiar and unfamiliar infant distress signals, Infant Behavior and Development, 4:281

Zeskind, P. S., 1987, Perceptions of cries of low- and high-risk infants, Child Development, 54:1119.

Zeskind, P. S., and Huntington, L., 1984, The effects of within-group and between-group methodologies in the study of perceptions of infant crying, Child Development, 55:1658.

Zeskind, P. S., and Lester, B. M., 1978, Acoustic features and auditory perceptions of the cries of newborns with prenatal and perinatal complications, Child Development 49:580.

Zeskind, P. S. and Marshall, T. R., 1988, The relation between variations in pitch and natural perceptions of Infant crying Child Development, 59, 193.

INDEX

DATE DUE

DEMCO NO. 38-298